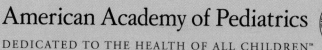

American Academy of Pediatrics

DEDICATED TO THE HEALTH OF ALL CHILDREN™

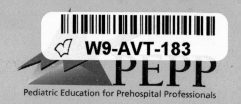

PEPP

Pediatric Education for Prehospital Professionals

Pediatric Education for Prehospital Professionals

SECOND EDITION

JONES AND BARTLETT PUBLISHERS

Sudbury, Massachusetts

BOSTON   TORONTO   LONDON   SINGAPORE

Ronald A Dieckmann, MD
Editor

To children everywhere, our most priceless and most vulnerable resource

Jones and Bartlett Publishers

World Headquarters
40 Tall Pine Drive
Sudbury, MA 01776
978-443-5000
info@jbpub.com
www.jbpub.com

Jones and Bartlett Publishers Canada
2406 Nikanna Road
Mississauga, Ontario L5C 2WG
Canada

Jones and Bartlett Publishers International
Barb House, Barb Mews
London W6 7PA
United Kingdom

American Academy of Pediatrics
DEDICATED TO THE HEALTH OF ALL CHILDREN™

Managing Editor: *Jodi Turner,* Manager, Life Support Programs
Charles W Linder, MD, FAAP, AAP Board Reviewer
Robert Perelman, MD, FAAP, Director, Department of Education
Wendy Simon, MA, CAE, Director, Life Support Programs
Eileen Schoen, Manager, Life Support Programs
Kristy Goddyn, Life Support Records Assistant
Bonnie Molnar, Life Support Assistant
Tina Patel, Life Support Assistant
Kimberly Townsend, Division Coordinator

American Academy of Pediatrics
141 Northwest Point Boulevard
Post Office Box 927
Elk Grove Village, IL 60009-0927
847-434-4795
www.aap.org

Production Credits

Chief Executive Officer: Clayton E Jones
Chief Operating Officer: Donald W Jones, Jr.
President, Higher Education and Professional Publishing: Robert W Holland, Jr.
V.P., Sales and Marketing: William J Kane
V.P., Production and Design: Anne Spencer
V.P., Manufacturing and Inventory Control: Therese Connell
Publisher, Public Safety Group: Kimberly Brophy
Editor: Jennifer L Reed

Production Editor: Susan Schultz
Associate Production Editor: Karen Ferreira
Senior Photo Researcher: Kimberly Potvin
Director of Marketing: Alisha Weisman
Text and Cover Design: Anne Spencer
Composition: Shepherd, Inc.
Cover Photograph: © Steve Smith Photography
Text Printing and Binding: Courier Kendallville
Cover Printing: John Pow Company

Jones and Bartlett's books and products are available through most bookstores and online booksellers. To contact Jones and Bartlett Publishers directly, call 800-832-0034, fax 978-443-8000, or visit our web site, www.jbpub.com.

Substantial discounts on bulk quantities of Jones and Bartlett's publications are available to corporations, professional associations, and other qualified organizations. For details and specific discount information, contact the special sales department at Jones and Bartlett via the above contact information or send an e-mail to specialsales@jbpub.com.

This material is made available as part of the professional education programs of the American Academy of Pediatrics. No endorsement of any product or service should be inferred or is intended. The Academy has made every effort to ensure that contributors to the *Pediatric Education for Prehospital Professionals (PEPP)* materials are knowledgeable authorities in their fields. Readers are nevertheless advised that the statements and opinions are provided as guidelines and should not be construed as official Academy policy. The recommendations in this publication or the accompanying resource manual do not indicate an exclusive course of treatment. Variations taking into account individual circumstances, nature of medical oversight, and local protocols may be appropriate. The Academy and the publisher disclaim any liability or responsibility for the consequences of any actions taken in reliance on these statements or opinions.

Notice: The patients described in the case studies throughout this text are fictitious.

Additional credits appear on page 404 which constitutes a continuation of the copyright page.

Library of Congress Cataloging-in-Publication Data
Pediatric Education for Prehospital Professionals / American Academy of Pediatrics;
Ronald A Dieckmann, editor. – 2nd ed.
p. ; cm.
Includes bibliographical references and index.
ISBN 0-7637-2654-0
1. Pediatric emergencies. 2. Pediatric emergency services. I. Dieckmann, Ronald A II. American Academy of Pediatrics. III. Pediatric Education for Prehospital Professionals (Program)
[DNLM: 1. Emergencies—Child. 2. Emergency Medical Services—methods. 3. Pediatrics. WS 205 P3709 2005]
RJ370.P425 2005
618.92'0025—dc22
2004056910

Printed in the United States of America
09 08 07 06 05   10 9 8 7 6 5 4 3 2 1

Brief Contents

Contents

Resource Preview

Pediatric Education for Prehospital Professionals (PEPP) represents a comprehensive source of prehospital medical information for the emergency care of infants and children. PEPP is designed to give prehospital professionals the education, skills, and confidence they need to effectively treat pediatric patients. Developed by the American Academy of Pediatrics, PEPP specifically teaches prehospital professionals how to better assess and manage ill or injured children.

PEPP combines complete medical content with dynamic features and an interactive course to better prepare prehospital professionals for the field. This textbook is the core of the PEPP program with features that will reinforce and expand on the essential information. These features include:

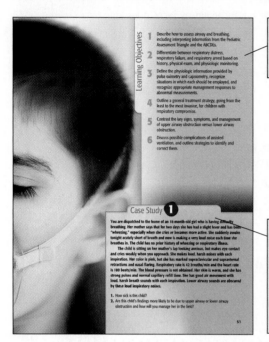

Learning objectives: Learning objectives are placed at the beginning of the chapter to highlight what providers should learn from the chapter.

Blips: Blips are placed throughout the chapter to warn providers about things they should avoid.

Case study: Each chapter opens with a case study to make providers start thinking about what they might do if they encountered a similar case in the field. Additional case studies can be found within the chapter, and answers can be found in the chapter review section at the end of the chapter.

Tips: Tips are placed throughout the chapter and provide advice from masters of the trade.

ALS icon: A bar is used to flag content that applies only to ALS providers.

Key terms: Terms are easily identifiable within the chapter and define important terminology the provider must know. A comprehensive glossary of key terms is found at the end of the textbook.

Controversies: Controversies highlight issues that may be under debate in the EMS community.

Key medications: Medications are easily identifiable within the chapter. Providers are directed to the Pediatric Medication Formulary which provides in-depth information on the recommended dose, maximum dose, use, precautions, and adverse reactions.

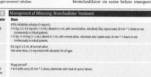

Key procedures: Procedures are easily identifiable within the chapter. Providers are directed to the visual, step-by-step Procedures found at the end of the textbook.

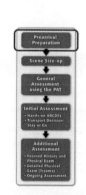

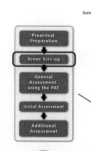

Patient assessment flowchart: The flowchart provides a quick, visual reference for the patient assessment process.

Pediatric Assessment Triangle (PAT): This triangle represents the essence of the PEPP patient assessment method, which includes assessing appearance, work of breathing, and circulation to the skin.

Chapter review: This section provides answers to the case studies and suggests additional resources that may supplement the chapter content.

Procedures: There are 23 procedures in the textbook. Each procedure provides a step-by-step guide to the most critical prehospital skills. Specific features include:

- Introduction and Rationale: These sections tell the student why the procedure is useful in emergency care situations.

- Preparation and Procedure: These sections guide the students step-by-step through the actual process.

- Indications, Contraindications, Equipment, and Complications: These are highlighted for quick and easy reference.

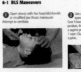

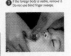

Resource Preview

The PEPP program is supported by a complete teaching and learning system. This system includes the textbook plus the following resources:

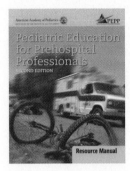

Resource Manual–ISBN: 0-7637-3703-8

An invaluable source of information, the Resource Manual contains:

- Helpful tips and guidelines for teaching a PEPP Course.
- Lecture outlines that offer a script for the PowerPoint presentations.
- Skill station strategies and activities.
- Scenarios that will keep providers engaged in group discussions.
- Administrative forms for the Course Coordinator's convenience.

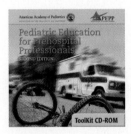

Toolkit CD-ROM - ISBN: 0-7637-3704-6

Preparing for a PEPP Course is easy with the resources found on this CD-ROM including:

- Lecture outlines that summarize the topics covered in the text.
- PowerPoint presentations that correspond with the lecture outlines.
- Image bank providing you with the most important images and tables found in the textbook.
- Administrative forms for the Course Coordinator's convenience.

Videos

ALS Video (VHS) – ISBN: 0-7637-3706-2
BLS Video (VHS) – ISBN: 0-7637-3707-0
ALS and BLS DVD – ISBN: 0-7637-3705-4
Containing real-life footage of the field, emergency departments, and operating rooms, these videos will captivate students and show them skills they could only learn by watching a real procedure.

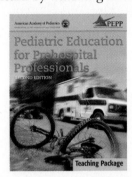

Teaching Package–ISBN: 0-7637-3700-3

This teaching package combines the PEPP textbook, Resource Manual, ToolKit CD-ROM, and VHS videos, and DVD in one convenient box.

www.PEPPsite.com

Make full use of today's teaching and learning technology with www.PEPPsite.com, a community of PEPP users and providers. This site has been specifically designed to complement PEPP and is regularly updated.

Acknowledgments

Editor: Ronald A Dieckmann, MD, MPH, FAAP, FACEP

Authors

Terry A Adirim, MD, MPH, FAAP

Amy L Baxter, MD, FAAP

David J Burchfield, MD, FAAP

James M Callahan, MD, FAAP, FACEP

Douglas S Diekema, MD, MPH, FAAP

Karen Frush, MD, FAAP

Susan Fuchs, MD, FAAP, FACEP

Patti Kunz-Howard, PhD, RN, CEN

Susan McDaniel Hohenhaus, RN, BS

Michael D Panté, NREMT-P

Chief Stephen G Simon, BS, NREMT-P

Paul Sirbaugh, DO, FAAP, FACEP

Donald J Wood, MD

George A Woodward, MD, MBA, FAAP, FACEP

Robert A Wiebe, MD, FAAP, FACEP

Senior Contributors

Dena Brownstein, MD, FAAP

Susan Fuchs, MD, FAAP, FACEP

Marianne Gausche-Hill, MD, FAAP, FACEP

Robert A Wiebe, MD, FAAP, FACEP

Reviewers

Angie Bowen, RN, BSN, NREMT-P
    Regional Coordinator, Emergency Medical Services
        for Children (EMSC)
    East Tennessee Children's Hospital
    Knoxville, Tennessee

Sharon Chiumento, BSN, EMT-P
    EMS QA/QI Coordinator
    Office of Prehospital Care/Monroe-Livingston EMS
        Council/University of Rochester
    Rochester, New York

Ramon Johnson, MD, FACEP
    Director of Pediatric Emergency Medicine
    Emergency Department
    Mission Hospital
    Laguna Niguel, California

Amy Marsh, BA, NREMT-P
    Program Coordinator
    South Dakota Emergency Medical Services for
        Children
    Sioux Falls, South Dakota

Gene McDaniel, BS, NREMT-P
    Firefighter/Paramedic, Phoenix Fire Department
    Resident Faculty, Phoenix College
    Phoenix, Arizona

Brian Moore, MD
    Pediatric Medical Director
    Mayo Medical Transport
    Assistant Professor of Pediatrics
    Rochester, Minnesota

Peter R. Morris, RN
    Pediatric Clinical Educator
    Utah Emergency Medical Services for Children
    Salt Lake City, Utah

Brian Pio, EMT-P
    Prehospital Education Coordinator
    Cincinnati Children's Hospital
    Cincinnati, Ohio

Larry Vandegriff, BS, NREMT-P, CCTP
    Paramedic Instructor
    Bartow County EMS
    Cartersville, Georgia

A tribute to Pam Baker

Pam's contributions to pediatric emergency care were widespread. She spent hours pondering a curriculum that was progressive, on target, and challenging. Pam was proud of the PEPP course and often stated that she thought this was the course that would make a difference in the lives of providers who cared for children and most importantly, the children that they cared for.

Preface

The first edition of the PEPP Course enjoyed unprecedented popularity. It was a long-awaited product, crafted out of ten years of collaboration, imagination, and dedication by thousands of physicians, nurses, prehospital professionals, and educators. The popularity of the textbook is an astonishing testimonial to the broadly based support for high quality pediatric services within our EMS systems. Over 5,000 PEPP Course Coordinators are now teaching the program in every state, as well as in nine foreign countries.

The course itself, the PEPPSite web site, the *PEPP Talk* newsletter, and the online PEPP refresher module have blazed new trails in life support education and in continuing pediatric education for prehospital professionals in firehouses and EMS training centers across the country. In a poignant affirmation of the significance of this project to our national goals for children's emergency care, in 2001, PEPP received the "National Heroes Award" from the US Maternal and Child Health Bureau's EMSC Program, as the most innovative educational program in pediatrics. Indeed, PEPP has touched a very sensitive nerve in modern EMS, and our dream for excellent prehospital care of children is now steadily coming to reality.

Since the implementation of the original PEPP program five years ago, there has been much progress in the world of EMS and in pediatric prehospital care. The original PEPP pediatric assessment triangle (PAT)—developed by Doctors Dieckmann, Brownstein, and Gausche-Hill—has been universally adopted by all American pediatric life support courses. We have learned a lot from the day-to-day feedback from our "PEPP family" and from a focused, comprehensive review of the PEPP.

The second edition of PEPP builds on the basic concepts and innovations of PEPP, but goes far beyond. Improving scientific principles, enhanced technology, better instructional strategies, and critical refinements in prehospital care and training overall have fostered this edition of PEPP, affectionately named "PEPP 2." PEPP 2 embodies all of the science generated in prehospital pediatrics and EMS over the last five years, and attempts to respond to the rising call for evidence-based treatment recommendations. In general, our PEPP 2 modifications reflect a more cautious philosophy to field care that emphasizes accurate assessment, family and child communications, error reduction in drug delivery and procedures, and pediatric-specific transport decision-making. All drug therapies and procedural approaches have undergone careful review. Advanced breathing techniques have been added, along with a more descriptive drug formulary, and expanded resuscitation algorithms. Many new subjects have been integrated into this version as well, such as children in disasters, transportation considerations, patient safety, pain assessment, and computer-based drug dosing and equipment sizing.

The PEPP Steering Committee has been instrumental in the development of a national collaborative workgroup seeking to identify and standardize terminology and clinical concepts among all pediatric life support courses. Consensus terminology is intended to minimize confusion and error, as children are treated in our emergency and critical care settings by a wide variety of medical professionals: prehospital professionals, nurses, and physicians. Standardization of terms and concepts is also intended to facilitate teaching, communication among professionals, and evaluation of emergency care and critical care pediatrics.

PEPP has flourished as a dynamic educational program since its creation in California in 1990 and its early cultivation under national ACEP and the Florida EMSC community. Its successes reflect the constant vigilance and commitment of so many friends and colleagues—especially the PEPP Steering Committee, the AAP, and Jones & Bartlett Publishers. In particular, Linda Lipinsky, formerly of the AAP and a principle architect of PEPP, Jodi Turner, our highly capable AAP Life Support Manager, Wendy Simon, the AAP Director of the Division of Life Support Programs, and Kimberly Brophy and Jennifer Reed, our tireless friends from Jones and Bartlett, deserve our highest commendations for their devotion, diligence, and belief in this project. However, the real future of PEPP rests with the street level prehospital professionals who have been our strongest champions and advocates from the very beginning 15 years ago. Much still needs to be done. It was from the pleas of our prehospital colleagues for better out-of-hospital pediatric care that PEPP originally arose. It is because of their invaluable support and trust that we now proudly present PEPP 2.

Ronald A Dieckmann, MD, MPH, FAAP, FACEP
Editor and Cochair
AAP Steering Committee
San Francisco, 2005

1

Pediatric Assessment

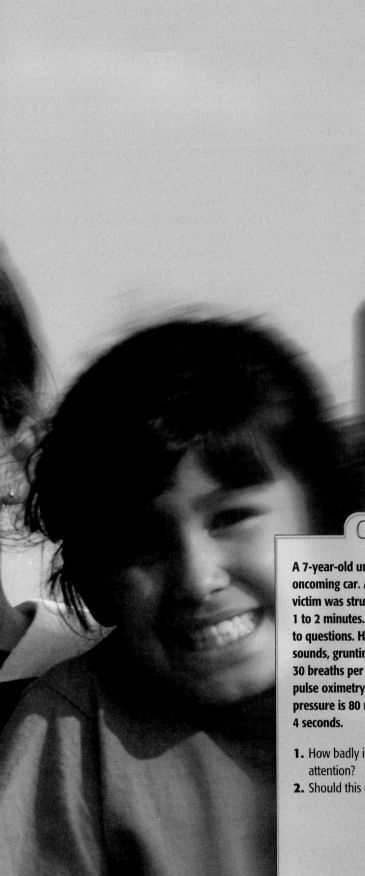

1 Introduce *Pediatric Education for Prehospital Professionals* (PEPP) as a program that meets national education priorities in emergency care of children.

2 Discuss the special challenges for the prehospital professional in pediatric assessment.

3 Present the key features of prearrival mental preparation and the scene size-up.

4 Differentiate the three elements of the Pediatric Assessment Triangle (PAT), or the general assessment.

5 Describe the important pediatric considerations for each step in the hands-on ABCDE sequence of the initial assessment.

6 Recognize clinical situations requiring pain assessment and management.

7 Discuss guidelines for when to stay on scene and treat, and when to immediately transport an ill or injured child.

8 Outline the unique considerations in the additional assessment of a child: the focused history and physical exam, the detailed physical examination, and the ongoing assessment.

Case Study 1

A 7-year-old unhelmeted boy rode his bicycle out of his driveway into the path of an oncoming car. According to witnesses, the car was moving about 30 mph (50 kph), the victim was struck and thrown approximately 15 feet (4.5 m), and was unconscious for 1 to 2 minutes. On your arrival, he is crying and anxious, but responds appropriately to questions. He is complaining that his stomach hurts. He has no abnormal airway sounds, grunting, flaring, or retracting. His skin is pale. The respiratory rate is 30 breaths per minute and there is good tidal volume, equal breath sounds, and a pulse oximetry of 98% on room air. His heart rate is 150 beats/min and the blood pressure is 80 mm Hg/palp. The brachial pulse is weak, and capillary refill time is 4 seconds.

1. How badly injured is this child and what physiologic process requires your emergent attention?

2. Should this child's pain be treated?

Introduction

CARING FOR A critically ill or injured infant or child is one of the most stressful duties in the career of the prehospital professional. Key history may be unreliable or unknown because the patient may be too young to have descriptive language, or the child may be afraid and unable to accurately recount the key events. The caregiver may be sobbing, frightened, and anxious for reassurance. Examination may be limited because of the child's small size and resistance to hands-on evaluation. Vital signs may be deceptive because of normal age-based variations, and difficulty obtaining them accurately. It is the job of the prehospital professional to bring comfort to the child, caregiver or family, and order to the chaos on scene, while simultaneously conducting an accurate assessment and delivering effective emergency treatment to the child.

The *Pediatric Education for Prehospital Professionals (PEPP) Course*, developed by the American Academy of Pediatrics (AAP), provides the core cognitive knowledge and skills to prepare prehospital professionals for comprehensive assessment and management of critically ill and injured infants and children. The PEPP materials are designed to meet the objectives of the national standard curricula for all levels of emergency medical technicians, as established by the United States Department of Transportation's National Highway Traffic Safety Administration (NHTSA), for both basic life support (BLS) and advanced life support (ALS) providers.

Effective emergency care for children involves many professionals, both inside and outside of the community's hospitals. Two of the most important concepts for comprehensive and high-quality out-of-hospital pediatric emergency care are teamwork and prevention. Teamwork involves professionals working together to develop and implement comprehensive clinical services and appropriate administrative oversight specifically for children. Prevention involves professionals recognizing the limitations of an emergency care system oriented toward treatment *after* an illness or injury occurs, and working to change potentially dangerous conditions *before* an illness or injury event. Of all community activities that can improve children's overall health and well-being, prevention of acute injury and illness is by far the most cost-effective. "Making a Difference," as described in detail in Chapter 15, involves new roles for prehospital professionals in injury and illness prevention, both in their professional day-to-day duties and as part of their activities as community leaders and health advocates.

Accurate assessment of a child with a serious illness or injury requires special knowledge and skills. For patients of all ages, the prehospital professional's evaluation includes five steps: (1) prearrival preparation; (2) scene size-up; (3) general assessment using the Pediatric Assessment Triangle (PAT); (4) initial assessment (primary assessment); and (5) additional assessment (secondary assessment). The initial assessment and additional assessment both have well-defined components that follow the same sequence used for adult patients. However, all five steps in assessment have important pediatric modifications. In the emergency department (ED), physicians and nurses perform an optional step, diagnostic testing, often with the benefit of ancillary tests.

Summary of Assessment Flowchart

This chapter introduces a flowchart that reflects the sequence of pediatric assessment taught by the PEPP Course. The flowchart reinforces the interconnecting relationships of the different assessment components. Sometimes the assessment sequence must be stopped after the general and initial assessment to allow the prehospital professional to treat potentially life-threatening problems and initiate transport. For example, when a child has a critical injury, the additional assessment—including the focused history and physical exam and the detailed physical exam—must be deferred until after the child is resuscitated and stabilized. Ongoing assessment, however, is required in every case to monitor response to treatment, guide further interventions, and assist with transport and triage decisions. Diagnostic testing is the hospital-based evaluation that often requires specialized tools, such as laboratory tests and x-rays.

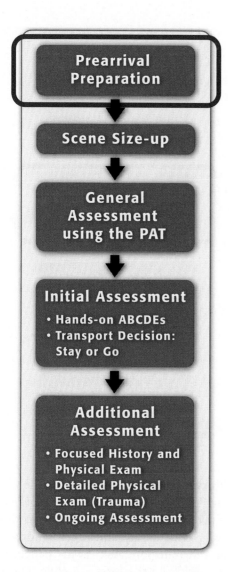

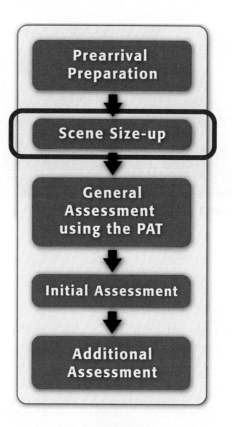

Prearrival Preparation

The prehospital professional's pediatric assessment begins at the time of the initial dispatch. On the way to the scene, prepare mentally for approaching and treating an infant or child, and for interacting with a distressed family. This means planning for a pediatric scene size-up, pediatric equipment and medication requirements, and age-appropriate physical assessment. The information from dispatch on age and gender of the child, location of the scene, and chief complaint or mechanism of injury (or both) is the basis for prearrival mental preparation.

Tip

On the way to the scene, mentally rehearse your approach to the assessment and treatment of an infant or child, and the expected interaction with a caregiver or family. Dispatch information, when available, about the child's age can be helpful to mentally prepare for age-appropriate developmental considerations and for anticipating equipment and medication requirements for assessment and treatment.

Scene Size-up

At the scene, begin the size-up by looking for possible safety threats to the child, caregiver, bystanders, or prehospital professionals. Examples of safety threats might include spilled toxins, open containers of alcohol, drug paraphernalia, weapons, or fire. The child herself may be a safety threat, if she has an infectious disease such as <u>varicella</u> or <u>meningococcemia</u>.

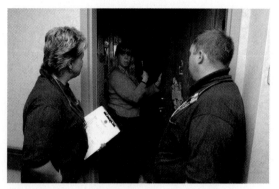

Figure 1-1 Environmental assessment.

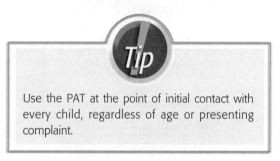

Tip

Use the PAT at the point of initial contact with every child, regardless of age or presenting complaint.

Next, do an <u>environmental assessment</u>. The environmental assessment will give important information on chief complaint, number of patients, mechanism of injury, and ongoing health risks. Evaluating the setting includes an inspection of the physical environment and watching the family-child and/or caregiver-child interactions (**Figure 1-1**). For example, documenting observations of dangerous scene conditions, and inappropriate statements from caregivers will greatly assist child protective services if the child is later determined to be a victim of inflicted injury. On the scene, be like a sponge; soak up as much useful information as possible to assure scene safety, secure valuable <u>etiological</u> information, and deliver timely care.

General Assessment: The Pediatric Assessment Triangle

After the scene size-up, do a general assessment of the child. The general assessment must have a developmentally appropriate approach. This assessment is the visual and

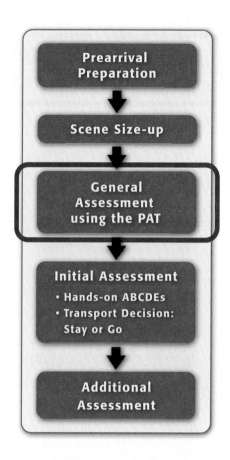

auditory "general impression" of the child, or the Pediatric Assessment Triangle (PAT).

Speedy assessment is essential to determine level of acuity and urgency for treatment and transport. Ask "is the patient sick or not sick?" In the case of a child who is a victim of trauma with a known mechanism of injury, or a child with clear-cut complaints of pain in a specific anatomic location, the assessment may be straightforward. Still, careful evaluation is needed to identify less obvious, but potentially serious injuries or <u>physiologic</u> instability. For a child with an illness, the assessment may be much trickier. The prehospital professional must elicit information on the onset, duration, severity, and progression of symptoms, often in a child who cannot accurately provide such history. Moreover, illness complaints may be vague and less specific to an anatomic region. Whether the child has an injury or an illness, the PAT will help to identify physiologic instability, help direct resuscitation priorities, and determine the timing of transport.

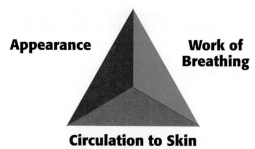

Figure 1-2 Pediatric Assessment Triangle (PAT).

The elements of the PAT are auditory and visual clues obtained from "across the room" without threatening an anxious child.

Developing a General Impression: The PAT

The PAT is an easy tool for the rapid, initial assessment of any child (**Figure 1-2**). It allows the prehospital professional to develop a first general impression of patient's status with only visual and auditory clues. By using the PAT at the point of first contact with the patient, the prehospital professional will immediately establish a level of severity, determine urgency for life support, and identify the general type of physiologic problem. Continued use of the PAT gives the prehospital professional a way to track response to therapy and determine timing of transport. It also allows for communication among medical professionals about the child's physiologic status and for accurate radio reporting.

There are three components of the PAT that together reflect the child's overall physiologic status: (1) appearance; (2) work of breathing; and (3) circulation to skin. The PAT is based on listening and seeing, and does not require a stethoscope, blood pressure cuff, cardiac monitor, or pulse oximeter. The PAT can be completed in less than 30 seconds and is designed to systematize a time-honored process of "across the room assessment"—an intuitive process that experienced pediatric providers do instinctively.

The PAT

Together, the physical characteristics of the PAT provide an accurate initial picture of the child's underlying cardiopulmonary status and level of consciousness. While the PAT does not necessarily lead to a diagnosis, it will identify the general category of the physiologic problem and establish urgency for treatment and/or transport. The PAT does not replace traditional vital signs and the ABCDEs, which are part of the initial assessment in the next phase of physical evaluation.

The patient characteristics emphasized by the three arms of the PAT did not originate with PEPP. Experienced healthcare providers have intuitively used these characteristics to obtain a rapid first "general impression" of ill or injured children based upon observation alone. What is unique about the PAT is its systematic approach to making, integrating, and communicating these observations. The PAT is the cornerstone of the PEPP Course. Use the PAT in every encounter with every child. Over time, it will become the basic method for making a rapid initial "sick or not sick" assessment of ill or injured children of all ages.

Appearance

Characteristics of Appearance The child's general appearance is the most important factor in determining the severity of the illness or injury, the need for treatment, and the response to therapy. Appearance reflects the adequacy of ventilation, oxygenation, brain perfusion, body homeostasis, and central nervous system (CNS) function. There are many characteristics of appearance; the most important are summarized in the "tickles" (TICLS) mnemonic: tone, interactiveness, consolabilty, look/gaze, and speech/cry (**Table 1-1**).

Identifying abnormal appearance is a better way to detect subtle abnormalities in behavior than the conventional AVPU scale (Alert, responsive only to Verbal stimuli,

Table 1-1	Characteristics of Appearance: The "Tickles" (TICLS) Mnemonic
Characteristic	**Features to look for**
Tone	Is she moving or resisting examination vigorously? Does she have good muscle tone? Or is she limp, listless, or flaccid?
Interactiveness	How alert is she? How readily does a person, object, or sound distract her or draw her attention? Will she reach for, grasp, and play with a toy or exam instrument, like a penlight or tongue blade? Or is she uninterested in playing or interacting with the caregiver or prehospital professional?
Consolability	Can she be consoled or comforted by the caregiver or by the prehospital professional? Or is her crying or agitation unrelieved by gentle reassurance?
Look/Gaze	Does she fix her gaze on a face, or is there a "nobody home," glassy-eyed stare?
Speech/Cry	Is her cry strong and spontaneous, or weak or high-pitched? Is the content of speech age-appropriate, or confused, or garbled?

Blip

In assessing patients with mild to moderate illness or injury, numerical "scoring" methodologies and severity scales for levels of consciousness are rarely useful. These classical neurologic evaluation systems work best in patients with severe injury or illness and serious brain dysfunction.

Blip

Never ignore the pale infant, the "nobody home stare," or the infant who doesn't respond appropriately to stimulation.

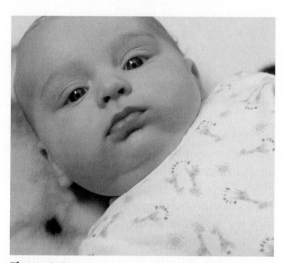

Figure 1-3 A child making good eye contact is not very sick.

responsive only to Pain, Unresponsive) or the Pediatric Glasgow Coma Scale for neurologic evaluation. Most children with mild to moderate illness or injury are "Alert" on the AVPU or "15" on the Pediatric Glasgow Coma Scale, although some may have an abnormal appearance, and a potentially serious underlying problem. Therefore, assessing a child's appearance is the most useful first thing to do in evaluating every pediatric patient.

Techniques to Assess Appearance Assess the child's appearance from the doorway. This is Step 1 in the PAT. Techniques for assessment of a conscious child's appearance include observing from a distance, allowing the child to remain in the caregiver's lap or arms, using distractions such as bright lights or toys to measure the child's ability to interact, and kneeling down to be at eye level with the child. An immediate "hands-on" approach may cause agitation and crying, and may complicate the assessment. Unless a child is unconscious or obviously critically ill, get as much information as possible by observing the child before touching or taking vital signs.

One example of a child with a normal appearance might be an infant with good muscle tone, good eye contact, and good color (**Figure 1-3**). An example of an infant with a worrisome appearance might be a toddler who makes poor eye contact with the caregiver or prehospital professional and is pale and listless (**Figure 1-4**).

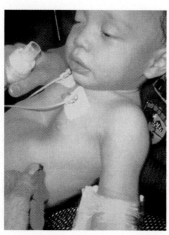

Figure 1-4 A limp, pale child unable to make eye contact or a child with retractions may be critically ill or injured.

An abnormal appearance may be due to many causes: inadequate oxygenation, ventilation, or <u>brain perfusion</u>; systemic abnormalities such as poisoning, infection, or <u>hypoglycemia</u>; or acute or chronic brain injury. Regardless of the cause, a child with grossly abnormal appearance is seriously ill or injured and needs immediate life support efforts to increase oxygenation, ventilation, and perfusion while the prehospital professional is completing the initial assessment.

While an alert, interactive child is usually not critically ill, there are some cases where a child may have life-threatening problems despite an initially normal appearance. Toxicologic or traumatic emergencies are good examples:

1. A child with <u>acetaminophen</u>, iron, or <u>cyclic antidepressants</u> overdose may not show symptoms immediately after ingestion. Despite the child's normal appearance, she may develop deadly complications in the coming minutes or hours.
2. A child with blunt trauma and solid organ injury may be able to maintain adequate <u>core perfusion</u> despite internal bleeding by increasing cardiac output and systemic vascular resistance and therefore, may appear normal on initial assessment. However, when these <u>compensatory mechanisms</u> fail, the

child may acutely "crash," with rapid progression to <u>decompensated shock</u>. Pallor may be the only finding on the PAT that suggests impending disaster.

A benign appearance should never justify a denial of transport. However, a normal appearance usually means that a transport with "lights and siren" is not necessary.

Age differences are associated with important developmental differences in psychomotor and social skills. Therefore, "normal" appearance and behavior varies by age group, as discussed in Chapter 2. Children of all ages engage their environment: newborns do this through energetic sucking and crying; older infants, by smiling or tracking a light; toddlers through physical exploration; and adolescents through speech. Knowledge of normal child development through the age groups will guide the assessment of appearance and result in more accurate treatment and transport decisions. While appearance reflects the severity of illness or injury, it does not define the cause. Appearance is the "screening" portion of the PAT. The other elements of the PAT—work of breathing and circulation to skin—provide more specific information about the type of physiologic derangement while giving additional clues about severity.

Work of Breathing

Characteristics of Work of Breathing In children, <u>work of breathing</u> is a more accurate indicator of oxygenation and ventilation than respiratory rate or chest sounds on auscultation, the standard measures of breathing effectiveness in adults. Work of breathing reflects the child's attempt to compensate for abnormalities in oxygenation and ventilation and therefore, it is a proxy for the effectiveness of gas exchange. This component of the PAT requires listening carefully for abnormal airway sounds and looking for signs of increased breathing effort. It is another "hands-off" evaluation method that does not require a stethoscope or pulse oximeter. **Table 1-2** summarizes the key characteristics of work of breathing.

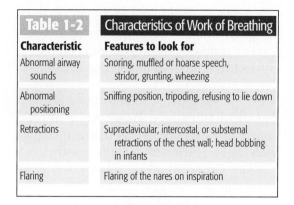

Table 1-2	Characteristics of Work of Breathing
Characteristic	**Features to look for**
Abnormal airway sounds	Snoring, muffled or hoarse speech, stridor, grunting, wheezing
Abnormal positioning	Sniffing position, tripoding, refusing to lie down
Retractions	Supraclavicular, intercostal, or substernal retractions of the chest wall; head bobbing in infants
Flaring	Flaring of the nares on inspiration

Tip

The child's general appearance is the single most important feature when assessing severity of illness or injury, need for treatment, and response to therapy.

Blip

While an alert, interactive child is usually not critically ill, there are some exceptions to the reliability of general appearance as an indicator of stable cardiopulmonary and neurologic function. The most common exceptions are ingestions with delayed physiologic effects, and blunt injury with slow internal bleeding.

Abnormal Airway Sounds Examples of abnormal airway sounds that can be heard without a stethoscope are snoring, muffled or hoarse speech, stridor, grunting, and wheezing. Abnormal airway sounds provide information about the physiology and anatomic location of the breathing problem.

Snoring, muffled or hoarse speech, and stridor suggest an upper airway obstruction. Snoring or gurgling occurs when the <u>oropharynx</u> is partially obstructed by the tongue and soft tissues. Muffled or hoarse speech reflects inflammation of the <u>glottis</u> or <u>supraglottic</u> structures. <u>Stridor</u> is a high-pitched sound

heard on inspiration, or during both inspiration and expiration, reflecting an obstruction at the level of the glottis or subglottic trachea. All of these sounds reflect an abnormal airflow across partially obstructed upper airway structures. Obstruction of upper airway passages can occur in a variety of illnesses and injuries, including <u>croup</u>, foreign body <u>aspiration</u>, bacterial upper airway infections, or as a result of bleeding or edema.

Abnormal lower airway sounds that may be heard in the PAT include <u>grunting</u> and <u>wheezing</u>. Grunting is a form of "auto-PEEP" (positive end-expiratory pressure), a way to distend lower respiratory air sacs or <u>alveoli</u> to promote maximum gas exchange. Grunting involves exhaling against a partially closed glottis. This short, low-pitched sound is best heard at the end of the exhalation and is easily mistaken for whimpering.

Grunting is often present in children with moderate to severe <u>hypoxia</u>, and it reflects poor gas exchange because of fluid in the lower airways and alveoli. Conditions that cause hypoxia and grunting are <u>pneumonia</u>, <u>pulmonary contusion</u> (bruising of the lungs), and <u>pulmonary edema</u> (fluid in air sacs).

Wheezing is the result of movement of air across partially blocked small airways. At first, wheezing may occur during <u>exhalation</u> and can be heard only by <u>auscultation</u>. As the airway obstruction increases and breathing requires more work, wheezing is present during both inhalation and exhalation. With more obstruction, wheezing is audible without a stethoscope. Finally, if respiratory failure develops, work of breathing may diminish and the wheezing may not be heard at all. The most common cause of wheezing in childhood is <u>asthma</u>, although wheezing may also be associated with <u>bronchiolitis</u> (a viral respiratory infection in infants) and lower airway foreign body aspiration.

Visual Signs of Increased Work of Breathing There are several useful visual signs of increased work of breathing. These signs reflect an increased breathing effort by the

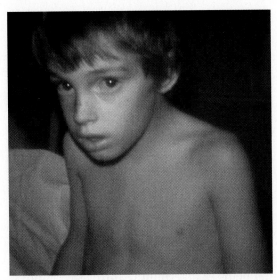

Figure 1-5 The sniffing position opens up the airways to improve patency.

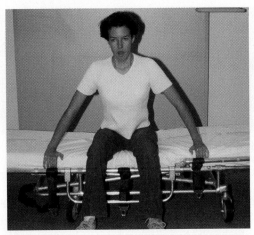

Figure 1-6 The abnormal tripod position indicates the patient's attempts to maximize accessory muscle use.

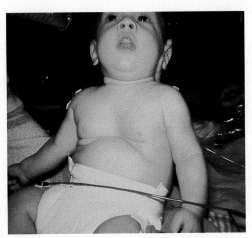

Figure 1-7 Retractions indicate increased work of breathing and may occur in the supraclavicular, intercostal, and substernal areas.

Tip

Abnormal airway sounds provide excellent anatomic and physiologic information about breathing effort, type and anatomic location of the breathing problem, and degree of hypoxia.

child to improve oxygenation and ventilation. The presence of certain physical features—abnormal positioning, retractions, and nasal flaring—reflect overall illness or injury severity. Abnormal positioning is usually evident from the doorway. There are several types of abnormal postures that indicate that the child is struggling to improve airflow. A child who is in the <u>sniffing position</u> is trying to align the axes of the airways to improve patency and increase airflow (**Figure 1-5**). This position is usually the result of severe upper airway obstruction. The child who refuses to lie down or who leans forward on outstretched arms (<u>tripoding</u>) is creating optimal mechanical advantage to utilize accessory muscles of respiration (**Figure 1-6**). The sniffing position and tripoding are abnormal and indicate airway obstruction, increased work of breathing, and severe respiratory distress.

<u>Retractions</u> are physical signs of increased work of breathing. Retractions represent the recruitment of accessory muscles of respiration to provide more "muscle power" to move air into the lungs in the face of airway or lung disease or injury. To optimally observe retractions, expose the child's chest. Retractions are a more useful measure of work of breathing in children than in adults because a child's chest wall is less muscular, and the inward excursion of skin and soft tissue between the ribs is more apparent. Retractions may be in the <u>supraclavicular</u> area (above the clavicle), the <u>intercostal</u> area (between the ribs), or the <u>substernal</u> area (under the sternum), as illustrated in **Figure 1-7**. Another

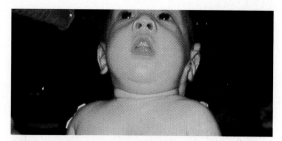

Figure 1-8 Nasal flaring indicates increased work of breathing and moderate to severe hypoxia.

form of retractions seen only in infants is "head bobbing," the use of neck muscles to help breathing during severe hypoxia. The infant extends the neck as she inhales, and then allows the head to fall forward as she exhales.

Nasal flaring is another sign of accessory muscle use that reflects significant increased work of breathing (**Figure 1-8**). Nasal flaring is the exaggerated opening of the nostrils during labored inspiration and indicates moderate to severe hypoxia. It reflects the child's extra effort to breathe during a hypoxic stress from conditions such as croup, pneumonia, asthma, bronchiolitis, or pulmonary contusion.

Techniques to Assess Work of Breathing
Step 2 in the PAT is assessing work of breathing. Begin by listening carefully from a distance for abnormal airway sounds. Next, look for key physical signs. Note if the child has abnormal posture, especially the sniffing position or tripoding. Next, have the caregiver uncover the chest of the child for direct inspection or have the child undress on the caregiver's lap. Look for intercostal, supraclavicular, and substernal retractions, and note if there is head bobbing in infants. After examining for retrac-

tions, inspect for nasal flaring. This stepwise process is critical for gathering accurate information. Once an infant or child begins to cry, assessment of work of breathing is more difficult.

Children may have increased work of breathing because of abnormalities anywhere in their airways, alveoli (air sacs), pleura (membrane surrounding the lungs and lining the walls of the pleural cavity), or chest wall. The *type* of abnormal airway sounds gives an important clue to the anatomic location of the illness or injury process, whereas the *number and type* of physical signs of increased work of breathing helps in determining the degree of physiologic stress.

Combining assessment of appearance and work of breathing can also help establish the severity of the child's illness or injury. A child with a normal appearance and increased work of breathing is in respiratory distress. An abnormal appearance and increased work of breathing suggests respiratory failure. An abnormal appearance and abnormally decreased work of breathing implies impending respiratory arrest.

Circulation to Skin

Characteristics of Circulation to Skin The goal of rapid circulatory assessment is to determine the adequacy of cardiac output and core perfusion, or perfusion of vital organs. The child's appearance is one indicator of brain perfusion, but abnormal appearance may be caused by other conditions unrelated to circulation, such as hypoxia, brain injury, or intoxication. For this reason, other signs of adequacy of perfusion must be added to the evaluation of appearance to assess the child's true circulatory status.

An important sign of core perfusion is circulation to skin. When cardiac output is inadequate, the body shuts down circulation to nonessential anatomic areas such as skin and mucous membranes in order to preserve blood supply to the most vital organs (brain, heart, and kidneys). Therefore, circulation to skin reflects the overall status of core circulation. Pallor, mottling, and cyanosis are

Tip

Head bobbing is a form of accessory muscle use and increased work of breathing that is specific to infants.

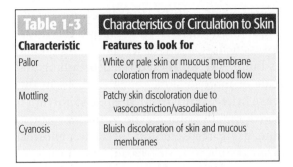

Table 1-3	Characteristics of Circulation to Skin
Characteristic	**Features to look for**
Pallor	White or pale skin or mucous membrane coloration from inadequate blood flow
Mottling	Patchy skin discoloration due to vasoconstriction/vasodilation
Cyanosis	Bluish discoloration of skin and mucous membranes

key visual indicators of reduced circulation to skin and mucous membranes. **Table 1-3** summarizes these characteristics.

Pallor may be the first sign of poor skin or mucous membrane perfusion. Pallor may be the only visual sign in a child with compensated shock and indicates reflex peripheral vasoconstriction to shunt blood away from the skin to the core. Pallor may also be a sign of anemia or hypoxia. Mottling is another sign of inadequate skin perfusion, reflecting vasomotor instability (abnormal blood vessel tone) in the capillary beds of the skin. Mottled skin has patchy areas of <u>vasoconstriction</u> (pallor) mixed with areas of <u>vasodilation</u> (cyanosis or erythema). Mottling may also be a normal physiologic response in a child exposed to cold environmental temperatures.

<u>Cyanosis</u> is blue discoloration of the skin and mucous membranes. It is the most extreme visual indicator of poor perfusion or poor oxygenation. Do not confuse <u>acrocyanosis</u>—or blue hands and feet in a newborn or infant less than 2 months of age—with true cyanosis. Acrocyanosis is a normal finding when a young infant is cold, and it reflects <u>vasomotor</u> instability rather than hypoxia or <u>shock</u>. True cyanosis is a late finding of respiratory failure or shock. A hypoxic child is likely to show other physical abnormalities long before turning blue. These abnormalities may include abnormal appearance with agitation or lethargy and increased work of breathing. A child in shock may also have pallor or mottling. Never wait for cyanosis to begin treatment with supplemental oxygen. However, the presence of cyanosis is always a critical sign

that requires immediate intervention with breathing support.

Abnormal circulation to skin in combination with abnormal appearance suggests shock. However, the abnormalities in appearance in early phases of compensated shock may be subtle, and some children may remain alert. As perfusion worsens and compensatory mechanisms fail, appearance will become abnormal, reflecting inadequate delivery of oxygen and glucose to the brain. Another clue to the presence of shock is <u>effortless tachypnea</u>, or <u>tachypnea</u> without signs of increased work of breathing. Effortless tachypnea is a reflex mechanism of blowing off carbon dioxide to compensate for the metabolic <u>acidosis</u> caused by poor peripheral perfusion (<u>lactic acidosis</u>). <u>Hypocarbia</u> (low blood CO_2 levels) generates a respiratory alkalosis and helps to restore normal pH (blood acid-base balance). Effortless tachypnea is different from the rapid and *labored* respirations that are present with illnesses and injuries associated with initial airway or lung pathology.

Techniques to Assess Circulation to Skin Step 3 in the PAT is evaluating circulation to skin. Be sure the child is exposed long enough for visual inspection, but not long enough to become cold. A cold child may have normal core perfusion, but abnormal circulation to skin. Cold circulating air temperature is the most common reason for misinterpretation of skin signs, and a young infant if undressed may become hypothermic quickly, even at normal ambient temperatures.

Inspect the skin and mucous membranes for pallor, mottling, and cyanosis. Look at the face, chest, abdomen, and extremities, and then inspect the lips for cyanosis. In dark skinned children, circulation to skin is sometimes more difficult to assess, and the lips, mucous membranes, and nail beds may be the best places to look for pallor or cyanosis (**Figure 1-9**).

Using the PAT to Evaluate Severity and Illness or Injury The PAT provides a general impression of the pediatric patient. The PAT

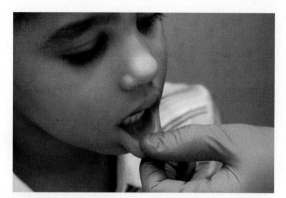

Figure 1-9 In dark skinned children, circulation to skin is sometimes more difficult to assess, and the lips, mucous membranes, and nail beds may be the best places to look for pallor or cyanosis.

Tip

By combining the three components of the PAT, the prehospital professional can answer three critical questions: (1) How sick or injured is the child? (2) What is the most likely physiologic abnormality? (3) What is the urgency for treatment?

uses pediatric-specific observations in combination with the scene size-up and chief complaint. The intent is to provide a standardized approach to the "general impression" and an instant picture of the child's physiologic status. By combining the three components of the PAT, the prehospital professional can answer three critical questions: (1) How severe is the child's illness or injury? (2) What is the most likely physiologic abnormality? (3) What is the urgency for treatment? This information will help the prehospital professional select her most important actions: how fast to intervene, what type of general and specific treatment to give, and how soon to transport.

The three elements of the PAT work together and allow a rapid assessment of the child's overall physiologic stability. For example, if a child is interactive and pink, but has mild intercostal retractions, the prehospital professional can take time to

approach the child in a developmentally appropriate manner to complete the initial assessment. On the other hand, if the child is limp, with unlabored rapid breathing and pale or mottled skin, shock is likely. In this case, the prehospital professional must move rapidly through the initial assessment and begin resuscitation, because abnormal appearance and decreased circulation to skin means shock. A child who has an abnormal appearance, but normal work of breathing and normal circulation to skin, probably has a primary brain dysfunction or a major metabolic or systemic problem, such as <u>postictal</u> state, <u>subdural hemorrhage</u>, brain <u>concussion</u>, intoxication, hypoglycemia, or <u>sepsis</u>.

The PAT has two important advantages. First, it allows the examiner to quickly obtain critical information about the child's physiologic status before touching or agitating the child. Second, the PAT helps set priorities for the rest of the hands-on initial assessment. The PAT takes only seconds, and it helps to identify the need for life saving interventions, and blends into the next phase of hands-on physical assessment.

The three components of PAT—appearance, work of breathing, and circulation to skin—can be assessed in any sequence, unlike the ordered ABCDEs of resuscitation discussed below.

Initial Assessment

Hands-on ABCDEs

The initial assessment follows the general assessment (PAT), and has two main parts: the hands-on physical assessment of the ABCDEs and the transport decision. The initial assessment is an ordered, hands-on, physical evaluation of the ABCDEs. It provides a prioritized sequence of life-support interventions to reverse critical physiologic abnormalities. As in adults, there is a specific order for treating life-threatening problems as they are identified, before moving to the next step. The steps are also the same as with adults, but there are important pedi-

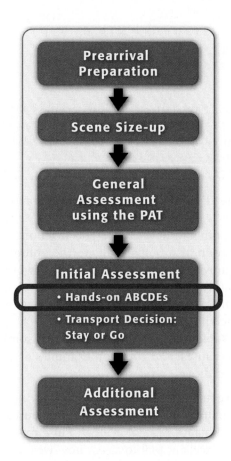

Table 1-4	Normal Respiratory Rate for Age
Respiratory Rate	**Age (breaths/min)**
Infant	30–60
Toddler	24–40
Preschooler	22–34
School-aged child	18–30
Adolescent	12–16

atric differences in anatomy, physiology, and signs of distress. ABCDE assessment involves the following components:

1. Airway
2. Breathing
3. Circulation
4. Disability
5. Exposure

Airway

The PAT may identify the presence of an airway obstruction, based on the presence of abnormal airway sounds. However, the loudness of the stridor or wheezing is not necessarily related to the amount of airway obstruction. For example, asthmatic children in severe distress may have little or no wheezing. Similarly, children with an upper airway foreign body below the <u>vocal cords</u> may have minimal stridor. Abnormal positioning and retractions will provide further information about the degree of obstruction, as will the quality of air entry on ausculta-

tion during the hands-on assessment of breathing.

If the airway is open, ensure that the chest rises with breathing. If gurgling is present, there may be mucus, blood, or a foreign body in the mouth or airway, or abnormal upper airway muscle tone. Based upon these simple observations, the prehospital professional can determine if the child's airway is patent (open), partially obstructed, or totally obstructed.

Breathing

Respiratory Rate Verify the respiratory rate per minute by counting the number of chest rises in 30 seconds, then doubling that number. Interpret the respiratory rate carefully. Normal infants may show "periodic breathing," or variable respiratory rate with short (< 20 second) periods of apnea. Therefore, counting for only 10 to 15 seconds may give a falsely low respiratory rate.

The significance of respiratory rates may be confusing. Rapid respiratory rates may simply reflect high fever, anxiety, pain, or excitement. Normal rates, on the other hand, may occur in a child who has been breathing rapidly with increased work of breathing for some time and is now becoming fatigued. Finally, interpretation requires knowledge of normal values for age (**Table 1-4**).

Serial assessment of respiratory rates may be especially useful and the trend is sometimes more accurate than any single value. A sustained increase or decrease in respiratory rate is usually significant.

Pay close attention to extremes of respiratory rate. A very rapid respiratory rate (more than 60 breaths/min for any age), especially with abnormal appearance or marked retractions, indicates respiratory distress and possibly respiratory failure. An abnormally slow respiratory rate is always worrisome because it might mean respiratory failure. Red flags are respiratory rates less than 20 breaths/min for children under 6 years of age and less than 12 breaths/min for children under 15 years of age. A normal respiratory rate alone never guarantees adequate oxygenation and ventilation. The respiratory rate must be interpreted along with appearance, work of breathing, and air movement.

Auscultation Listen with a stethoscope over the mid-axillary line to hear abnormal lung sounds, in inhalation and exhalation, such as crackles and wheezing (**Figure 1-10**). Inspiratory crackles indicate disease in the alveoli (air sacs) themselves. Often crackles are not heard on auscultation, even when the child has a pathologic condition such as pneumonia. The younger the child, the

Red flags respiratory rates are less than 20 breaths/min for children under 6 years of age and less than 12 breaths/min for children under 15 years of age.

more difficult it is to appreciate abnormal sounds on auscultation. Expiratory wheezing points to lower airway obstruction. Auscultation also helps evaluate the volume of air movement and effectiveness of work of breathing. A child with increased work of breathing and poor air movement may be in impending respiratory failure.

Table 1-5 lists abnormal breath sounds, their causes, and common examples of associated disease processes.

Oxygen Saturation After determining the respiratory rate and before forming auscultation, obtain pulse oximetry. Pulse oximetry is an excellent tool to assess how well a child is breathing (**Figure 1-11A**). **Figure 1-11B** illustrates the technique of placing a pulse oximetry probe on a young child. A pulse oximetry reading above 94% saturation on room air indicates good oxygenation. Be careful not to underestimate respiratory distress in a child with a reading above 94%. Sometimes the child can compensate for hypoxia by significantly increasing work of breathing and respiratory rate, and pulse oximetry may not reflect the true severity or urgency of the respiratory problem. As with any other measure-

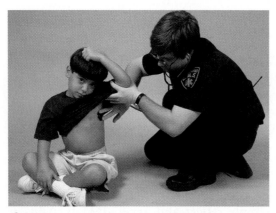

Figure 1-10 Listen for air movement over the mid-axillary line.

Table 1-5	Interpretation of Abnormal Breath Sounds	
Sound	**Cause**	**Examples**
Stridor	Upper airway obstruction	Croup, foreign body aspiration, retropharyngeal abscess
Wheezing	Lower airway obstruction	Asthma, foreign body, bronchiolitis
Expiratory grunting	Inadequate oxygenation	Pulmonary contusion, pneumonia, drowning
Inspiratory crackles	Fluid, mucus, or blood in the airway	Pneumonia, pulmonary contusion
Absent breath sounds despite increased work of breathing	Complete airway obstruction (upper or lower airway)	Physical barrier to transmission of breath sounds, foreign body, severe asthma, hemothorax, pneumothorax, pleural fluid, pneumonia, pneumothorax

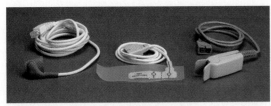

A

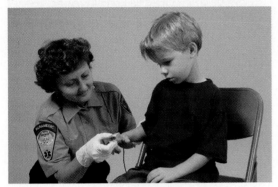

B

Figure 1-11 (A) Various pulse oximeter probes wrap around or clip onto a digit or earlobe. (B) Pulse oximetry is an excellent tool for assessing the effectiveness of breathing.

> **Tip**
>
> A rapid initial respiratory rate may simply reflect high fever, anxiety, pain, or excitement, and not any real physiologic or anatomic problem. Noting a trend of an abnormal respiratory rate is more useful for indicating true **pathology**.

ment, interpret pulse oximetry in the context of the "big picture," including work of breathing, appearance, and circulation.

While pulse oximetry is quite helpful in identifying a child with moderate respiratory distress, it will also help identify the child in respiratory failure. When the pulse oximetry reading is below 90% saturation in a child on 100% oxygen by a nonrebreathing mask, this usually represents respiratory failure requiring assisted ventilation. On the other hand, sometimes a child in severe respiratory distress or early respiratory failure may maintain her measured oxygen saturation by increasing

work of breathing and respiratory rate. This child may not appear to be critically ill by pulse oximetry alone. Interpret pulse oximetry together with the rest of the assessment to accurately evaluate the degree of respiratory distress or failure.

Circulation

The PAT provides important visual clues about circulation to skin. Observations from the hands-on evaluation of heart rate, pulse quality, skin temperature, capillary refill time, and blood pressure will give further information on the adequacy of perfusion.

Heart Rate Methods used to assess adult circulatory status—heart rate and blood pressure—have important limitations in children. First, normal heart rate varies with age, as noted in **Table 1-6.** Second, tachycardia may be an early sign of hypoxia or poor perfusion, but it may also reflect less serious conditions such as fever, anxiety, pain, and excitement. Like respiratory rate, interpret heart rate within the overall history, PAT, and initial assessment. A trend of increasing or decreasing heart rate may be

Case Study ❷

A 2-year-old male toddler was found face down in the family swimming pool. He was under water for no more than 1 minute and required cardiopulmonary resuscitation (CPR) by the mother to get him breathing again. On arrival of EMS, the child is alert, pink, and clinging to his mother. Respirations appear regular and non-labored, at 26 per minute. When you attempt to examine him further, he screams and fights you. You are unable to obtain a blood pressure, heart rate, or assess lung sounds. Mother is sobbing and frightened.

1. How useful is the Pediatric Assessment Triangle (PAT) in evaluating severity of illness and urgency for care?
2. In what ways is the PAT different than the ABCDEs in the initial assessment?

Table 1-6	Normal Heart Rate for Age
Age	**Heart Rate (beats/min)**
Infant	100–160
Toddler	90–150
Preschooler	80–140
School-aged child	70–120
Adolescent	60–100

Be careful not to underestimate respiratory distress in a child with a pulse oximetry reading above 94%, who may be using increased work of breathing and **tachypnea** to compensate for a serious hypoxic stress.

Interpret heart rate in the context of the overall history, PAT, and entire physical assessment.

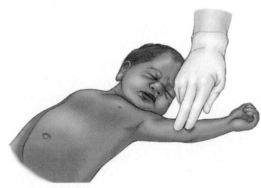

Figure 1-12 The anatomic position of the brachial pulse is medial to the biceps muscle.

quite useful, and may suggest worsening hypoxia or shock, or improvement after treatment. When hypoxia or shock becomes critical, the heart rate falls, leading to frank bradycardia. <u>Bradycardia</u> means *critical* hypoxia and/or ischemia. With tachycardia above 180 beats/min, an electronic monitor is necessary to accurately determine heart rate.

Pulse Quality Feel the pulse to obtain heart rate. Normally, the brachial pulse is palpable medial to the biceps in the <u>antecubital fossa</u> (**Figure 1-12**). Note the quality as either weak or strong. If the brachial pulse is strong, the child is probably not hypotensive. If a peripheral pulse cannot be felt, attempt to find a central pulse. Check the femoral pulse in infants and young children, or the carotid pulse in an older child or adolescent. If there is no pulse, start CPR.

Skin Temperature and Capillary Refill Time Next, do a hands-on evaluation of circulation to skin. While children with normal circulation may have cool hands and feet, the skin should be warm above the wrists and ankles. With decreasing perfusion, the

extremities become cooler proximally. Check capillary refill time in a fingertip, toe, heel, or on the pads of the fingertips. Normal capillary refill time is less than 2 to 3 seconds. The value of measuring capillary refill time is controversial for several reasons: peripheral perfusion may vary in some children at baseline; environmental factors such as cold room temperature may complicate interpretation; and it may be difficult for the prehospital professional to accurately count seconds under critical circumstances. The capillary refill time is just one element of the assessment of circulation. It must be evaluated in the context of the PAT and other perfusion characteristics such as heart rate, pulse quality, and blood pressure.

Signs of circulation to the skin (skin temperature, capillary refill time, and pulse quality) are tools to assess a child's circulatory status, especially when performed consecutively on a child who is not cold.

Blood Pressure Blood pressure determination and interpretation may be difficult in children because of the lack of patient cooperation, confusion about proper cuff size, and problems remembering normal values for age. **Figure 1-13A** illustrates the different sizes of blood pressure cuffs, and **Figure 1-13B** demonstrates the technique for getting a cor-

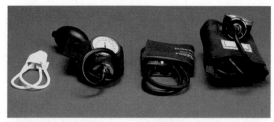

A

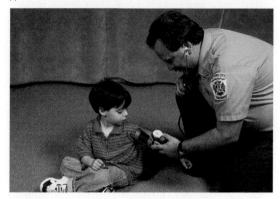

B

Figure 1-13 (A) There are several different blood pressure (BP) cuff sizes: neonatal, infant, child, and adult. (B) To obtain an accurate BP reading, use a cuff that is two-thirds the length of the child's upper arm.

Table 1-7	Normal Blood Pressure for Age
Age	Minimal Systolic Blood Pressure (mm Hg)
Infant (birth to 12 mos.)	> 60
Toddler (1–3)	> 70
Preschooler	> 75
School-aged child	> 80
Adolescent	> 90

Tip

For patients less than 3 years of age, the value of obtaining a blood pressure in the field may be outweighed by the technical difficulties of getting an accurate measurement.

Blip

Do not depend on blood pressure readings to diagnose shock. A "normal" blood pressure frequently exists in compensated shock.

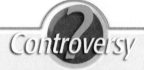

Controversy

The value of capillary refill time is controversial. Peripheral perfusion may be variable in some children, and environmental factors such as ambient temperature may have a strong influence on capillary refill time.

rect blood pressure in the arm or thigh. Always use a cuff with a width of two-thirds the length of the upper arm or thigh. For patients 3 years of age or less, technical difficulties reduce the value of a blood pressure in the field. When shock is suspected in this age group based on other assessments (e.g., history, mechanism, PAT), consider attempting blood pressure once on scene, but do not delay treatment or transport. For patients over 3 years of age, try one blood pressure measurement in the field, then move on to the rest of the assessment.

For children above one year of age, an easy formula for determining the lower limit of acceptable blood pressure by age is: minimal systolic blood pressure = 70 + (2 × age, in years). For example, a 2-year-old toddler with a systolic blood pressure of 65 mm Hg is in decompensated shock. **Table 1-7** shows approximate normal minimal systolic blood pressure values for different ages. High blood pressure is not a clinical problem for children in the field. Assume that a blood pressure is within normal limits if an infant or young child is agitated, crying, has pink skin, and easily palpable peripheral pulses. In a patient with this clinical profile, do not delay transport to obtain a blood pressure. Remember, a normal blood pressure measurement may be misleading. Although a low blood pressure definitely indicates decompensated shock, a "normal" blood pressure frequently exists in children with compensated shock.

Assessment of Pain—A New Vital Sign

It is easy for the prehospital professional to ignore, underestimate, or misinterpret the signs and symptoms of pain in infants and young children. Children are much less likely to receive effective pain medications than adults. Studies have demonstrated reluctance by all levels of emergency care personnel to administer drugs to children for control of pain and anxiety. The younger the child, the less likely the child will receive effective **analgesia** and **anxiolysis**. Yet, both adult and pediatric experience has validated the effectiveness of analgesia in the prehospital setting to decrease pain, without causing respiratory depression or interference with the accuracy of physical assessment.

Pain is present with most types of injury and with many illnesses. Inadequate treatment of pain has many adverse effects on the child and family. Pain itself causes significant morbidity and misery for the child and caregivers, and interferes with the prehospital professional's accurate assessment of physiologic abnormalities. Children who do not receive appropriate analgesia are more likely to have exaggerated pain responses to subsequent painful procedures. Even neonates have demonstrable chronic changes in pain perception when they are subjected to painful procedures without the benefit of analgesia. Post-traumatic stress is also more common among children who experience pain during acute illness and injury, and do not receive pharmacologic relief. Hence, just as with adults, it is essential to carefully assess pain in all children and to consider effective methods to provide relief from suffering when appropriate.

Local EMS protocols are now requiring that prehospital professionals assess and manage pain as a part of the initial assessment. Indeed, evaluation of pain is becoming a new vital sign in all ages, including

Tip

Evaluation of pain is becoming a new vital sign. Pain management will not only relieve distress of the child and family and greatly facilitate communication and physical assessments, but it will also assist in timely provision of necessary interventions and in the ease of transport.

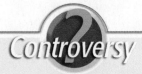

Controversy

While "self report" pain scales have not yet been extensively employed in the prehospital environment, they have been validated in other clinical settings as a method to provide an immediate evaluation of intensity of pain, and to monitor response to treatment.

children. Appropriate pain management will relieve distress of the child and family, and facilitate communication, physical assessment, and ease of transport.

Assessment of pain must take into consideration the developmental age of the patient. The ability to recognize pain will improve with the age of the child. For example, crying and agitation in a preverbal infant who is inconsolable when held by the caregiver may be due to hunger, hypoxia, or pain. In infants, further assessment is essential to identify sources of pain before administration of analgesia. In contrast, verbal children over 3 years of age are usually quite vocal about pain. Therefore, in older children, pain scales using pictures of facial expressions (Wong-Baker FACES Scale) or **visual analogue scores** may be helpful in assessing the need for pharmacologic relief of pain. **Figure 1-14** illustrates the Wong-Baker FACES Scale. While such "self report" scales have not yet been extensively employed in the prehospital environment, they have been validated in other settings to provide an immediate evaluation of intensity of pain, and to monitor response to treatment.

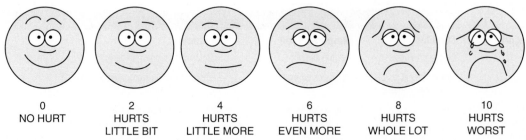

0	2	4	6	8	10
NO HURT	HURTS LITTLE BIT	HURTS LITTLE MORE	HURTS EVEN MORE	HURTS WHOLE LOT	HURTS WORST

Figure 1-14 Wong-Baker FACES Pain Rating Scale for self-assessment of pain.

Table 1-8	Methods of Prehospital Analgesia and Anxiolysis	
Non-pharmacologic	**Pharmacologic**
Calm manner	Morphine
Caregiver assistance through presence or holding	Fentanyl Nitrous oxide
Distraction techniques, with "toolbox" of toys	Benzodiazepines
Ice	12%–25% sucrose for neonates
Visual imagery	
Pacifier	
Music	

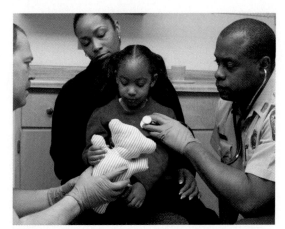

Figure 1-15 Use distraction techniques to help reduce the child's pain.

There is much overlap between the management of fear and anxiety, and the management of pain in infants and young children. Many non-pharmacologic and pharmacologic methods will relieve anxiety and reduce the perception of pain, as summarized in **Table 1-8.** Remaining calm, and providing quiet professional reassurance to both parents and child is the first important step. *A calm parent will help to make his/her child calm and more at ease.* Distraction techniques may be extremely helpful in reducing pain. Many prehospital providers learn to use toys, "magic tricks," or engaging stories to provide distraction. Some EMS systems use a "toolbox" with distraction equipment to facilitate pain relief (**Figure 1-15**). Keeping the caregiver with the child, and sometimes holding the child, are also useful strategies.

In older children, visual imagery techniques can often be helpful. Ask the child where she would most prefer to be at the present time; then assist her in visualizing the more tranquil or enjoyable environment while closing her eyes. Music is also a very effective distraction. Sucrose pacifiers are valuable in reducing pain in neonates. A 12% to 25% sucrose solution prior to a painful procedure is a useful technique that is known to reduce pain perception.

Pharmacologic methods for reducing pain are becoming a standard of prehospital care. Opiates, benzodiazapines, and nitrous oxide are available to prehospital professionals in many EMS systems. Intramuscular medications are less effective because children fear needles, and injection site pain may last for days. Analgesic and anxiolytic drugs may be easily delivered through inhalation technique, the transmucosal (e.g., sublingual, rectal) route, or by the transdermal route, although experience is still limited. Several techniques, such as inhaled nitrous oxide and rectal diazepam, have had excellent success in prehospital pediatric care. The fastest method for

Table 1-9	AVPU Scale		
Category	**Stimulus**	**Response Type**	**Reaction**
Alert	Normal environment	Appropriate	Normal interactiveness for age
Verbal	Simple command or sound stimulus	Appropriate/Inappropriate	Responds to name /Nonspecific or confused
Painful	Pain	Appropriate/Inappropriate/ Pathological	Withdraws from pain/Sound or motion without purpose or localization of pain/Posturing
Unresponsive			No perceptible response to any stimulus

Tip

Analgesic and anxiolytic drugs may be easily delivered through inhalation, transmucosal (e.g., sublingual, rectal) routes, or transdermal routes. Several techniques, such as inhaled nitrous oxide and rectal **diazepam**, have had excellent success in prehospital pediatric care.

administration of analgesia and anxiolysis is through the IV route. IV delivery provides the most effective, and the most controllable or <u>titratable</u> method, but it does involve establishing vascular access, which is usually painful. Also, the child's response to pain and anxiolytic medication is sometimes unpredictable, and must be carefully weighed against unwanted side effects. Medications to reduce pain also cause sedation and can result in respiratory depression, bradycardia, <u>hypoxemia</u>, <u>hypotension</u>, and even loss of protective airway reflexes. Occasionally, anxiolytic drugs cause a paradoxical worsening of agitation.

Assessment of pain has become a "vital sign," and management of pediatric pain and anxiety must be a routine part of field care in all EMS systems. This entails a thorough understanding of available non-pharmacologic techniques, drugs, potential drug contraindications and complications, and management of those complications.

Disability

Assessment of disability or neurologic status involves quick evaluation of the two main parts of the central nervous system: the <u>cerebral cortex</u> and the <u>brain stem</u>. First, assess neurologic status, which is controlled by the cortex, by looking at appearance as part of the PAT and then at level of consciousness using the AVPU scale (**Table 1-9**). Evaluate the brain stem by checking the responses of each pupil to a direct beam of light. A normal pupil constricts after a light stimulus. Pupillary response may be abnormal in the presence of drugs, ongoing seizures, hypoxia, or <u>impending brain stem herniation</u>. Next, evaluate motor activity. Look for symmetrical movement of the extremities, seizures, posturing, or <u>flaccidity</u>.

AVPU Scale The AVPU scale is a conventional way of assessing the level of consciousness in all patients. It categorizes motor response based on simple responses to stimuli. The patient is either alert, responsive to verbal stimuli, responsive only to painful stimuli, or unresponsive.

Abnormal Appearance and the AVPU Scale Assessment of appearance with the PAT provides different information than the AVPU scale. A child with an altered level of consciousness (ALOC) on the AVPU scale will always have abnormal appearance in the PAT because such a child will almost always have a serious or critical condition. However, a child with a mild to moderate illness or injury may be alert on the AVPU scale but have an abnormal appearance. *Assessing appearance using the PAT may give an earlier indication of the presence of serious illness and injury.*

The accuracy of the AVPU scale is controversial and it has an important limitation. While its ability to predict the extent of neu-

Neither the AVPU scale nor the Pediatric Glasgow Coma Scale allows assessment of restless or agitated behavioral states.

rologic compromise has not been well tested in children, it is easy to remember (there are no numbers to recall) and to use.

Indeed, the simplicity of the AVPU scale is a major advantage. One limitation of the AVPU scale, however, is in the evaluation of children with restless or agitated states. The scale only addresses *decreased* levels of responsiveness—a problem common to all of the current prehospital methods for disability assessment.

The more complicated Pediatric Glasgow Coma Scale (GCS) involves memorization and numerical scoring—tasks that may be hard to remember and apply in critical situations. Recent data suggest that the motor component of the GCS alone is the best predictor of neurological outcome. The much simpler-to-administer motor component of the GCS may be adequate for mental status evaluation in the field. The motor categories of the GCS are: (1) no response; (2) <u>extensor posturing</u>; (3) <u>flexor posturing</u>; (4) withdraws; (5) <u>localizes</u>; (6) obeys instructions (when age-appropriate). Like the AVPU scale, the GCS does not address degrees of neurologic disability in children who are restless, agitated, or combative.

Exposure

Proper exposure of the child is necessary for completing the initial physical assessment. The PAT requires that the caregiver remove part of the child's clothing to allow careful observation of the face, chest wall, and skin. Completing the ABCDE components of the initial assessment requires further exposure, as needed, to fully evaluate physiologic function, anatomic abnormalities, and unsuspected injuries. Be careful to avoid heat loss, especially in infants, by covering the child up as soon as possible.

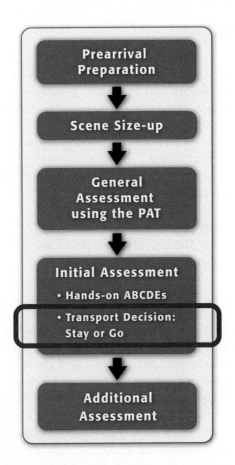

The Transport Decision: Stay or Go?

After completing the general and initial assessments and beginning resuscitation when necessary, the prehospital professional must make a crucial decision: Should she immediately transport the child to the ED, or should she continue with the additional assessment and treatment on scene? This decision process will be different for each child and for each EMS system.

BLS System

In a BLS system, field treatment options are limited. A request for ALS backup or early transport is appropriate if the scene is unsafe for the child, caregiver, or prehospital professional or when a child has:

- A serious mechanism of injury
- A history compatible with serious illness
- A physiologic abnormality noted on initial assessment
- A potentially serious anatomic abnormality
- Significant pain

ALS System

In an ALS system with more extensive treatment options, the transport decision is often complex. Major factors to consider include:

- The type of clinical problem (injury versus illness)
- The expected benefits of ALS treatment in the field
- Local EMS system treatment and transport policies
- The ALS provider's comfort level
- Transport time

The Clinical Problem

If the 9-1-1 call is for trauma, and if the child has a serious mechanism of injury, a physiologic abnormality, a potentially significant anatomic abnormality, or if the scene is unsafe, immediate transport is imperative. In these cases, stabilize the spine, manage the airway and breathing, stop external bleeding, and then transport. Attempt vascular access on the way to the ED. Examples of such patients include a child with an abnormal appearance after a closed head injury from a fall, or a child struck by a car who has a painful, deformed femur.

If the 9-1-1 call is for illness, the decision to stay or go is less clear cut and depends on the following factors: expected benefits of treatment, EMS system regulations, comfort level, and transport time.

Expected Benefits of Treatment

Time to operative care in the hospital has a major effect on the outcomes of children with serious injuries. Therefore, rapid transport after initial stabilization of the cervical spine, airway, and breathing is extremely important. Time to hospital care may also significantly affect the outcomes of children with certain medical illnesses. For example, a child in cardiogenic shock will benefit most from rapid transport to definitive care, because the hospital is the best place for life-saving treatments of this rare and complex condition.

On the other hand, some critically ill children will benefit from ALS treatment on scene. For example, for a child who is seizing, early treatment with a benzodiazepine is the best hope for getting the seizure under immediate control, and avoiding additional <u>anticonvulsant</u> administration and endotracheal intubation. Similarly, the risk of brain injury is decreased if <u>glucose</u> is administered to the unconscious diabetic child at the time that the prehospital professional documents hypoglycemia with a bedside test.

EMS System Regulations

The decision to stay or go will often be defined by EMS system regulations about treatment and transport. For example, some systems allow prehospital professionals to treat a child in cardiopulmonary arrest with ALS interventions until either the resuscitation is successful or death is declared. Other systems require transport after initial resuscitation is underway, with the decision to discontinue efforts left to the ED staff.

Comfort Level

Whenever a prehospital professional feels that the illness or injury requires a higher level of care, it is best to initiate transport quickly. Moreover, whenever the prehospital professional feels uncomfortable with a critical intervention, it is best to transport and attempt the intervention on the way to the ED, rather than on scene. For example, a child with decompensated hypovolemic shock usually deserves one attempt at vascular access on scene, then fluid administration on the way to the ED. The time spent on multiple IV attempts on scene might be better spent in transporting the child to definitive care, where the underlying cause of shock can be addressed.

Transport Time

The time to the nearest ED is another key factor. A shorter transport time will ordinarily support a shorter scene time. For example, if a child has ingested a potentially lethal poison, immediate transport is prudent if the ED is close by because of the complications of delay to definitive care. However, if transport time is long, consider initiating treatment on scene.

Summary of General and Initial Assessment

The initial components of pediatric assessment include the general assessment and the hands-on ABCDEs. The pediatric assessment triangle (PAT) is the basis for the general assessment. It includes evaluation of characteristics of appearance, work of breathing, and circulation to skin, and uses clues obtained by listening and looking from across the room. The initial assessment includes a hands-on evaluation of pediatric-specific indicators of cardiopulmonary or neurologic abnormalities. Although vital signs can be useful in the initial assessment, they can also be misleading. They must be interpreted in the context of age and the overall initial assessment. Interventions may be necessary at any point in the ABCDE sequence. Assessment and treatment of pain is an important addition to the initial assessment. After the ABCDEs, another crucial decision is whether to stay on scene and begin treatment or transport immediately. The type of clinical problem, the expected benefits of earlier transport, the local EMS policy, the prehospital professional's comfort level, and the transport time are key elements in the transport decision.

Additional Assessment

Focused History and Physical Exam

The focused history and physical exam has three objectives and is performed on both medical and trauma patients.

1. To obtain a complete description of the main complaint
2. To determine the mechanism of injury or circumstances of illness
3. To perform additional physical exam of specific anatomic locations

If the child appears to be physiologically unstable based on the initial assessment, the prehospital professional may decide to transport immediately and defer the focused his-

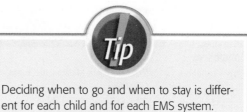

Tip

Deciding when to go and when to stay is different for each child and for each EMS system.

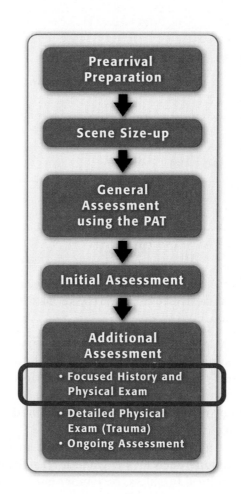

tory and physical exam. If the child is stable and the scene is safe, perform the focused history and physical exam and perform the detailed physical exam on trauma patients on scene, prior to transport. As opposed to the initial assessment—which focuses on *physiologic* problems that may be immediately life-threatening—the additional assessment focuses on *anatomic* abnormalities which are rarely life-threatening.

To obtain the focused history, use the SAMPLE mnemonic, as suggested in **Table 1-10.**

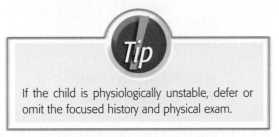

Table 1-10	Pediatric SAMPLE Components
Component	**Explanation**
Signs/Symptoms	Onset and nature of symptoms or pain or fever Age-appropriate signs of distress
Allergies	Known drug reactions or other allergies
Medications	Exact names and doses of ongoing drugs Timing and amount of last dose Timing and dose of analgesic/antipyretics
Past medical problems	Previous illnesses or injuries Immunizations History of pregnancy, labor, delivery (infants and toddlers)
Last food or liquid	Timing of the child's last food or drink, including bottle or breastfeeding
Events leading to the injury or illness	Key events leading to the current incident Fever history

Tip

If the child is physiologically unstable, defer or omit the focused history and physical exam.

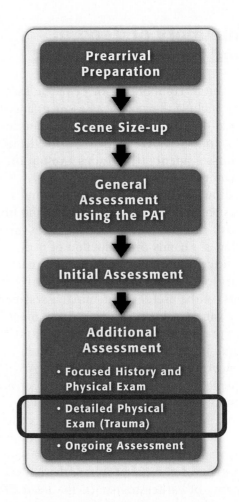

- Prearrival Preparation
- Scene Size-up
- General Assessment using the PAT
- Initial Assessment
- Additional Assessment
  - Focused History and Physical Exam
  - Detailed Physical Exam (Trauma)
  - Ongoing Assessment

After getting the focused history and physical exam, reassess the physical findings based on the additional information. In trauma patients, after the detailed physical exam, reconsider the need for immediate transport.

If a child has an apparently minor condition—such as low-grade fever, feeding difficulties, fussiness, or minor trauma—be careful not to overlook clues to possible serious underlying conditions. Ingestions, metabolic problems, and systemic infections may present with nonspecific findings in infants and toddlers. Consider child maltreatment when the physical findings are not logically related to the complaint leading to the call, or if the history is implausible.

Detailed Physical Exam—Trauma

If the child with traumatic injuries is stable on scene and does not need treatment after the focused history and physical exam, or if she is on the way to the hospital but does not require ongoing treatment, perform a detailed physical exam. This physical evaluation must include all anatomic areas and builds on the findings of the initial assessment and focused history and physical exam.

Often this portion of the assessment is not possible because of transport and treatment priorities. Sometimes, it is unnecessary because the problem has been fully evaluated in earlier phases of the assessment or the complaint and history are minor or well localized (e.g., a laceration, twisted ankle).

Use the toe-to-head sequence for the detailed physical examination of infants, toddlers, and preschoolers. This approach allows the prehospital professional to gain the child's trust and cooperation, and will increase the accuracy of the physical findings. Ask for the assistance of the caregiver in the detailed exam.

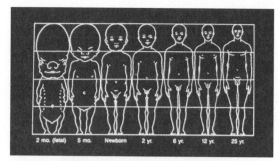

Figure 1-16 The relationship of the head to the body changes with advancing age.

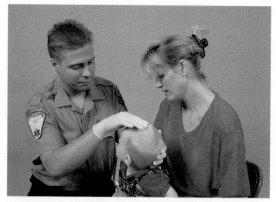

Figure 1-17 The anterior fontanelle of the infant is a window to the central nervous system.

Note the following special anatomic characteristics of children when performing the detailed examination.

General Observations
Observe the clothing for any unusual odors or for stains that might suggest a poison. If poisoning is suspected, remove soiled or dirty clothing and save it, and wash the child's skin with soap and water.

Skin
Observe the skin carefully for rashes and for bruising patterns that may suggest maltreatment, as discussed in Chapter 12. Look for bite marks; straight line marks from cords or straps; pinch marks; or hand, belt, or buckle pattern bruises. Inspect for non-blanching <u>petechiae</u> or <u>purpuric</u> lesions, and look for any new lesions during transport.

Head
The younger the infant or child, the larger the head is in proportion to the rest of the body, increasing the risk for head injury with deceleration (such as in motor vehicle crashes) (**Figure 1-16**). Look for bruising, swelling, and <u>hematomas</u>. Significant blood can be lost between the skull and scalp of a small infant. Assessment of the anterior <u>fontanelle</u> in infants less than 9- to 18-months-old can provide information (**Figure 1-17**). A bulging and <u>nonpulsatile fontanelle</u> suggests elevated intracranial pressure due to <u>meningitis</u>, <u>encephalitis</u>, or <u>intracranial</u> bleeding. A sunken fontanelle suggests dehydration.

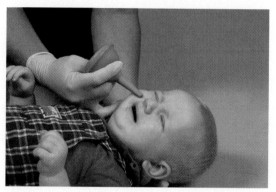

Figure 1-18 Gentle bulb suction may bring relief to the infant.

Eyes
A thorough evaluation of pupil size, reaction to light, and symmetry of <u>extraocular</u> muscle movements may be difficult to perform in infants. Gently rocking infants in the upright position will often get them to open their eyes. A colorful distracting object can then be used to look at eye movements.

Nose
Young infants preferentially breathe through their nose, so nasal congestion with mucus can cause marked respiratory distress. Gentle bulb or catheter suction of the nostrils may bring relief (**Figure 1-18**). Leaking blood (<u>cerebrospinal fluid [CSF]</u>, <u>rhinorrhea</u>) suggests a <u>basilar skull fracture</u>.

Ears
Look for any drainage from the ear canals. Leaking blood (<u>CSF otorrhea</u>) suggests a basilar skull fracture. Check for bruises

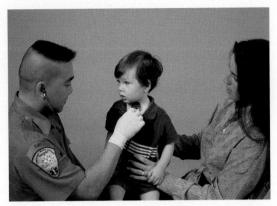

Figure 1-19 Listen at the trachea to distinguish the origin of abnormal airway sounds.

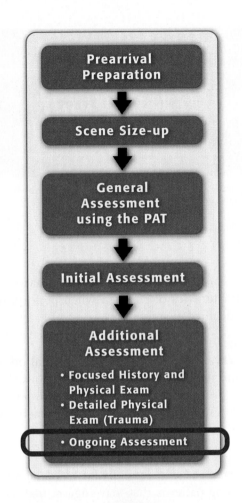

behind the ear or <u>Battle sign</u>, another sign of basilar skull fracture. The presence of <u>pus</u> may indicate an ear infection or perforation of the ear drum.

Mouth

In the trauma patient, look for active bleeding and loose teeth. Note the smell of the breath. Some ingestions are associated with identifiable odors, such as <u>hydrocarbons</u>. <u>Acidosis</u>, as in <u>diabetic ketoacidosis</u>, may impart a sweet smell to the breath.

Neck

Examine the <u>trachea</u> for <u>edema</u>, or bruising. Listen with a stethoscope over the trachea at the midline (**Figure 1-19**). This is a quick and easy way to differentiate between very proximal airway obstruction (usually mucus in the nose) and true wheezing or stridor.

Chest

Reexamine the chest for penetrating injuries, lacerations, bruises, or rashes. If the child is injured, feel the <u>clavicles</u> and every rib for tenderness and/or deformity.

Back

Inspect the back for lacerations, penetrating injuries, bruises, or rashes.

Abdomen

Inspect the abdomen for <u>distention</u>. Gently palpate the abdomen and watch closely for guarding or tensing of the abdominal muscles, which may suggest infection, obstruction, or <u>intra-abdominal</u> injury. Note any tenderness or masses.

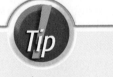

Always do the ongoing assessment to track problems and monitor response to treatment.

Extremities

Assess for <u>symmetry</u>. Compare both sides for color, warmth, size of joints, and tenderness. Put each joint through full range of motion while watching the eyes of the child for signs of pain, unless there is obvious deformity of the extremity suggesting a fracture.

Ongoing Assessment

Perform ongoing assessment of all patients to observe the response to treatment and to track the progression of identified physiologic and anatomic problems. New problems may also be identified on reassessment. Data from the reassessment will guide ongoing treatment.

The elements in the ongoing assessment are:

1. The PAT
2. The ABCDEs with repeat vital signs
3. Assessment of positive anatomic findings
4. Review of the effectiveness and safety of treatment

The elements in the ongoing assessment are also the basis for determination of an appropriate transport destination, and for accurate, pediatric-specific, radio or telephone communications with medical oversight or the ED.

Radio Reporting

Proper radio reporting promotes a seamless transfer of care from the out-of-hospital to ED settings, maximizing the ability of all clinicians to provide efficient and effective care. A good radio report transmits vital data completely and concisely, highlighting pediatric-specific information to allow the ED team to best prepare for the patient's arrival. For a step-by-step explanation see

(Field Reporting, Procedure 1).

Diagnostic Testing

Diagnostic testing usually begins when the child reaches the ED. Although in reality, the prehospital professional can perform some types of specific testing in the field, with rapid glucose determinations, 12-lead ECG monitoring, and pulse oximetry. This part of the assessment frequently requires ancillary testing, such as laboratory and radiographic evaluations. Diagnostic testing is usually part of in-patient assessment in the hospital pediatric ward or pediatric intensive care unit.

Summary of Additional Assessment and Diagnostic Testing

After the initial assessment and resuscitation, the prehospital professional must determine the severity of the illness or injury, and make a decision regarding timing of the transport. If additional evaluation is appropriate, perform a focused history and physical exam and a detailed physical exam (for the injured child) either on scene or on the way to the ED. These additional phases of assessment are not indicated if there is an acute life-threatening or limb-threatening problem. The detailed physical exam is more for detection of anatomic problems than for evaluation of physiologic abnormalities. Always perform ongoing assessments to observe the response to interventions and to guide changes in treatment, transport, and triage. Diagnostic testing refers to laboratory and radiographic evaluation to determine causation, and mainly occurs after arrival in the ED and during hospitalization for admitted patients.

Case Study 3

You are called to the home of a 2-month-old infant boy who stopped breathing and turned blue according to his babysitter. He reportedly had a fever all day. The infant is lying supine; his skin is pale and mottled. When touched, the infant becomes extremely irritable and exhibits a high-pitched, screeching cry. When left alone he appears lethargic and poorly responsive. There is no abnormal positioning, abnormal airway sounds, stridor, flaring, or grunting. The respiratory rate is 60 breaths/min and unlabored. The heart rate is 200 beats/min. Peripheral pulses are weak and the extremities are cool to the touch. Capillary refill is approximately 5 seconds.

1. Does this infant's appearance suggest a serious problem?
2. Is this infant in shock?

Chapter Review

Case Study Answers

Case Study ❶ page 3

Beware of the pale child! Consider any child who has experienced significant trauma, and who is pale at the scene, to have significant blood loss until proven otherwise. Children are able to compensate for blood loss and hypovolemia through catecholamine surges, which cause tachycardia and peripheral vasoconstriction. These reflexes shut down the circulation to the skin and result in a pale patient. Although this child appears to have had a significant head injury, his level of consciousness is reasonably normal, so the initial issue needing emergent attention is hemorrhagic shock. Abdominal injuries with blunt trauma to the liver and spleen can result in significant internal bleeding without external signs of injury. Many children with internal bleeding do not even have abdominal tenderness. This child requires timely transport to a trauma center with pediatric capabilities.

The most important physiologic process needing emergent attention is hemorrhagic shock. Indicators of suspected hemorrhagic shock are mild tachycardia, weak pulses, delayed capillary refill, and a borderline low blood pressure (80 mm Hg/palp). Rapid transport is necessary. Delay vascular access until the child is en route to the hospital.

This child is clearly in pain. However, weigh the benefits of pharmacologic therapy to relieve pain against the potential for circulatory collapse, delay in transport, and the need to effectively assess appearance. Do not use opiate analgesics, such as morphine, in patients with suspected compensated hemorrhagic shock.

Case Study ❷ page 17

The PAT is an accurate tool to evaluate severity of illness and the urgency for providing life saving care. On arrival at the scene of this patient, it is quite reassuring to find the toddler alert, pink, and with non-labored respirations. His vigorous responses make it difficult to perform the conventional ABCDE assessment! Since this child clearly has no serious cardiorespiratory problems, is alert and awake, and fights your examination, there is no need for transport with lights and siren. Transport every infant or child who has had a submersion injury to a hospital for observation of progression of symptoms. However, the findings on the PAT allow the prehospital professional to slow the pace, get more information on scene, withhold resuscitative interventions, and avoid the risk of "lights and siren" transport.

Anytime there is an unwitnessed submersion event, consider a traumatic injury. The usual mechanism of a toddler pool drowning involves falling less than 3 feet (1 meter) into a body of water. In this scenario, it is unlikely that he has sustained a significant head or spinal injury. Furthermore, if he is moving his neck without apparent discomfort while in his mother's arms, but then vigorously screams and fights when you attempt to examine him, it is unlikely that spinal stabilization will be helpful. Local protocols govern this decision. Treatment and transport in this patient are not emergent. However, ongoing assessment during transport is necessary as pulmonary complications of submersion, primarily hypoxia, may have a delayed presentation.

Case Study **3** page 29

Any infant who has an acute life-threatening event, who stopped breathing or turned blue, deserves EMS transport, regardless of their appearance on your arrival. In this case, the need for urgent treatment and transport is obvious. The PAT indicators of shock in this infant include altered appearance. While that finding could be due to causes other than poor brain perfusion (e.g., infection, trauma, toxins, hypoxia), the presence of effortless tachypnea and mottled skin support the diagnosis of shock. Alternating lethargy and irritability may progress to unresponsiveness, as perfusion worsens.

Hands-on examination confirms the suspicion of shock. This patient's heart rate is rapid at 200 beats/min, with weak peripheral pulses, cool extremities, and delayed capillary refill. Even without a blood pressure, the abnormal appearance and skin findings suggest that he should be treated for decompensated shock. Although the cause of shock is unknown, treatment of any type of decompensated shock includes vascular access and 20 mL/kg boluses of <u>crystalloid fluid</u>. Make one attempt at vascular access on scene and then rapidly transport this patient to definitive care. Reassess his response to therapy frequently en route.

Suggested Readings

Textbooks

American Academy of Orthopaedic Surgeons: *Emergency Care and Transportation of the Sick and Injured,* 9th Edition. Sudbury, MA, Jones and Bartlett Publishers, 2005.

American Academy of Pediatrics and the American College of Emergency Physicians: *APLS: The Pediatric Emergency Medicine Resource,* 4th Edition. Sudbury, MA, Jones and Bartlett Publishers, 2004.

Anne M, Agur A, Dalley A: *Grant's Atlas of Anatomy,* 11th Edition. Lippincott Williams & Wilkins, 2004.

Bledsoe B, Porter R, Cherry R: *Essentials of Paramedic Care.* New Jersey, Prentice Hall, 2003.

Hazinski M, Zaritsky A, Nadkarni V, et al: *PALS Provider Manual.* American Heart Association, 2002.

Zitelli B, Davis H: *Atlas of Pediatric Physical Diagnosis,* 4th Edition. Philadelphia, Mosby, 2002.

Articles

Gausche M. Out-of-hospital care of pediatric patients. *Pediatr Clin North Am.* Dec 1999; 46(6):1305–27.

Warren J. Guidelines for the inter- and intrahospital transport of crtically ill patients. *Crit Care Med.* Jan 2004; 32(1):256–62.

Using a Developmental Approach

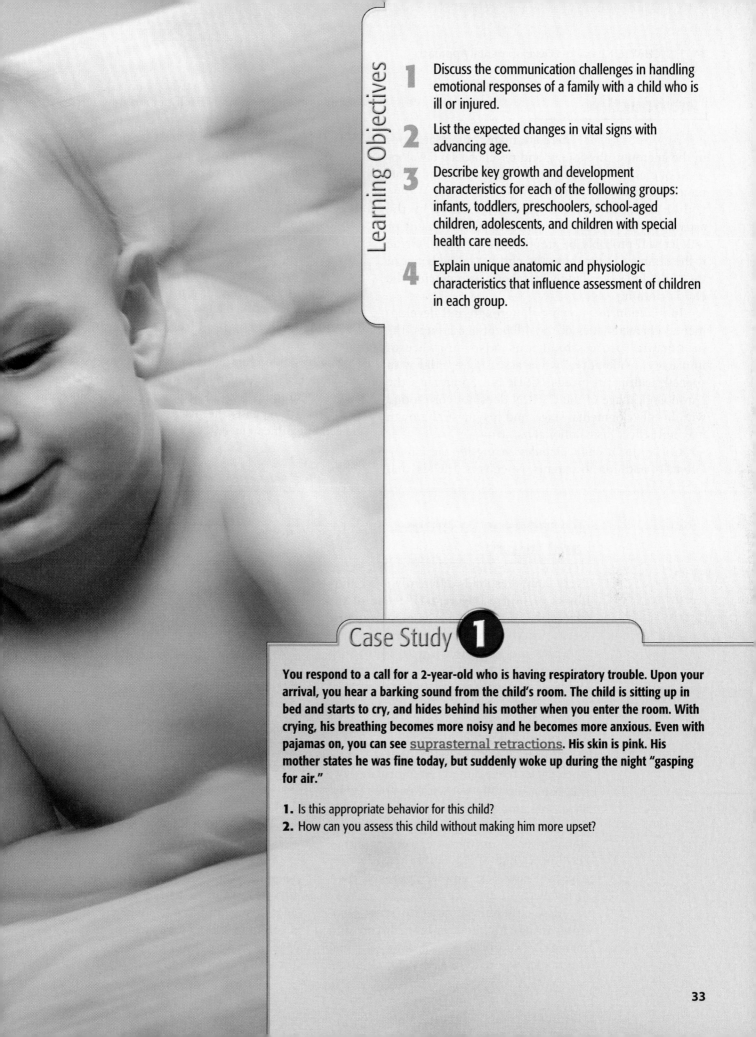

Learning Objectives

1 Discuss the communication challenges in handling emotional responses of a family with a child who is ill or injured.

2 List the expected changes in vital signs with advancing age.

3 Describe key growth and development characteristics for each of the following groups: infants, toddlers, preschoolers, school-aged children, adolescents, and children with special health care needs.

4 Explain unique anatomic and physiologic characteristics that influence assessment of children in each group.

Case Study **1**

You respond to a call for a 2-year-old who is having respiratory trouble. Upon your arrival, you hear a barking sound from the child's room. The child is sitting up in bed and starts to cry, and hides behind his mother when you enter the room. With crying, his breathing becomes more noisy and he becomes more anxious. Even with pajamas on, you can see <u>suprasternal retractions</u>**. His skin is pink. His mother states he was fine today, but suddenly woke up during the night "gasping for air."**

1. Is this appropriate behavior for this child?
2. How can you assess this child without making him more upset?

Introduction

CHILDREN ARE SPECIAL! There are many unique features in the anatomy, physiology, and psychosocial development of children that affect their assessment and treatment. Each age requires different considerations. Unlike the adult, who is usually reassured by the arrival of the prehospital professional, the infant or toddler will probably be afraid. This is especially true if the stranger is touching the child, coming between the child and other family members, or removing the child's clothing.

In addition to knowing the growth and developmental characteristics of the different age groups, the prehospital professional must also be aware of unusual considerations when assessing a child with special health care needs (CSHCN). Sometimes the chronological age of the CSHCN does not correspond with his developmental stage, and his physical growth may not reflect his emotional maturity.

Caring for a child includes caring for the family. Often, in addition to parents, caregivers, friends, and siblings may be present. Each person may have a different response to the child who is ill or injured, and the prehospital professional must be prepared to care for the entire "extended" family of friends and relatives. Communication skills are often as important as assessment and treatment skills in establishing an atmosphere of trust and comfort. Creating such an atmosphere requires that the prehospital professional have a confident and efficacious attitude toward children's care, and employ age-appropriate pediatric skills. Communication skills become especially important in the event of a mass casualty incident or natural disaster (see Chapter 8, *Children in Disasters*).

This chapter will address age-specific growth characteristics and assessment techniques for physiologically stable children from infancy to adolescence, and for CSHCN. Chapter 1 addresses general assessment techniques for the acutely ill or injured child. Chapter 10 expands the discussion on children with special health care needs.

Responses to Illness and Injury

Every family responds differently to a child's illness or injury (**Figure 2-1**). Some of the factors that determine the family's response are: the child's developmental level; the family's previous experience with the health care system; coping strategies; culture; availability of support systems; and the nature of the emergency. **Table 2-1** summarizes some of the common ways in which adults behave under family illness or injury stress.

While some caregivers' responses in emergencies may seem too emotional or illogical, listen carefully to their concerns. Establishing an atmosphere of collaboration, rather than dismissal, allows the prehospital professional to draw on the caregivers' expertise and knowledge of the child, because they usually know best how to approach their own child.

Also, children are quick to sense emotions in adults such as fear, anger, and shame. A calm professional demeanor and appearance will help to gain the trust of the

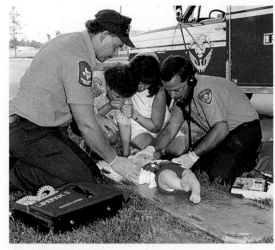

Figure 2-1 Every family responds differently to a child's illness or injury.

caregivers, which many times helps to calm the child and gain his trust.

The ill or injured child may also respond to a stressful situation in a variety of ways, often by acting younger than his age. It is helpful to tell caregivers that this is a common and temporary response. An adolescent may exhibit responses similar to those of the caregivers.

Table 2-1	Common Responses of Caregivers to Acute Illness or Injury in a Child
Response	**Description**
Disbelief	Caregivers may be struggling with the child's illness or injury. They may seem too calm or unconcerned.
Guilt	Caregivers may be horrified that they were unable to recognize the serious nature of their child's condition or because they were unable to prevent an injury. They may focus their attention on what should have been done, rather than on the child's immediate situation.
Anger	Caregivers may show their consternation as anger, and they may direct their anger at the prehospital professional. Caregivers may become hostile when the prehospital professional makes efforts to stabilize the child. They may attempt to refuse transport.
Physical symptoms	Caregivers may have tachycardia, nausea, headache, chest pain, sweaty palms, dry mouth, or hyperventilation.

A family's response to a child's illness or injury will be influenced by the child's developmental level, previous experience with the medical system, coping strategies, culture, availability of support systems, and the nature of the emergency.

Table 2-2	Normal Respiratory Rate for Age
Age	**Respiratory Rate (breaths/min)**
Infant	30–60
Toddler	24–40
Preschooler	22–34
School-aged child	18–30
Adolescent	12–16

Communication skills are often as important as assessment and treatment skills.

Summary of Communication Skills

Children, families, and caregivers all respond differently to the emotional effects of illness and injury. The child's development level, previous experience with the medical system, coping strategies, culture, availability of support systems, and the nature of the emergency all influence reactions. The prehospital professional must appreciate the spectrum of psychological responses and be prepared to communicate effectively with patients and families under many different circumstances. Effective communication is a cornerstone of effective out-of-hospital care.

Vital Signs Through the Ages

A common challenge in evaluating infants and children is determining normal vital signs based on the age of the patient. Respiratory rate, heart rate, and blood pressure are all influenced by age, the presence or absence of fever, anxiety, or pain as well as the child's activity level. In ill or injured children, the prehospital professional must attempt to distinguish the impact of these "generic" factors on vital signs from changes due to pathologic processes. Chapter 1 presents key physical characteristics and assessment techniques that will assist the prehospital professional in separating the "sick" child from the "not sick" child.

Respiratory Rate

While normal values for vital signs vary with age, there are a variety of physiologic or anatomic bases for these changes. The normal range of respiratory rate slows with age due to an increasing number of <u>alveoli</u>, and increasing lung volume and lung compliance with linear growth. **Table 2-2** lists the normal respiratory rate by age.

Sometimes there is a problem with accurate counting of the rate, especially if the

In infants, observe abdominal excursions and count rate for 30 to 60 seconds to obtain an accurate respiratory rate.

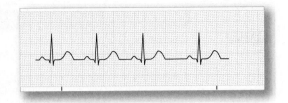

Figure 2-2 ECG of a sinus arrhythmia.

count is done in a 15 second interval. In infants, observe and count <u>abdominal excursions</u> for 30 to 60 seconds to obtain an accurate respiratory rate. As a child grows, breathing becomes less dependent on abdominal muscles and the diaphragm and more dependent upon the chest muscles. Observing <u>thoracic excursions</u> for 15 to 30 seconds will provide an accurate respiratory rate in an older child.

Heart Rate

The baseline heart rate of infants and children slows with age, reflecting increasing control of the heart rate by the <u>vagus nerve</u>. The vagus nerve transmits <u>cholinergic impulses</u>, which slow the beating of the heart. **Table 2-3** lists normal heart rates for age. In addition, by 2 years of age a <u>circadian rhythm</u> in heart rate is present, manifested by a fall of 10 to 20 beats/min while the child is asleep. One confusing factor in assessing a child's heart rate during different phases of the sleep-wake cycle, or during different phases of respiration, is that the child's rhythm is more irregular than an adult's. This <u>sinus arrhythmia</u> is more prominent in toddlers to school-aged children and is also due to immature vagus nerve control (**Figure 2-2**).

Table 2-3	Normal Heart Rates for Age
Age	**Heart Rate (beats/min)**
Infant	100–160
Toddler	90–150
Preschooler	80–140
School-aged child	70–120
Adolescent	60–100

Table 2-4	Normal Blood Pressure Values for Age
Age	**Minimal Systolic Blood Pressure (mm Hg)**
Infant (birth–12 mos)	> 60
Toddler (1–3)	> 70
Preschooler	> 75
School-aged child	> 80
Adolescent	> 90

Blood Pressure

A child's <u>blood pressure</u> increases with age (**Table 2-4** lists normal blood pressure values for age). The measured blood pressure is affected by equipment size. A cuff that is too small will give falsely elevated readings, while one that is too large will give readings that are too low. If <u>diastolic pressure</u> cannot be <u>auscultated</u>, obtain a systolic pressure by palpating the pulse. This value is approximately 10 mm Hg lower than an auscultated pressure because of the relative insensitivity of <u>palpation</u> in appreciating initial pulsations as the cuff is deflated.

Temperature

Body temperature also varies with age, and site of measurement. Newborn temperatures are often higher than older children, averaging 37.5°C (99.5°F) during the first 6 months of life. After 3 years of age, the temperature falls to below 37.2°C (99°F), and finally to 36.7°C (98°F) by 11 years of age. There is also a circadian rhythm to body temperature that develops by 5 years of age. This results in a lower temperature at night and a higher temperature during the day. In infants, when

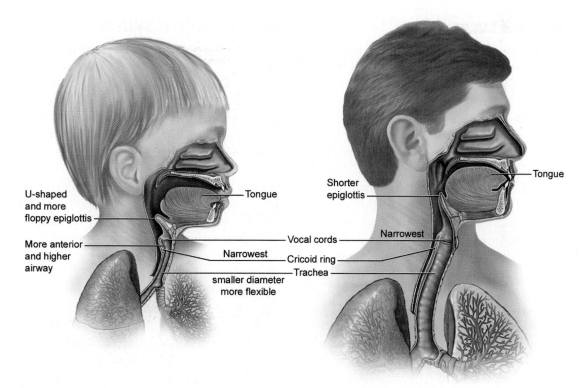

Figure 2-3 The epiglottis changes from a U shape to the longer and thinner adult structure.

a recorded temperature is important to the assessment, and the child is stable, ask the caregiver to obtain a rectal temperature. A rectal temperature is the gold standard. A tympanic temperature may be acceptable in older children (>1 year) but is not as accurate as a rectal temperature. An axillary temperature is approximately 2°F (1°C) lower than the rectal temperature. Normal body temperature decreases with increasing distance from the central circulation.

Growth Rates

Physical growth of infants and children includes body (somatic) growth as well as organ system growth. Skeletal and muscular growth has two spurts, the first from birth to 4 years of age and the second in adolescence (ages 9–14 for females, ages 10–16 for males). Brain, spinal cord, and nerve growth occurs maximally in the first few years of life, and reaches adult proportions by 10 years of age.

The presence or absence of key secondary sex characteristics, especially pubic hair, marks a key physiologic turning point for children. Genital growth begins about 8 years of age in females and 9 years of age in males, but there is significant variation. *When children have visible pubic hair, they have usually attained adult physiology.*

Anatomical Changes

Neck/Airway

The neck is short in infancy and elongates during childhood due to vertebral growth. As this occurs, anatomic landmarks also change in shape, size, and location. The epiglottis changes from a U shape to the longer and thinner adult structure (**Figure 2-3**). It also moves in location from the level of the C-1 vertebra to the C-3 vertebra. At birth, the larynx is only 1/3 the adult size. It becomes wider and longer until 3 years of age, and undergoes another growth spurt during puberty. At birth, the trachea is 1/3 the adult length, and increases in anteroposterior (AP) and lateral diameters 300% by puberty.

Chest and Lungs

At birth, the chest wall is round (AP diameter equals lateral diameter). As the infant grows, it flattens out (lateral growth exceeds AP growth). Because an infant's chest wall is thin, heart and lung sounds are also transmitted throughout the chest. Breath sounds are often audible on inspiration and expiration (<u>bronchovesicular</u>). In addition, secretions present anywhere in the respiratory tract are often heard throughout the chest. In an infant, respirations are mainly abdominal, due to the greater role of the <u>diaphragm</u> in breathing mechanics. By 6 years of age, breathing becomes more thoracic in origin, due to the development of chest wall musculature.

The lung tissue itself also changes with age. At birth, an infant has only 8% of the adult number of <u>alveoli</u>. The number of alveoli increases until 8 years of age, after which they increase in size but not number.

Heart

At birth, the right <u>ventricle</u> is the same size as the left ventricle, a function of the demands of fetal circulation. This accounts for a right axis on <u>electrocardiograms (ECGs)</u> in infants. However, the left ventricle quickly grows in size and muscle mass, and greatly outsizes the right ventricle with age. The left ventricle reaches adult proportions of 2:1 by 1 year of age.

Abdomen

A newborn infant has a protuberant abdomen for numerous reasons. The liver is relatively large, the stomach is more horizontal, and the lungs expand downward with movement of the diaphragm. The stomach capacity increases from 30 to 90 mL at birth, to 210 to 360 mL by 1 year of age, and 500 mL by 2 years of age. It assumes a more vertical position during childhood, and reaches an adult volume of 750 to 900 mL. The abdomen also seems protuberant in toddlers due a normal lumbar <u>lordosis</u> (curvature) of the spine. The abdomen becomes more <u>scaphoid</u> (flat) in school-age children.

Musculoskeletal System

In infants and young children, new longitudinal bone growth occurs in secondary centers of <u>ossification</u> at the end of the long bones, <u>vertebral bodies</u>, and the <u>cranium (physeal plates)</u>. These <u>cartilaginous growth plates</u> are relatively weak, and are vulnerable to fractures exclusive to childhood. Bone growth ends with the ossification of the growth cartilage and union of the <u>epiphysis</u> and <u>diaphysis</u>. Growth in children is asymmetric, with the lower extremities, especially the <u>distal extremities</u> (e.g., feet), growing prior to puberty, and the trunk during puberty.

Muscle growth includes an increase in the size of muscle cells. There is a growth spurt in the number of muscle cells at 2 years of age, with a maximal increase during puberty. The proportions of muscle mass to body weight changes during childhood, going from 1:5 at birth to 1:3 in adolescence.

Nervous System

The growth of the nervous system occurs rapidly during infancy. It is 25% the adult size at birth, 50% by 1 year of age, 80% by 3 years of age and 90% by 7 years of age. This includes growth of <u>glial cells</u>, <u>dendrites</u>, and <u>synaptic connections</u>. This growth is associated with the rapid increase in fine motor, gross motor, and language skills of infants and toddlers. These changing competencies impact the type of assessment techniques appropriate for evaluating children of different ages.

Summary of Changes in Vital Signs and Anatomy Through Childhood

Vital signs are useful for assessment but are sometimes difficult to obtain and difficult to interpret. Not only do normal vital signs change significantly with age, but respiratory and heart rates are especially sensitive to <u>adrenalin</u> release due to fear, pain, anxiety, cold, or high activity level. Other anatomic changes in the airway, chest, heart, abdomen, musculoskeletal system, and nervous system occur throughout childhood and require adaptations in assessment techniques.

Infants

Developmental Characteristics

Infants are vulnerable and have a limited number of behaviors (**Figure 2-4**). Infants less than 2 months of age spend most of their time sleeping or eating. They are not yet able to tell the difference between parents and other caregivers or strangers. They need to be kept warm, dry, and fed. They experience the world through their bodies. Being held, cuddled, or rocked soothes the infant. Hearing is also well developed at birth, and calm and reassuring talk is often helpful.

Infants between 2 and 6 months of age are more active, which makes them easier to evaluate. They spend more time awake, they

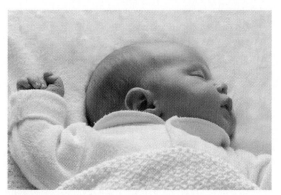

Figure 2-4 Infants are vulnerable creatures, with a limited number of behaviors.

begin to make eye contact, and they recognize caregivers. Healthy infants in this age group will have a strong suck, active extremity movement, and a vigorous cry. They may follow a bright light or toy with their eyes, or turn their heads toward a loud sound or the caregiver's voice.

Between the ages of 6 and 12 months, most infants learn to talk or babble, sit unsupported, reach for toys, move objects from one hand to another, and put things in their mouths. At approximately 1 year of age, most infants start to scoot or crawl, pull to a stand, "cruise" furniture, and may start to walk.

At 7 to 8 months, infants show a clear preference for their parents or caregivers, and by the age of 9 to 10 months demonstrate stranger anxiety, making separation of the child and caregiver for the purposes of assessment or transport especially problematic. They are most easily comforted by their parent or by a familar adult.

Table 2-5 summarizes anatomic and physiologic differences that are important in the assessment and care of the infant.

The infant's capacity to interact with his environment is limited, and the signs and symptoms of illness are not always easy to appreciate. Because of these factors, always take the caregiver's perception that "something is wrong" seriously. *An infant in the first 3 months of life who is reported to be fussier than usual, feeding poorly, or sleeping excessively, or who has a temperature greater than 38°C must be seen by a physician.* It is important to find out if there has been a recent history of trauma, how

Table 2-5	Anatomic and Physiologic Features of Infants

- Infants are nose breathers for the first several months of life. Obstruction of the nose from secretions, blood, or edema may cause respiratory distress.
- The muscles of the infant's chest wall are not yet developed, and the abdominal muscles are the main muscles used for breathing. "Belly breathing" is normal in infants and may become exaggerated as breathing becomes more rapid.
- Retractions are easily seen in the infant with respiratory distress.
- A faster metabolic rate increases the need for oxygen and nutrients.
- Due to immature temperature regulation and high body surface to mass ratio, infants are at risk for heat loss and hypothermia if left undressed.
- The head is large (**Figure 2-5**) and may be a potential source of significant heat loss.

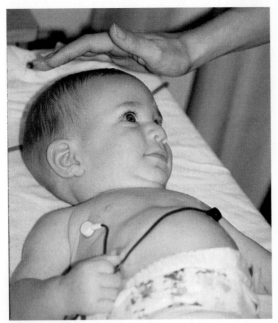

Figure 2-5 The infant's head is disproportionately large compared to older children and adults. The head may be a source of significant heat loss.

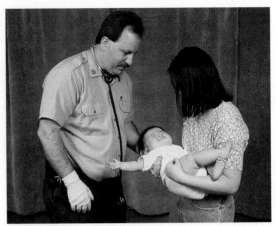

Figure 2-6 Approaching an infant: Observe the infant in the caregiver's arms before palpating or auscultating.

Tip

An infant under 3 months of age who is reported to be fussier than usual, feeding poorly, or sleeping excessively, or who has a temperature greater than 38°C must be seen by a physician.

the infant was acting prior to the event, and if the infant has been healthy since birth. Find out if the infant was born at term and if there were any problems during pregnancy, labor, delivery, or immediately after the birth.

In the first few months of life, excessive irritability or sleeping, fever, and poor feeding may be symptoms of a very serious illness, such as <u>sepsis</u> or <u>congenital heart disease</u>. <u>Apnea</u> is a common chief complaint in the infant period. Apnea may be a sign of infection, heart disease, seizure activity, head injury, or a metabolic problem such as <u>hypoglycemia</u>. As the infant grows older and the behavioral repertoire expands, making the "sick" versus "not sick" decision becomes easier.

Assessment of the Infant

Conduct the assessment of the infant using the following principles:

- Ask the caregiver the infant's name and use it.
- Observe, auscultate, and palpate in this order to get the most information with the least amount of stress to the infant (**Figure 2-6**).
- Approach the infant slowly and calmly because loud voices and quick movements may frighten him.
- Squat down or sit at "baby level."
- Observe the interaction of the infant with the caregiver(s). It is often helpful to assess the infant while the caregiver is holding him. This is especially true for the infant older than 7–8 months, who may have stranger anxiety. An infant who is happily snuggled in a caregiver's arms may become fussy and cry when unwrapped and placed on cold sheets.
- If the infant begins to cry, a pacifier, blanket, or favorite toy may help to calm him. Avoid feeding the infant who is seriously ill or injured.
- Perform the assessment based on the infant's activity level. For example, if the infant is calm, get the respiratory rate and auscultate lung sounds at the beginning of the assessment.

- Make non-threatening physical contact first, such as touching an extremity to assess warmth and capillary refill. Perform the most upsetting parts of the exam last.
- Use a warmed stethoscope and warm hands, and handle the infant gently. Talk in a monotonous, soothing voice.
- Avoid doing anything potentially painful or distressing until after the assessment is completed. It is difficult to assess heart and lung sounds or to palpate the abdomen when the infant is crying.
- Consider offering the infant a toy as a distraction.
- In the older infant who may have stranger anxiety, have the caregiver remove the baby's clothing. Remove one item of clothing at a time, and then replace it, if possible, to avoid heat loss and hypothermia.
- Praising the infant's appearance and behavior will promote a positive interaction with the caregiver, who is a key ally in assessing the baby!

Toddlers

Developmental Characteristics

Toddlers (ages 1–3 years) experience rapid changes in growth and development. By about 18 months of age, the toddler is able to run, feed himself, play with toys, and communicate with others. The toddler begins making his own decisions and asserting his independence. The "terrible two" stage actually begins at about 1 year of age and often lasts into the third year. Toddlers are mobile, opinionated, and may be terrified of strangers. They are illogical by nature, and are intensely curious but lack a sense of danger. Problem solving is concrete, as toddlers cannot reason abstractly. Learning is done by trial and error, with little anticipation of consequences. Toddlers are playful, magical thinkers, and are tremendously self-centered. They understand ownership and will label things (toys, etc.) as "mine."

Language capabilities vary widely. Some toddlers will utter only single words while others may speak in paragraphs. They often understand what is being said, even if they cannot respond with words. Older toddlers may remember earlier experiences with doctors or nurses, such as vaccinations or stitches, and be fearful about being examined.

The toddler's anatomy and physiology are much like the infant's, notably a large head and use of abdominal muscles to breathe. Thermoregulation is better, and limb muscles are more developed.

Case Study 2

You receive a 9-1-1 call about a fussy infant. Upon your arrival, a frantic mother meets you at the door with her 4-week-old daughter in her arms. The infant is crying inconsolably. She has no retractions, but her skin is mottled, both on the trunk and extremities. Her arms and legs are cool. The baby has been fussy all day, vomiting all of her feedings, and her mother thinks her stomach looks big. She had a brief episode of limpness and pallor, and her mother gave her several rescue breaths before calling 9-1-1.

1. How do you assess and treat this child, and address her mothers' concerns?
2. What are the worrisome findings in this infant?

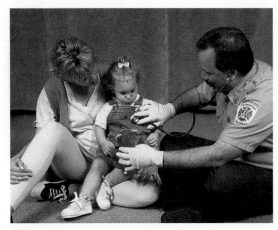

Figure 2-7 Approaching a toddler: Offer a toy or distraction tool to help with the assessment.

Do not separate the older infant or toddler from the caregiver.

Assessment of the Toddler

Conduct the assessment of the toddler using the following principles:

- Approach the toddler slowly and keep physical contact to a minimum until he is familiar with you. Watch the toddler's activity level and behavior as you approach.
- Sit or squat and use a quiet, soothing voice. Allow the toddler to remain on the caregiver's lap.
- Use play and distraction tools, such as a penlight or teddy bear, to help with the assessment (**Figure 2-7**). Introduce equipment slowly and encourage him to hold it.
- Talk to the toddler, preferably about himself. Admire his shoes; ask about pets or recent events. A toddler is the center of his universe.
- Give him limited choices, such as "Do you want me to listen to your belly or your heart first?" This provides the toddler with a sense of control.

- Avoid questions that the toddler can answer with "no."
- Praise the toddler to get cooperation.
- Use simple, concrete terms. Provide a lot of reassurance and praise.
- Perform the most critical parts of the assessment first: "toe-to-head," with the head and neck last.
- Ask for caregiver assistance with the assessment. The toddler is often less upset if the caregiver removes his clothes or administers oxygen.
- If necessary, ask the caregiver to gently palpate the toddler's extremity to test for pain.
- Do not expect toddlers to sit still and cooperate. Be flexible but thorough.
- In certain situations, the toddler may be extremely difficult to examine. If he is alert but resists the exam, determine the need for transport based on history. Use of lights and sirens during transport may increase the toddler's level of fear.

Preschoolers

Developmental Characteristics

Preschoolers (ages 3–5 years) are creative and illogical thinkers (**Figure 2-8**). They are not always able to know the difference

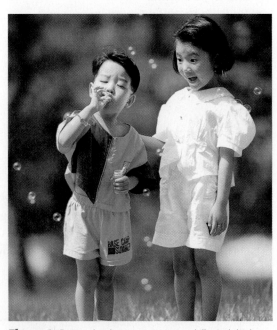

Figure 2-8 Preschoolers are creative and illogical thinkers.

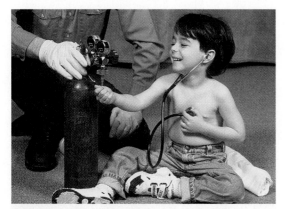

Figure 2-9 When approaching a preschooler, allow the child to handle the equipment.

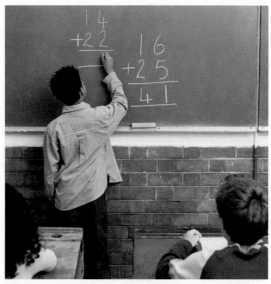

Figure 2-10 School-aged children are talkative, analytical, and able to understand the concept of cause-and-effect.

between fantasy and reality, and they have many misconceptions about illness, injury, and bodily functions. For example, a preschooler might think of a cut as "my insides leaking out." If you tell a preschooler you are going to take his pulse, he may ask, "Where are you going to take it and will I get it back?" Common fears for this age group include body mutilation, loss of control, death, darkness, and being left alone. Attention span is short.

Assessment of the Preschooler

Conduct the assessment of the preschooler using the following principles:

- Use simple terms to explain procedures.
- Choose words carefully, using language that is age-appropriate.
- Clarify any apparent misconceptions.
- Use dolls or puppets, if available, to explain what you are doing.
- Allow the child to handle equipment (**Figure 2-9**).
- Ask for his help.
- Set limits on behavior; for example, "You can cry or scream, but don't bite or kick."
- Praise good behavior. Use games or distraction tools. Use dressings or bandages freely.
- Focus on one thing at a time.

Tip

Preschoolers are creative thinkers who fear loss of control. Explain procedures in simple terms, allow them to handle equipment, and assess from toe to head.

School-aged Children

Development Characteristics

School-aged children are talkative, analytical, and able to understand the concept of cause-and-effect (**Figure 2-10**). They feel a sense of accomplishment as they acquire new skills. Their knowledge of how bodies work may be sketchy and they have limited ability to gauge the seriousness of a particular illness or injury. With careful choice of words, they can understand simple explanations about their bodies and like to be involved in their own care.

Common fears include separation from parents and friends, loss of control, pain, and physical disability. They are often afraid to talk about their feelings and be unable to put their feelings into words. As they become more mobile and more independent, they begin to take more risks. They

Tip

School-aged children fear separation from care-givers, loss of control, pain, and physical disability. Explain procedures and anticipate questions, provide privacy, and conduct assessment from head-to-toe.

Blip

Offering choices that aren't really there violates the child's sense of trust. Tell the school-aged child what you are going to do, and do it!

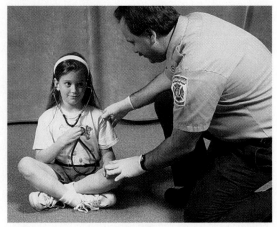

Figure 2-11 Approaching a school-aged child: Let the child be involved in her own care.

live in the present. Belonging and peer group support are important.

The anatomy and physiology of a child is similar to an adult's by about 8 years of age.

Assessment of the School-aged Child

Conduct the assessment of the school-aged child using the following principles:

- Speak directly to the child, and then include the caregiver.
- Anticipate the child's questions and fears, and discuss them immediately.
- Explain in simple terms what is wrong and how it will affect them. For example, when speaking to a 5-year-old, you may explain, "Your arm-bone is broken, but the doctor will be able to fix it good as new. We'll give you some medicine in your arm to help stop it from hurting so much."
- Be careful not to offer too much information.
- Explain procedures immediately before doing them. Never lie to a child, telling

them that something won't hurt or that you are almost finished if this is not true. Remember that the child may not ask questions, even if they have real concerns.
- Ask the older school-aged child if he would like to have the caregiver present.
- Provide privacy. Children in this age group are modest. Expose the child for physical assessment as necessary and cover him up when done.
- If physical restraint is necessary to complete a procedure or to guarantee the safety of the child or crew, tell the child what is going to happen and then do it.
- Don't negotiate unless the child really has a choice. For example, it is okay to ask the child if he would like the IV in the right or left hand but not to ask if it is okay to start an IV when it must be done.
- Let the child be involved in the care. Children in this age group are afraid of being out of control (**Figure 2-11**).
- Reassure the child that being ill or injured is not a punishment.
- Praise the child for cooperating. Be careful not to be irritable if the child does not cooperate.
- The physical assessment can usually be done in the head-to-toe format.

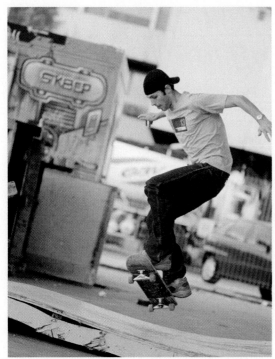

Figure 2-12 Adolescence is a time of experimentation and risk-taking behaviors.

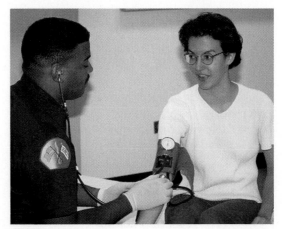

Figure 2-13 When approaching an adolescent, speak to her directly.

Adolescents

Growth and Development Characteristics

Adolescents sometimes seem to share some characteristics of toddlers: they are very mobile but may lack common sense! But adolescents are, in reality, rational, understand cause-and-effect, and able to express themselves with words. Adolescence is a time of experimentation and risk-taking behaviors (**Figure 2-12**). Adolescents often feel that they are free from danger, that they are "indestructible." They gradually shift from relying on family to relying on friends for psychological support and social development.

Adolescents struggle with independence, loss of control, body image, sexuality, and peer pressure. Anything that makes them different from their peers causes anxiety. Psychosomatic complaints are common in this age group. They may have mood swings, or depression, and, when ill or injured, may act younger than their age, leaving a scared child in an adult body.

Assessment of the Adolescent

Conduct the assessment of the adolescent using the following principles:

- Provide accurate information about the illness or injury, normal body functions, and interventions. Explain what you are doing and why.
- Encourage him to ask questions and to be involved in his own care.
- Show respect. Speak directly to the adolescent. Do not turn to the caregiver for initial information (**Figure 2-13**).
- Respect the adolescent's privacy and confidentiality unless it places him at risk.
- Be honest and nonjudgmental.
- Don't be misled by the adolescent's size, or make assumptions about his comprehension of events. He may misinterpret the seriousness of the situation. Adolescents may also have many fears about permanent injury, disfigurement, or "being different" as a result of the illness or injury. Give the adolescent accurate information, and anticipate their questions or fears.
- Avoid becoming frustrated or angry if the adolescent does not talk or is uncooperative.
- Enlist his friends to help persuade him to cooperate with the assessment or treatment, if he resists.

Adolescents struggle with independence, loss of control, body image, sexuality, and peer pressure. Provide concrete information, respect their privacy, and speak to them directly.

Don't assume that a child with physical disability is cognitively impaired. Always ask the caregiver to clarify the child's normal level of functioning and interaction.

Tip

Even if a disabled child cannot talk or interact, show your respect by introducing yourself, explaining what you are doing, and providing verbal reassurance.

Children with Special Health Care Needs

Growth and Development Characteristics

When working with children with special health care needs (CSHCN), it is important to consider developmental age, rather than chronological age.

Assessment of a CSHCN

Children with special health care needs (CSHCN) may have any type of chronic condition that affects health, normal growth and development. This may include physical disability, developmental or learning disability, technologic dependency, and chronic illness. The child who is technology dependent may have a home ventilator, tracheostomy, gastric feeding tube, or long-term intravenous access device. The developmental or learning disability may include mental retardation, difficulties in communication, sensory impairment, or limitations in physical activity. Specific categories of patients and methods of assessment and treatment are discussed in Chapter 10.

The number of children in the community with special needs is growing. Prehospital professionals must be familiar with the conditions and types of technology used in assessing and treating CSHCN. These children may require transport and care for exacerbation of their illness or for an unrelated illness or injury.

Conduct the assessment of the CSHCN using the following principles:

- Get a careful history from the caregiver. He can provide detailed information about the child's medical history, medications, and current complaints. He is also aware of how best to approach the child, and of typical responses and behaviors.
- Ask the caregiver what he thinks of the child's condition, activity, and behaviors. Find out if the caregiver feels that the child is "not acting right."
- Include the impressions of the caregiver in chart documentation.
- Approach the child with a developmental delay gently and using techniques appropriate to his developmental level, not his chronological age. Use language and techniques tailored to the child's cognitive level to communicate.
- Do not assume that the child with a physical disability is mentally impaired (**Figure 2-14**). Ask the caregiver about the child's level of function and interaction with others. To get at baseline functional level you might query, "What would Johnny be doing right now, if he were feeling well?"

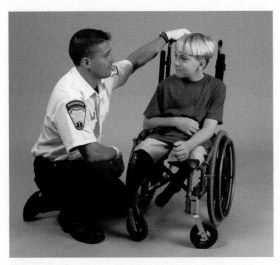

Figure 2-14 Approaching the child with special health care needs: Obtain a thorough history and identify developmentally appropriate approaches that work best with the child.

- Use polite, professional behavior, acknowledge the caregivers' expertise, and take their concerns seriously. Families of chronically ill children usually have had extensive experience with the medical system. If most of their experiences have been good, they will very likely perceive the prehospital professional as an ally. However, if they have had bad experiences, they may feel a need to be very vigilant in protecting their child and be perceived as difficult or controlling.
- Keep in mind the amount of stress that the caregiver of a CSHCN may be experiencing and be sympathetic.

Summary

Understanding the characteristics of growth and development for each age group is essential for accurate assessment and treatment of the child in the out-of-hospital environment. Good field care requires good communication with the child and family. The family may include a large number of people, all of whom become "patients." CSHCN pose additional challenges in assessment, but their caregivers can be a great asset in guiding field evaluation and management.

Case Study 3

You respond to the scene of a bike versus automobile crash. The bike rider is a 14-year-old male, who is now walking around the scene. He was wearing a helmet, and denies any loss of consciousness. His only complaints are that his wrist hurts, the front wheel of his bike is bent, and he will be late to meet his friends. He doesn't want to be examined, definitely doesn't want to go to the hospital, and starts to leave the scene as you approach him.

1. Is this teenagers' reaction normal?
2. What techniques can help you adequately assess his injuries?

Chapter Review

Case Study Answers

Case Study ❶ page 33

Toddlers are often fearful of strangers, so enlisting the help of the parents/caregivers will make patient assessment much easier. Allow the child to remain with the parent. Sit on the bed, or crouch down to the child's eye level, and use a calm, soothing voice. You can use distractions such as a penlight, or ask about a stuffed animal on the bed, to gain the child's attention and to evaluate interactivity. Ask the parent to remove the child's pajamas, and observe the work of breathing, including suprasternal, subcostal, and/or intercostal retractions, and respiratory rate. Although your main concern is the child's respiratory status, you may have to perform other portions of the hands-on examination, such as touching or tickling his toes before you get to the chest. When listening to breath sounds, warm the stethoscope beforehand, and explain what you are doing. If the child resists, you may be able to listen to a stuffed animal first, and allow the child to do the same, before resuming your examination.

Your assessment reveals the child's respiratory rate is 32 breaths/min, and heart rate is 128 beats/min. You decide to give the child oxygen, but he refuses to keep the oxygen mask in place even with his mother's help, a response you recognize is typical of a toddler who is not seriously ill. For transport to the hospital, you secure the child on the gurney, allowing his mother to accompany you in the ambulance, and direct oxygen in his direction via blow-by.

Case Study ❷ page 41

Even though the mother is frantic, it is important to get additional history: Was the infant full-term? Did she have any problems with delivery or after birth? Has she had feeding problems or vomiting in the past? Any fever? Diarrhea?

Infants in the first few months of life have a limited range of behaviors, so anything out of the ordinary in the child's feeding, sleeping, or basic activity level is concerning for serious underlying illness or injury. Any infant who reportedly had an apneic episode that resulted in color change (pallor, <u>cyanosis</u>) or unresponsiveness may have had an <u>apparent life-threatening event (ALTE)</u>. Causes of ALTE include <u>sepsis</u>, congenital heart disease, metabolic abnormalities, seizures, <u>gastroesophageal reflux</u>, and brain injury. These diagnoses are impossible to establish in the out-of-hospital setting, and require emergency department evaluation.

Reassuring the mother is important, but this baby may be critically ill, and requires rapid assessment and transport. While an infant's extremities may be mottled due to cold, mottling of the trunk is an extremely worrisome sign, reflecting poor perfusion. The possibility of <u>hypovolemic shock</u> is supported by the baby's cool extremities and history of vomiting. Furthermore, though infants can develop abdominal distension due to crying and swallowing air, abdominal distension in association with vomiting, and signs of shock (abnormal appearance and abnormal circulation to skin) suggest serious pathology such as intestinal obstruction.

Move the baby quickly into the ambulance, explaining what you are doing and why to the mother. If local protocol permits, allow the mother to ride with you to the hospital. Treatment of this infant includes administration of oxygen by a face mask, and rapid transport to an Emergency Department. Prevention of heat loss by swaddling the baby and applying a hat is important, as <u>hypothermia</u> is a risk for a small infant. Consider vascular access en route, with a bolus of 20 mL/kg of crystalloid fluid.

Case Study 3 page 47

This teenager is asserting his independence but is not legally able to give consent or refuse care, unless he is emancipated. He may not realize the risks of occult injury. Show respect, be honest and non-judgmental, and speak directly to him. Explain why it is important to check him for potentially serious injuries, and offer him the privacy of the ambulance to conduct the exam. If he still refuses care, attempt to contact his parents or caregivers or enlist the assistance of police.

Suggested Readings

Textbooks
American Academy of Pediatrics and the American College of Emergency Physicians: *APLS: The Pediatric Emergency Medicine Resource,* 4th Edition. Sudbury, MA, Jones and Bartlett Publishers, 2004.
Behrman R, Kliegman R, Jenson H: *Nelson Textbook of Pediatrics,* 17th Edition. Philadelphia, Saunders, 2004.
Hazinski M, Zaritsky A, Nadkarni V, et al: *PALS Provider Manual.* American Heart Association, 2002.
Zitelli B, Davis H: *Atlas of Pediatric Physical Diagnosis,* 4th Edition. Philadelphia, Mosby, 2002.

Article
Loyacono T. Family-centered prehospital care. *Emerg Med Serv.* June 2001; 30(6):64–7.

3

Respiratory Emergencies

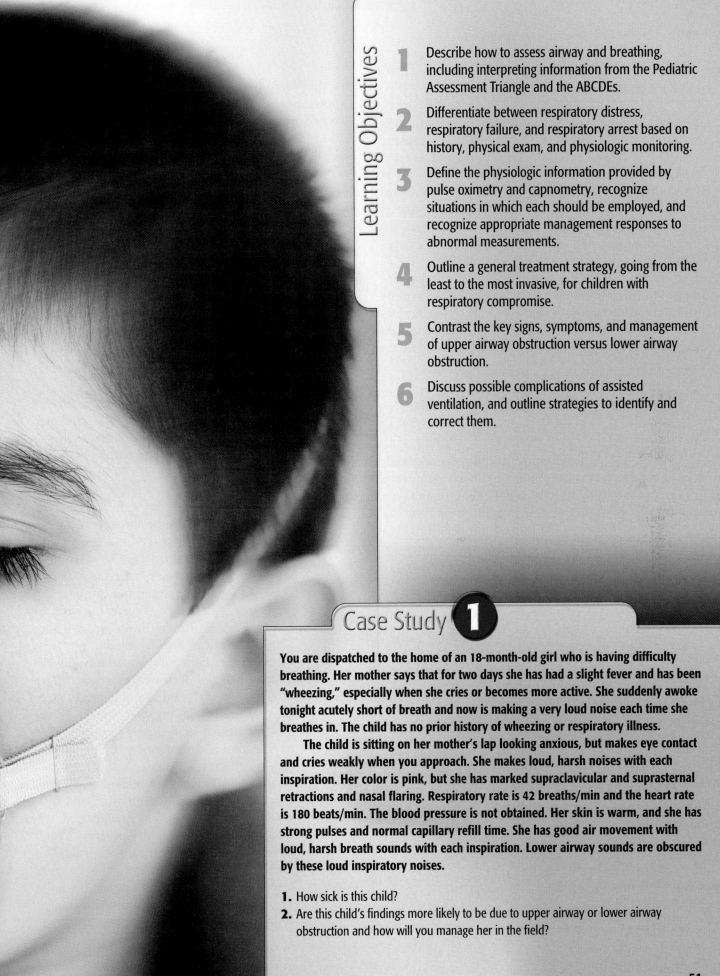

Learning Objectives

1 Describe how to assess airway and breathing, including interpreting information from the Pediatric Assessment Triangle and the ABCDEs.

2 Differentiate between respiratory distress, respiratory failure, and respiratory arrest based on history, physical exam, and physiologic monitoring.

3 Define the physiologic information provided by pulse oximetry and capnometry, recognize situations in which each should be employed, and recognize appropriate management responses to abnormal measurements.

4 Outline a general treatment strategy, going from the least to the most invasive, for children with respiratory compromise.

5 Contrast the key signs, symptoms, and management of upper airway obstruction versus lower airway obstruction.

6 Discuss possible complications of assisted ventilation, and outline strategies to identify and correct them.

Case Study **1**

You are dispatched to the home of an 18-month-old girl who is having difficulty breathing. Her mother says that for two days she has had a slight fever and has been "wheezing," especially when she cries or becomes more active. She suddenly awoke tonight acutely short of breath and now is making a very loud noise each time she breathes in. The child has no prior history of wheezing or respiratory illness.

The child is sitting on her mother's lap looking anxious, but makes eye contact and cries weakly when you approach. She makes loud, harsh noises with each inspiration. Her color is pink, but she has marked supraclavicular and suprasternal retractions and nasal flaring. Respiratory rate is 42 breaths/min and the heart rate is 180 beats/min. The blood pressure is not obtained. Her skin is warm, and she has strong pulses and normal capillary refill time. She has good air movement with loud, harsh breath sounds with each inspiration. Lower airway sounds are obscured by these loud inspiratory noises.

1. How sick is this child?
2. Are this child's findings more likely to be due to upper airway or lower airway obstruction and how will you manage her in the field?

Introduction

RESPIRATORY DISEASE IS the most frequent pediatric pre-hospital medical problem. Of all conditions causing respiratory disease in children, asthma is the most common. However, many other illnesses, as well as foreign bodies and trauma, cause respiratory problems in children. Good assessment and early intervention for pediatric respiratory problems can avert serious illness and preventable death, and may shorten treatment time in the emergency department (ED).

Focusing on certain key physical signs and symptoms will allow the prehospital professional to rapidly assess the effectiveness of gas exchange in the airways and lung alveoli. Using the PAT is an important first step in determining the severity of the disease, localizing the physiologic problem, and beginning treatment. Appearance reflects the overall state of ventilation and oxygenation. Increased work of breathing indicates either airway obstruction at some level or a problem in gas exchange at the alveolar level; it is often an early sign of hypoxia and/or hypercapnia. Fading respiratory effort is a sign of severe hypoxia and/or hypercapnia. Cyanosis of the skin or mucous membranes also indicates severe hypoxia.

In addition to the PAT, the initial assessment includes counting the respiratory rate, performing hands-on chest auscultation, and obtaining pulse oximetry. This assessment not only provides a picture of respiratory function, but also helps prioritize general and specific treatments as well as invasive interventions and timing of transport.

Respiratory Distress and Failure

Respiratory distress, failure, and arrest are three points on a continuum of physiologic response to different types of hypoxic stress. Causes of hypoxic stress are variable, and include asthma, bronchiolitis, croup, pneumonia, and chest wall injury. While these three points in the continuum (respiratory distress, failure, and arrest) have different clinical characteristics in theory, in reality they are all part of a spectrum that is not black or white. Respiratory distress is an abnormal physiologic condition identified by increased work of breathing. Increased respiratory rate, supraclavicular, suprasternal, intercostal or subcostal retractions, use of accessory neck muscles and nasal flaring are signs, which alone or together indicate increased work of breathing. These physical signs represent the patient's attempt to make up for decreased gas exchange in the lungs and airways and to maintain oxygenation and ventilation. The child in respiratory distress is effectively compensating. The brain is still getting enough oxygen, and the child's appearance is relatively normal.

Respiratory failure occurs when the infant or child exhausts his energy reserves or can no longer maintain oxygenation and ventilation. When the effects of the respiratory insult begin to overwhelm the child's ability to respond, she begins to decompensate. Respiratory failure may occur when chest wall muscles get tired after a long period of increased work of breathing (e.g., a child with severe asthma who is very tight and has been working hard to breathe for several hours), when the insult is severe and progressive (e.g., fulminant pneumonia), or when there is a failure of central respiratory drive (e.g., a child with a severe closed head injury). An abnormal appearance (severe agitation or lethargy) or cyanosis in a child with an increased work of breathing indicates probable respiratory failure. An abnormally low respiratory rate and decreased respiratory effort, usually with bradycardia, also indicates probable respiratory failure. Respiratory failure must be treated immediately to restore good oxygenation and ventilation, and to prevent respiratory arrest.

Respiratory arrest means absence of effective breathing. If ventilation and oxygenation are not immediately supported, respiratory arrest will rapidly progress to full cardiopulmonary arrest. Most episodes of cardiac arrest in pediatric patients begin as respiratory arrest. Intervening at this point will often prevent cardiac arrest. Early intervention in respiratory failure and arrest will have a far better chance of producing neurologically intact survivors than treatment of full blown cardiac arrest, which has an extremely low probability of survival.

Prearrival Preparation

Based upon dispatch information and while en route to the scene, whenever possible, prepare mentally for management of respiratory distress and failure by reviewing the appropriate assessment techniques and treatment options for the child's age. This includes recalling an age-based approach to assessment as outlined in Chapter 1, equipment needs, and the likely treatment and transport options. Also, anticipate the determinants of whether to stay on scene and treat or to manage the airway and transport immediately to the emergency department.

Scene Size-up

Be sure the scene is safe, and there are no obvious illness or injury threats. Assess the environment for noxious gases, fumes, chemicals, or smoke. Document scene conditions if environmental factors may be contributing to anticipated respiratory problems.

General Assessment: The PAT

Evaluating the Presenting Complaint

Find out the nature of the presenting complaint by asking several directed questions, as suggested in **Table 3-1**. After the initial

assessment, in patients with mild distress, there is time to get a more complete SAMPLE history (see **Table 3-9**) on scene as part of the focused history. If the child is in respiratory failure, do this later, if possible, while en route to the ED.

Assessment of Respiratory Status

Using the PAT

Begin the assessment with the PAT, as discussed in Chapter 1. Carefully evaluate appearance, work of breathing, and skin circulation. The PAT will help establish how sick the child is, the type of physiologic abnormality (respiratory distress or respiratory failure), the level of obstruction if present (upper or lower airway), and the urgency for treatment. Table 1-2 lists physical features in the child to help make these clinical distinctions by simple observation and listening.

Appearance

Appearance reflects the adequacy of oxygenation and ventilation in a child with difficulty breathing. If the child is compensating effectively for the respiratory insult, the appearance will be fairly normal, and the TICLS mnemonic (Table 1-1) will show an interactive child with good tone and color, and normal vocalizations, who will lock gaze. If the child is not compensating, the appearance will be abnormal, and the child will have abnormal findings in the TICLS mnemonic because her brain will be impaired due to hypoxia and/or hypercapnia. Abnormal appearance is a spectrum of clinical states, so that the severity of respiratory failure will

Table 3-1	Key Questions about the Presenting Complaint	
Key Question	**Possible Medical Problem**
Has your child ever had this kind of problem before?	Asthma, chronic lung disease
Is this the first time that he has had trouble breathing?	
Is your child taking any medications?	Asthma, chronic lung disease, congenital heart disease
Has your child had a fever?	Pneumonia, bronchiolitis, croup
Did your child suddenly start coughing/choking/gagging?	Foreign body aspiration or ingestion
Has your child had an injury to his chest?	Pulmonary contusion, pneumothorax

determine how abnormal the child appears. Also, assessing appearance will guide urgency of BLS versus ALS treatment.

Advanced Life Support

Example 1: A 3-year-old child who has stridor and retractions, but is running around the room and has a normal appearance, requires general noninvasive treatment and transport. The child is compensating effectively and is only in respiratory distress.

Example 2: An 8-year-old child who is agitated or inconsolable, with wheezing and increased work of breathing, has an abnormal appearance, and is probably hypoxic. The child is beginning to decompensate and is in early respiratory failure. In addition to general noninvasive treatment, this child requires immediate specific ALS treatment on scene with a <u>bronchodilator</u>, then rapid transport to an ED.

Example 3: A 3-year-old child who has been working hard to breathe and is now sleepy or poorly responsive has a strongly abnormal appearance. Her altered level of consciousness is the result of severe hypoxia or hypercapnia, reflecting late respiratory failure, and impending respiratory arrest. She requires immediate assisted ventilation with bag-mask ventilation on scene, and possibly endotracheal intubation in certain circumstances.

Work of Breathing

Look for signs of increased work of breathing:

1. Abnormal positioning (tripoding, "sniffing" position)
2. Abnormal airway sounds (such as snoring, stridor, wheezing, or grunting)
3. Retractions (or head bobbing in infants)
4. Nasal flaring

The significance of each of these findings is discussed in Chapter 1. These indicators of breathing effort will help to identify the anatomic location of the problem (upper airway, lower airway, or lung alveoli), the severity of the physiologic dysfunction (respiratory distress, failure, or arrest), and the urgency for treatment (immediate resuscitation, general treatment only on scene with specific treatment en route, general and specific treatment on scene). In addition to abnormal airway sounds (stridor, wheezing, and grunting), retractions and the use of accessory muscles may help localize the site of airway problems. Use of the accessory muscles of the neck and suprasternal and supraclavicular retractions occurs more often with upper airway obstruction. Predominant subcostal and intercostal retractions and the use of abdominal muscles tends to localize an obstructive process to the lower airways.

Circulation to Skin

Finally, evaluate skin color. Cyanosis is an ominous sign, signaling profound hypoxia and the need for assisted ventilation. However, a child may have severe hypoxia without an obvious change in skin color. Pulse oximetry is very helpful, so use it whenever available in a child with respiratory distress or respiratory failure.

Initial Assessment: The ABCDEs

After the PAT, perform the second portion of the initial assessment, the hands-on ABCDEs. There are three parts to the "B" or breathing evaluation:

1. Respiratory rate
2. Auscultation for air movement and abnormal breath sounds
3. Pulse oximetry

Respiratory Rate

In the noncritical patient, determine respiratory rate by sitting the child in her caregiver's lap and exposing her chest. Count the rise and fall of the abdomen over 30 seconds, and then double that number. Normal respiratory rates vary in children of different ages (see Table 1-4). Always think about respiratory rates in the context of the PAT and the overall clinical assessment. Respiratory rate may be affected by level of activity, fever, anxiety, and metabolic state.

A respiratory rate of greater than 60 breaths/min is abnormal in a child of any age and should be a signal for careful evaluation for other signs of respiratory or circulatory problems. Even more dangerous is a rate that is too slow for age. A respiratory rate of less than 20 breaths/min in a sick child under 6 years of age, or a rate of less than 12 breaths/min in a sick child under 15 years of age may be a sign of respiratory failure and therefore, immediate intervention is required. A child who has normal appearance and good color, without increased work of breathing, has good breathing regardless of her respiratory rate.

Auscultation for Air Movement and Abnormal Breath Sounds

Assess air movement by placing the stethoscope and listening for the amount of air movement with each breath (**Figure 3-1**). Poor air movement may exist in children with respiratory problems for many reasons, as outlined in **Table 3-2**.

Assessing air movement, or the volume of air exchanged with each breath, allows clinical estimation of <u>tidal volume</u>. Tidal volume is one of two factors that determine minute ventilation: the volume of air exchanged per minute. <u>Minute ventilation</u> is the basis for gas exchange in the lungs.

Minute Ventilation = Tidal Volume × Respiratory Rate

This equation shows the connection between tidal volume and respiratory rate. A child may not have enough gas exchange if tidal volume is low, even with a normal or fast respiratory rate. Also, a normal or increased tidal volume does not mean there will be enough gas exchange if the respiratory rate is too slow.

While listening for air movement, also listen for abnormal breath sounds. Table 1-5 summarizes the types and causes of abnormal breath sounds. Stridor, which is usually inspiratory in nature at least initially, is indicative of upper airway obstruction whereas crackles and wheezes are associated with lower airway processes.

Pulse Oximetry

Pulse oximetry is a useful tool for detecting and measuring hypoxia. **Figure 3-2** illustrates possible sites for placement of the oximetry probe. ⬭Pulse Oximetry, Procedure 9⬭ explains how to use a pulse oximeter. The pulse oximeter emits red light of two different wavelengths. These are absorbed differently by saturated and desaturated hemoglobin. The sensor on the pulse oximeter measures the transmission of the two wavelengths of red light, and a computer in the machine then determines the percentage of hemoglobin that is saturated with oxygen. When properly applied, *and if there is a good arterial tracing,* a reading of 95% or higher means normal blood oxygen saturation. *A value of 94% or less on*

Table 3-2	Causes of Poor Air Movement in Children
Functional Problem	**Possible Causes**
Obstruction of airway	Asthma, bronchiolitis, croup
Restriction of chest wall movement	Chest wall injury, severe scoliosis or kyphosis
Chest wall muscle fatigue	Prolonged increased work of breathing, muscular dystrophy
Decreased central respiratory drive	Head injury, intoxication
Chest injury	Rib fractures, pulmonary contusion, pneumothorax

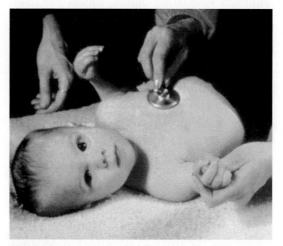

Figure 3-1 Assess air movement by placing the stethoscope and listening for the amount of air movement with each breath.

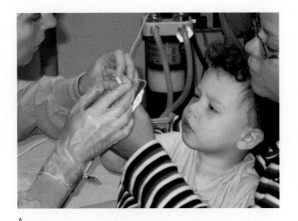

A

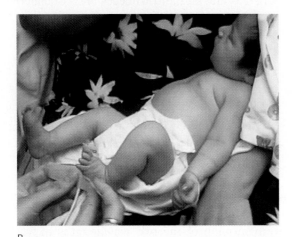

B

Figure 3-2 Possible sites for placement of the oximetry probe.

hypoxia becomes the stimulus to breath. Over-treating hypoxia disturbs this regulatory function, and may paradoxically decrease drive to breathe and make the child worse.

Be careful not to over-interpret low oxygen saturation. Pulse oximetry is an adjunct to physical assessment. Falsely low readings are common with pulse oximetry. Movement by the child, cold extremities, or a cold ambient temperature and interference by light in the child's surroundings all may cause inaccurate pulse oximetry readings. Check probe placement, the quality of the tracing, and the child's clinical state before treating. Inaccurate readings or the inability to obtain any reading may also occur in children in shock with poor perfusion. However, give these children oxygen even if they do not have respiratory distress and regardless of pulse oximeter readings. Also, do not under-interpret a normal pulse oximetry reading. *Sometimes an apparently normal oxygen saturation above 94% may be present in a child with significant respiratory distress, who is compensating by increased work of breathing.* Always use pulse oximetry in combination with physical assessment to assure accurate interpretation of adequacy of breathing.

room air is abnormal and is a signal to give supplemental oxygen. A reading of less than 90%, with the patient on 100% oxygen, usually indicates respiratory failure, unless the child has a chronic respiratory problem.

Occasionally, a child with a pre-existing chronic respiratory illness (e.g., cystic fibrosis) has a baseline abnormal pulse oximetry. In this type of patient, obtain the baseline value from the caregiver and attempt to provide enough oxygen to get the child to her baseline pulse oximetry level. Providing more oxygen than is needed to achieve the baseline pulse oximetry level may actually suppress ventilation by reducing the child's hypoxic drive to breathe. In normal children, hypercapnia or increased carbon dioxide pressure stimulates the drive to breathe, but in some children with chronic respiratory disease, hypercapnia is a constant state. In such cases,

Tip

Remember, the pulse oximeter does not tell you about adequacy of ventilation. A patient who is receiving supplemental oxygen may have a normal pulse oximeter reading but not have adequate ventilation. **Capnometry**, which quantitatively measures exhaled carbon dioxide, monitors carbon dioxide levels and adequacy of ventilation.

Blip

Be careful not to over-interpret low oxygen saturation. Match with the physical findings.

General Noninvasive Treatment

For every child in respiratory distress, begin general noninvasive treatment. *The general noninvasive treatment of every noncritical patient is the same—allow her to assume a position of comfort and supply oxygen, if tolerated* (**Figure 3-3**). This is the only treatment for patients in respiratory distress without upper or lower airway obstruction. If the child is in respiratory failure or arrest, perform assisted ventilation immediately.

Positioning

A child in respiratory distress will naturally move into the position that gives her the best air exchange—her "position of comfort." For example, a child with severe upper airway obstruction may get into the "sniffing position" to straighten the airway and open the air passages (**Figure 3-4**). A child with severe

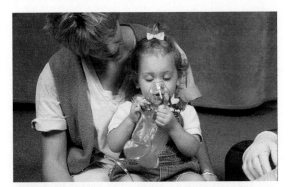

Figure 3-3 Always keep a child with respiratory distress in her position of comfort.

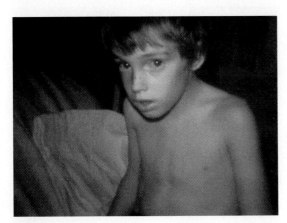

Figure 3-4 Sniffing position.

lower airway obstruction may voluntarily take the "tripod" posture—sitting up and leaning forward on outstretched arms—to help accessory muscles (**Figure 3-5**). Infants and toddlers may be most comfortable in their caregiver's arms or lap. Do not move a child from her position of comfort. This might worsen the respiratory distress. In the ambulance, keep the dyspneic child safely restrained in an upright position, unless she requires assisted ventilation or has other physiologic problems that require treatment in a supine position.

Oxygen

Treatment with high-flow oxygen is usually safe. If the child has chronic respiratory illness, be careful not to administer too much oxygen, as noted above. The prehospital professional must weigh the possible benefits of giving oxygen against the risks of agitating the child and worsening her respiratory distress. This is a special concern in a child with an unstable airway. Oxygen toxicity in newborns, especially premature newborns, is occasionally an issue in the prehospital setting. Newborns with respiratory distress, cyanosis, or other signs of respiratory disease require high-flow, 100% oxygen. But do not give oxygen to newborns without signs of hypoxia, as explained in Chapter 9.

Most children will accept oxygen therapy, especially if the prehospital professional is creative in the approach. This often means getting the help of the caregiver. If a child

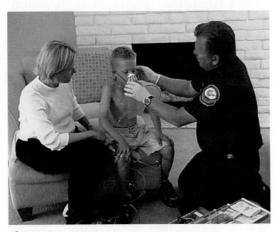

Figure 3-5 Tripod position.

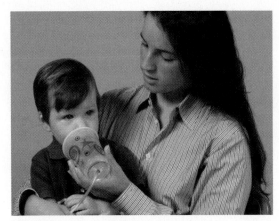

Figure 3-6 If the child resists application of a mask or nasal cannula, administer oxygen through a nonthreatening object such as a cup.

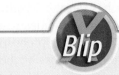

Do not move a child from her position of comfort.

resists the use of a mask or <u>nasal cannula</u>, have the caregiver give blow-by oxygen from the end of the oxygen tubing or from tubing inserted into a cup (**Figure 3-6**).

Oxygen Delivery

Give oxygen to any child with clinical signs of cardiopulmonary distress or failure, or with a history suggesting possible abnormalities in gas exchange. The delivery method should provide the concentration of oxygen most appropriate for the child's condition, degree of cooperation, respiratory effort, and age. For a step-by-step explanation of this procedure, see Oxygen Delivery, Procedure 3.

Summary of General and Initial Respiratory Assessment and General Noninvasive Treatment

The PAT is a good tool for determining the effectiveness of gas exchange, based on observation of appearance and work of breathing. If the PAT suggests respiratory distress, begin general noninvasive treatment with oxygen and keep the child in her position of comfort. The PAT will also identify the critical child in respiratory failure who requires immediate assisted ventilation. Obtaining respiratory rate, listening for air movement, and determining oxygen saturation by pulse oximetry will work in concert with the PAT. The initial assessment should allow an evaluation of severity and urgency for treatment, and establish if specific treatment for upper or lower airway obstruction is indicated.

Specific Treatment for Respiratory Distress

After completing the initial assessment, consider specific treatment. The PAT and ABCDE assessment will help determine whether the child has upper or lower airway obstruction, lung disease, or disordered control of breathing (from conditions such as brain or nerve injury, poisoning, or sepsis). Snoring or stridor indicates upper airway obstruction; wheezing indicates lower airway obstruction. It can be difficult to separate true stridor from upper airway noise due to nasal congestion. Breath sounds may also make it difficult to tell the difference between upper airway noise and true wheezing. Listen for breath sounds in the second or third intercostal space at the midaxillary line bilaterally (**Figure 3-7**). At this location, it is easier to distin-

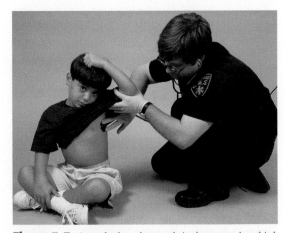

Figure 3-7 Listen for breath sounds in the second or third intercostal space at the midaxillary line bilaterally.

guish upper airway congestion from lower airway obstruction. When abnormal airway sounds are loudest with the stethoscope held near the child's nose rather than over the lungs, nasal congestion is the likely cause.

The absence of abnormal airway sounds in a child with hypoxia and increased work of breathing suggests lung disease, such as pneumonia. Lastly, a child with hypoxia and *decreased* work of breathing may have either respiratory failure from airway obstruction or lung disease or disordered control of breathing from another insult to her brain, nerves, or metabolic system.

Tip

When abnormal airway sounds are loudest with the stethoscope held near the child's nose rather than over the lungs, nasal congestion is the likely cause.

Upper Airway Obstruction

Proximal Airway Obstruction

In a patient with neurologic impairment, loss of oropharyngeal muscle tone may cause upper airway obstruction and stridor due to the tongue and <u>mandible</u> falling back and partially blocking the <u>pharynx</u>. This is a common problem in children during and after seizures. The head-tilt/chin-lift maneuver (**Figure 3-8**) or jaw thrust maneuver (**Figure 3-9**) may relieve this <u>proximal</u> airway obstruction. At times it may be help-

ful or even necessary to have two rescuers assist with the jaw thrust maneuver, especially in larger children, children who are actively seizing or in children receiving positive-pressure ventilation (**Figure 3-10**).

Sometimes secretions, blood, or foreign bodies block the proximal upper airway. This is an important concern in the child with closed head injury or seizures. Suctioning alone will often relieve the upper airway obstruction caused by fluids or occluding objects in the mouth, pharynx, or nose.

Maintenance of an adequate airway may require placement of an oropharyngeal airway, <u>nasopharyngeal airway</u>, or a endotracheal tube. The role of endotracheal intubation of children in the prehospital setting has been brought into question by recent data demonstrating significant failure rates, induced hypoxia, airway injury, and endotracheal tube dislodgement. *Bag-mask ventilation is the key life-saving technique that should be mastered by all prehospital providers*

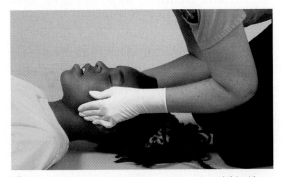

Figure 3-9 Use the jaw thrust maneuver in a child with possible spinal injury.

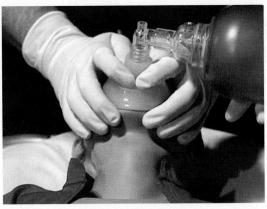

Figure 3-10 Two-rescuer technique for the jaw thrust maneuver and positive-pressure ventilation.

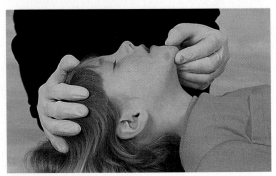

Figure 3-8 Use the head-tilt/chin-lift maneuver to place the airway in a neutral position.

and will provide adequate airway management for the vast majority of pediatric patients.

Airway Obstruction Above the Thoracic Inlet

Upper airway obstruction beyond the proximal upper airway may result from a variety of causes. It is not necessary to make an exact diagnosis in order to provide appropriate management to children with upper airway obstruction. In most of these cases, simply allow the child to maintain her position of comfort and provide supplemental oxygen by the least invasive and least threatening means possible. Causing the child to become more agitated or struggle may worsen her airway obstruction and precipitate the onset of a complete obstruction leading to respiratory failure or respiratory arrest.

In an awake, alert child, upper airway obstruction and stridor are usually due to croup, a viral disease with inflammation, edema, and narrowing of the larynx, trachea, or bronchioles. Croup usually affects infants and toddlers. Most children with croup have had several days of cold symptoms. The cold symptoms are followed by the development of a barking or "seal" cough, stridor, and various levels of respiratory distress. There is usually a low-grade fever, and symptoms are often worse at night. The severity of symptoms will vary widely among patients, but they usually progress over days, rather than hours.

Treatment Treat children with apparent croup with cool mist, either in the form of humidified oxygen or nebulized saline. Ask the caregiver to assist (**Figure 3-11**).

Advanced Life Support

Pharmacologic Treatment of Croup Nebulized <u>epinephrine</u> is a specific treatment for the upper airway inflammation associated with croup. Epinephrine is a potent alpha and beta <u>agonist</u>, and works through vasoconstriction to decrease the upper airway edema causing partial obstruction. If local EMS protocols permit, consider nebulized epinephrine therapy for children with stridor, increased work of

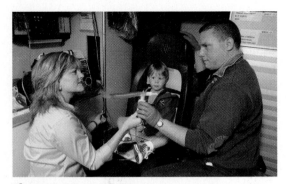

Figure 3-11 Use the caregiver to assist in the administration of oxygen or nebulized saline.

breathing, poor air movement, blood oxygen saturation less than 94%, or altered appearance.

Nebulized epinephrine has two formulations, and either is acceptable: <u>racemic</u> epinephrine and L-epinephrine.

Side effects of nebulized epinephrine include tachycardia, tremor, and vomiting. Children who receive nebulized epinephrine may need a period of observation in the ED because of possible return of stridor after the medicine wears off. Very few children with croup will require assisted ventilation in the prehospital setting. In the rare case of a child with croup and respiratory failure, begin assisted ventilation and reassess. Two-person bag-mask ventilation technique may be necessary.

Invasive Airway Management for Croup Perform endotracheal intubation only in the unusual case of the child with respiratory failure who does not respond to bag-mask ventilation. Preparation for intubation includes choosing an endotracheal tube that is one or two sizes smaller than normal for age or length. Inflammation of the trachea at the <u>subglottic</u> level makes it difficult or impossible to use an endotracheal tube of normal size. Do not use paralytics when attempting endotracheal intubation for upper airway obstruction.

Bacterial Upper Airway Infections

Bacterial infections may also cause upper airway obstruction in children. Unlike viral croup, these infections tend to progress rapidly

Stridor is often mistaken for wheezing. Stridor is an inspiratory sign of upper airway obstruction and may improve with an agent with vasoconstrictive properties, like nebulized epinephrine.

Position of comfort, humidified oxygen, and avoiding agitation are the best treatments for suspected croup.

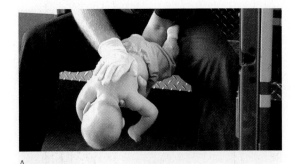

A

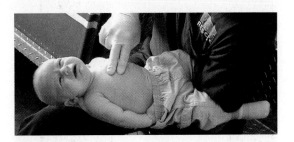

B

Figure 3-12 (A) Use five back blows, followed by (B) five chest thrusts in infants with complete airway obstruction.

with severe respiratory compromise developing over hours. The child with a bacterial upper airway infection usually is older than 12 months, appears ill or toxic, has pain on swallowing, and is often drooling. Stridor may be present, but the child may not have the barking cough that is common with croup.

There are several possible but even less common causes of bacterial upper airway infections. Epiglottitis, inflammation of the epiglottis, is now extremely rare due to widespread vaccination of infants against the bacteria *Haemophilus influenzae*, type B. Peritonsillar abscess, retropharyngeal abscess, tracheitis, and diphtheria are other possible causes of upper airway infection.

Treatment When a bacterial upper airway infection is suspected, give only general noninvasive treatment with high-flow oxygen in a position of comfort. Avoid agitating the child by trying to place an IV or attempting another maneuver, and quickly transport. If the child is in respiratory failure, initiate bag-mask ventilation and consider endotracheal intubation.

Foreign Body Aspiration

Foreign body aspiration may cause mechanical obstruction anywhere in the airway, from the pharynx to the bronchus. A retained esophageal foreign body can also cause respi-

ratory distress in an infant or young child. This happens because the trachea is pliable and can be compressed by the adjacent distended esophagus. A typical history of foreign body aspiration includes the sudden onset of coughing, choking, gagging, and shortness of breath in a previously well child without a fever or other symptoms of upper respiratory tract infection. Older infants and toddlers, who explore their world by placing things in their mouths, are at highest risk.

Treatment If the child can still cough, cry, or speak, the airway is only partially obstructed. Stridor is typical. Immediately transport such children, who have incomplete upper airway obstruction. Use only general noninvasive treatment, avoid agitating the child, and keep her in a position of comfort.

If the child has severe respiratory distress and is at risk for getting worse during transport, be prepared to perform foreign body airway obstruction maneuvers for complete obstruction, as illustrated in **Figures 3-12** and **3-13**. **Table 3-3** summarizes these maneuvers. Consider these foreign body airway obstruction maneuvers if the child cannot cough, cry, or speak. *Never perform foreign body airway*

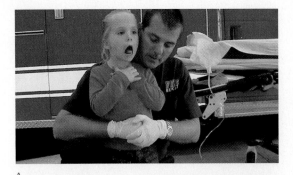

A

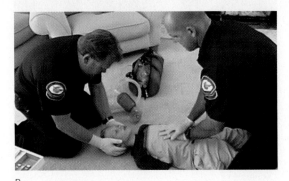

B

Figure 3-13 (A) Use five abdominal thrusts to treat complete airway obstruction in the conscious child in the standing position. (B) For the unconscious child with a suspected airway obstruction, use five abdominal thrusts with the patient in the supine position.

Table 3-3	Foreign Body Airway Obstruction Maneuvers
Age	**Technique**
Infant (< 12 months)	Five back blows followed by five chest thrusts
Child (> 1 year)	Five abdominal thrusts

obstruction procedures if the child has incomplete obstruction (i.e., can cough, cry, or speak).

Airway Obstruction/Foreign Body Removal

In the setting of complete airway obstruction, prehospital professionals can make the difference between life and death. Immediate removal of an airway foreign body can often be achieved using BLS procedures. Sometimes basic maneuvers are unsuccessful. In such cases, Magill forceps along with direct <u>laryngoscopy</u> may be the only option for removal. For a step-by-step explanation of this procedure, see

(Foreign Body Obstruction, Procedure 6).

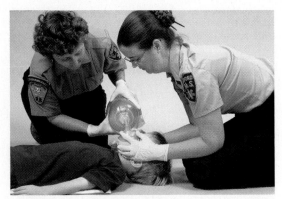

Figure 3-14 Two-person bag-mask ventilation technique.

Foreign Body Airway Obstruction Maneuvers If the child has complete obstruction and BLS maneuvers fail to dislodge the foreign body to the mouth where it can be easily removed, consider direct laryngoscopy. If the foreign body can be seen at or above the level of the larynx, remove it using pediatric Magill forceps. If the child has complete obstruction and neither foreign body airway obstruction maneuvers nor direct laryngoscopy relieve the obstruction, attempt bag-mask ventilation, using the two-person technique whenever possible (**Figure 3-14**). If bag-mask ventilation fails to achieve chest rise, perform endotracheal intubation.

Specific Treatment of Upper Airway Obstruction

When transporting any child with suspected incomplete upper airway obstruction, have airway equipment immediately available. Consider transporting the caregiver with any conscious child with airway obstruction, as this may keep the child calm. Also, the caregiver can help administer oxygen.

Lower Airway Obstruction

Bronchiolitis and asthma are the most common conditions causing lower airway obstruction in children. Foreign body aspiration is much less common and usually occurs in toddlers who have been otherwise well, and then suddenly start choking, coughing, or wheezing. *Wheezing is the clinical hallmark of lower airway obstruction of any cause.* Pneumonia can also cause lower airway disease but usually without obstruction. A specific diagnosis of lower airway obstruction in the field is not necessary, and many times it is impossible to tell which of the three main conditions the child is experiencing: bronchiolitis, asthma, or foreign body aspiration. Treatment for all forms of **bronchoconstriction** is similar, but asthma is much more likely to respond to bronchodilators than bronchiolitis.

Asthma

Asthma is the most common chronic disease of childhood, affecting almost 5 million children in the United States. The emergency department admission rate for asthmatics under 5 years of age is more than twice the national average for all ages, and the mortality rate for children is rising. Half of all pediatric asthma deaths occur in the out-of-hospital setting. The length of the final attack is less than 1 hour in many children, and less than 2 hours in half of asthmatic children who die. Common reasons for an asthma attack include upper respiratory infection and exercise. Exposure to cold air, emotional stress, and passive exposure to smoke may trigger attacks as well.

Asthma is a disease of small airway inflammation. The inflammatory reaction leads to bronchoconstriction, mucosal edema, and profuse secretions. These three factors in combination cause severe airflow obstruction and **ventilation-perfusion mismatch**. Clinically, children having an asthma attack will show different degrees of tachypnea, tachycardia, increased work of breathing, and wheezing on exhalation. Pulse oximetry may be normal or low.

Never perform airway obstruction procedures if the child has only incomplete obstruction and can still cough, cry, or speak.

Attempt BLS maneuvers first in a child with suspected foreign body aspiration and critical airway obstruction.

Carefully assess air movement by auscultation. The asthmatic complaining of shortness of breath, but without wheezing on auscultation, may have too much airway obstruction to wheeze. Aggressive bronchodilator treatment may improve airflow and increase audible wheezing. Beware of the following features of the initial assessment, which suggest severe bronchospasm and respiratory failure:

- Altered appearance
- Exhaustion
- Inability to recline
- Interrupted speech
- Severe retractions
- Decreased air movement

Case Study 2

A mother calls 9-1-1 because an 11-year-old asthmatic "can't breathe." The girl is on daily treatments with a metered dose inhaler (MDI). Her physician prescribed oral steroids yesterday for worsening asthma symptoms. The girl tells you using broken phrases that she was up all night, using her albuterol MDI every 1 to 2 hours. She is sleepy and pale, has audible wheezing and is in the tripod position. There are suprasternal, intercostal, and substernal retractions and nasal flaring. The respiratory rate is 32 breaths/min, the heart rate 154 beats/min, and the blood pressure is 138/84 mm Hg. Blood oxygen saturation is 86% on room air. On auscultation you hear minimal air movement and a prolonged expiratory phase.

1. What is this child's physiologic status and where is the level of her airway obstruction?
2. What is the most important treatment?

In the focused history, several things suggest that a severe or potentially fatal attack is to come. These include:

- Prior intensive care unit admissions or intubation
- More than three ED visits in a year
- More than two ED admissions in past year
- Use of more than one metered dose inhaler (MDI) canister in the last month
- Use of steroids for asthma in the past
- Use of bronchodilators more frequently than every 4 hours
- Progressive symptoms despite aggressive home therapy

Home therapy of asthma has several goals: preventing and controlling asthma symptoms, reducing the number of attacks and the severity of each one, and reversing existing air flow obstruction. Some children with a history of severe or frequent asthma attacks are on daily medications, but most children receive treatment only during serious attacks. **Table 3-4** lists the medications frequently used in home asthma therapy for quick relief. Some patients may think they will obtain quick relief from medications that do not have a quick onset of action and delay calling for help.

Treatment of Lower Airway Obstruction

For all children with lower airway obstruction, give general noninvasive treatment as the first field action.

Advanced Life Support

Asthma Treatment

Specific field treatment of wheezing includes either inhaled bronchodilators or subcuta-neous (SQ) epinephrine. **Figures 3-15, 3-16,** and **3-17** illustrate administration of inhaled bronchodilators.

Bronchodilators

Early bronchodilator therapy, on the scene and on the way to the ED, helps immediately open airways, relieve respiratory distress, and improve oxygen delivery in asthma. In unstable or critical patients, continuous inhaled treatment with a beta agonist is the preferred approach, although SQ bronchodilators are acceptable in some patients who cannot cooperate with inhalation therapy. For a step-by-step explanation of this procedure, see Bronchodilator Therapy, Procedure 7.

Pharmacologic Treatment of Wheezing

Albuterol (salbutamol) is the most popular inhaled bronchodilator. Because of its selective action on the bronchiole smooth muscles and its minimal effect on cardiac rate, the drug has a high margin of safety. In a critical child with wheezing, treat with the highest dose and give continuous treatment.

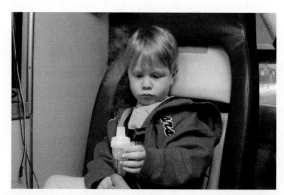

Figure 3-15 A nebulized bronchodilator can also be given without a mask using a blow-by technique.

Table 3-4	Asthma: Common Home Therapy Quick-Relief Medications for Acute Asthma Attacks	
Class of Medication	**Medication**	**Mechanism of Action**
Beta-2 agonists	Inhaled bronchodilators (albuterol [salbutamol]), levalbuterol	Relax bronchiole smooth muscle; prevent bronchospasm; rapid onset of action.
Anticholinergics	Inhaled anticholinergics (ipratropium)	Relax bronchiole smooth muscle; decrease secretions; rapid onset of action.
Anti-inflammatory medications	Oral corticosteroids (prednisone)	Block allergic response; reduce airway hyper-responsiveness; improve response to bronchodilators; delayed onset of action (2–12 hours).

Unit dose vials of albuterol (salbutamol) premixed with saline are used by most prehospital systems. These vials provide 2.5 mg of albuterol (salbutamol) in a total volume of 3 mL. One vial is an acceptable initial dose for almost all children and adolescents. For critical patients the nebulizer may be refilled continuously or two vials may be placed in the nebulizer initially and given immediately. <u>Levalbuterol</u> is an isomer of albuterol that has not been studied in the out-of-hospital setting, and may be an excellent alternative nebulized bronchodilator.

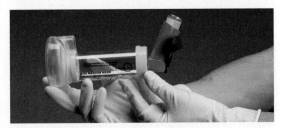

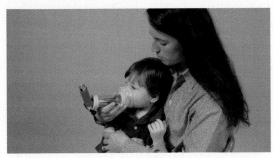

Figure 3-16 (A) A metered dose inhaler and spacer can be used with or without a mask. (B) An MDI with spacer and mask can be used in children as young as 6 months old.

Depending on local protocols, give ipratropium with albuterol (salbutamol). <u>Ipratropium</u> is an anticholinergic that may provide additional bronchodilation in addition to beta agonists. Precautions include sensitivity to the effects of ipratropium or <u>atropine</u>. Adverse reactions include dry mouth, headache, cough, hoarseness, blurred vision, tachycardia, and occasionally flushing. Add to a unit dose vial of albuterol (salbutamol) and administer together via nebulizer. Multiple doses of ipratropium probably provide added benefit in asthma exacerbations.

If a child cannot tolerate nebulized drug therapy, or is moving air so poorly that the drug is not being inhaled, give SQ epinephrine. Transport with cardiac monitoring if frequent nebulized treatments or SQ epinephrine is necessary. **Table 3-5** summarizes the drugs and doses for field bronchodilator therapy.

In most cases of known asthma, give a bronchodilator on scene before transport,

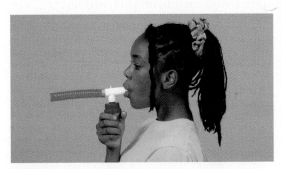

Figure 3-17 One method for delivering a bronchodilator is with an oxygen-powered nebulizer.

Table 3-5	Management of Wheezing: Bronchodilator Treatment
Bronchodilator	**Dose**
Albuterol (salbutamol)	Nebulized solution (1.25 mg/3 mL, 2.5 mg/3 mL, 5 mg/mL) Minimum dose: 2.5 mg every 20 minutes for 3 doses, repeat at dose of 0.15–0.3 mg/kg up to 10 mg every 1–4 hours as needed. Dilute in minimum of 2 to 3 mL of saline for adequate nebulization. May use continuously for status asthmaticus.
Ipratropium bromide inhalation solution	Nebulized solution (0.5 mg/2.5 mL) *Children < 12 years:* 0.25 mg nebulized every 20 minutes for 3 doses *Children > 12 years:* 0.5 mg nebulized every 20 minutes for 3 doses
Albuterol (salbutamol) metered dose inhaler	90 μg per puff 4–8 puffs every 15–20 minutes for 3 doses.

Tip

When a child has history of increased work of breathing, but now has altered appearance and a slow or normal respiratory rate without retractions, THINK RESPIRATORY FAILURE.

and then give additional doses en route, as indicated.

IM and SQ Injections

Intramuscular (IM) or subcutaneous (SQ) administration allows the medication to absorb slowly but steadily. The SQ route (e.g., for SQ epinephrine in bronchospasm) has few complications because it avoids contact with tendons, nerves, and blood vessels. The IM route may result in nerve damage, particularly if the injection is in the buttocks of infants and small children. For a step-by-step explanation of this procedure, see

Intramuscular and Subcutaneous Injections, Procedure 14 .

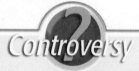

Controversy

The value of levalbuterol in pediatric out-of-hospital care of children with bronchospasm is unknown, but hospital studies suggest that it may be an excellent alternative to albuterol.

Advanced Life Support

Unit dose vials of 2.5 mg of albuterol (salbutamol) premixed with saline to a total volume of 3 mL may be used as an initial dose for children and adolescents of all ages. In critical patients, doses may be repeated continuously en route to the emergency department.

Assisted Ventilation Because of the severe air trapping associated with bronchospasm, assisted ventilation may be associated with many complications and death. Positive pressure ventilation requires very high inspiratory pressures and may result in pneumothorax or

pneumomediastinum. Consider bag-mask ventilation and endotracheal intubation of a wheezing child only if the child is in respiratory failure and has failed to respond to high-flow oxygen and maximal bronchodilator therapy. While assisting ventilation in any patient with lower airway obstruction, slow rates (12–15 breaths per minute in older children and adolescents and a maximum rate of 20–30 breaths per minute in infants) with long expiratory times are useful in minimizing barotrauma and complications.

Bronchiolitis

Bronchiolitis is a viral lower respiratory infection, which usually affects infants and children less than 3 years of age. Often caused by the respiratory syncytial virus (RSV), this disease is widespread in the winter months. The infection leads to destruction of the lining of the bronchioles, profuse secretions, and bronchoconstriction. Infants are particularly likely to catch the disease because of their small airway size, high resistance to airflow, and poor airway clearance. Airway edema and debris from sloughed cells and mucous are much more important in the pathophysiology of this disease than bronchospasm and smooth muscle contraction.

Presenting complaints of bronchiolitis include upper respiratory infection symptoms, fever, cough, vomiting, poor feeding, poor sleep, and trouble breathing. Assessment shows variable degrees of increased work of breathing, tachypnea, diffuse wheezing, inspiratory crackles, and tachycardia.

Historical risk factors for respiratory failure in infants with suspected bronchiolitis include age less than 2 months, history of prematurity, underlying lung disease, congenital heart disease, and immune deficiency. **Table 3-6** lists important clinical predictors of respiratory failure in children with suspected bronchiolitis.

Advanced Life Support

Treat bronchiolitis with nebulized epinephrine or albuterol (salbutamol), which may prevent the need for assisted ventilation.

Foreign Body Aspiration

Children with lower airway obstruction due to foreign body aspiration usually are only mildly

Table 3-6	Predictors of Respiratory Failure in Suspected Bronchiolitis

Respiratory rate > 60 breaths/min with increased work of breathing

Heart rate > 200 beats/min or < 100 beats/min

Poor appearance

Blood oxygen saturation < 90% on supplemental oxygen

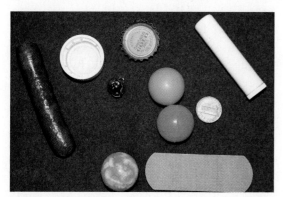

Figure 3-18 Examples of foreign bodies that can obstruct the airway.

Blip

The efficacy of treatment of bronchiolitis with bronchodilators is questionable. Begin transport of a wheezing infant and give a dose en route, but do not delay transport for scene treatment.

ill. Unlike foreign bodies in the upper airway, it is rare to develop respiratory failure or complete airway obstruction from a small foreign body in the lower airway. Foreign body aspiration is most common in older infants and toddlers (**Figure 3-18**). Often, there is an abrupt onset of coughing or choking that may be followed by a period of relatively few symptoms. Tachypnea, increased work of breathing, and wheezing or decreased breath sounds, which are usually unilateral unless the foreign body is in the trachea, may develop rapidly or over a period of hours to days. The absence of a history of asthma or the symptoms of an upper respiratory infection in a child of the right age should suggest the possibility of foreign body

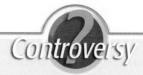

Controversy

Specific field treatment of infants with wheezing may include bronchodilation with nebulized beta agonists or nebulized epinephrine. The relative effectiveness of these treatments for bronchiolitis is controversial.

aspiration. General noninvasive treatment, including allowing the child to assume a position of comfort and providing oxygen if tolerated, should be given to all patients. A trial of inhaled bronchodilators is reasonable if the diagnosis is unclear, but do not delay transport. Additional diagnostic tests may be done after arrival at the emergency department.

Lung Disease

In children, most lung disease is pneumonia. Other causes, such as pulmonary edema or pulmonary contusion, are rare. Pneumonia may cause symptoms of lower airway disease and respiratory distress or failure in children. Almost all children with pneumonia will have fever or a history of fever at some point in their illness. The majority of pneumonias in children are due to viruses. These children generally have less severe symptoms and symptoms of a more gradual onset than children with bacterial pneumonia.

Bacterial pneumonia in children occurs following hematogenous seeding or aspiration of bacteria into the lung. This is followed by an acute inflammatory reaction leading to the accumulation of fluid within the airspaces of the lung. At times, this may be accompanied by the development of a pleural effusion or collection of fluid in the pleural space outside the lung parenchyma. Children with bacterial pneumonia usually have an abrupt onset of symptoms including fever, shaking, chills, tachypnea, and frequently nonspecific complaints including lethargy or irritability, poor appetite, and occasionally chest pain. Cough may not develop until after a period of other more nonspecific symptoms.

Physical findings include fever, rales or decreased breath sounds, and tachypnea or increased work of breathing. Grunting respirations are relatively common in young children with any form of lung disease. Wheezes may be heard, especially with viral infections, but are not as common as rales or decreased breath sounds. In the absence of underlying illness, disability, or very young age, it is unusual for a child to abruptly develop respiratory failure due to pneumonia. Mild respiratory distress is more likely.

Approach children with suspected pneumonia like any patient with symptoms of lower airway disease. Making the diagnosis is not as important as providing good supportive care. Give general, noninvasive treatment to all patients. If the patient has wheezing, try bronchodilators. Patients with signs of respiratory failure may need assisted ventilation. Respiratory failure from lung disease is more commonly seen in young infants, children with underlying neurologic or pulmonary disease, and children who have been ill for several days. There is no specific prehospital therapy for children with pneumonia.

Disordered Control of Breathing

Sometimes hypoxia and/or respiratory insufficiency is caused by problems in control of breathing. This category of respiratory disease includes brain injury, spinal injury, poisoning, metabolic problems (e.g., botulism, Guillan-Barre Syndrome), or sepsis. The hallmark of patients with disordered control of breathing is inadequate minute volume, from poor tidal volume and/or slow breathing rate. Treatment includes ventilatory support with oxygen, bag-mask ventilation, and occasionally endotracheal intubation.

Summary of Specific Treatment for Respiratory Distress

After identifying respiratory distress or failure and beginning general supportive measures, assess whether the anatomic level of the respiratory problem is in the upper or lower airway, using both the PAT and the hands-on ABCDEs. Stridor is the hallmark of upper airway obstruction, wheezing is the hallmark of lower airway obstruction, grunting is the hallmark of lung disease, and inadequate minute volume and decreased work of breathing are the clinical markers for disordered control of breathing.

The most common cause of upper airway obstruction is croup. Rarely, foreign bodies lodged at or above the vocal cords, may be the cause of stridor in infants and toddlers. Specific treatment of croup includes cool mist and nebulized epinephrine. Frequent causes of lower airway obstruction are asthma and bronchiolitis—a disease of infants. Asthma is the most likely reason for wheezing in all children from infancy to adulthood. A nebulized bronchodilator—delivered continuously if necessary—is the specific treatment for all causes of wheezing. Albuterol (salbutamol) and epinephrine have similar effectiveness as bronchodilators, and the anticholinergic ipratropium provides added benefit in asthma patients. Start treatment on scene in asthmatics.

Foreign body aspiration and pneumonia may present as lower airway problems, but there is no specific treatment for these conditions in the prehospital setting other than the general noninvasive measures for respiratory distress. Disordered control of breathing has many causes and requires general ventilatory support.

Management of Respiratory Failure

Regardless of the cause, initially treat every cooperative child in respiratory failure with general noninvasive measures. If upper or lower airway obstruction is present, attempt specific treatment. On the other hand, if the child has altered appearance or altered level of consciousness and has signs of increased or decreased work of breathing (e.g., flaring, grunting, gasping, apnea, or cyanosis), or if the child has a documented blood oxygen saturation of less than 90% on 100% non-rebreathing oxygen mask, the child is in respiratory failure or respiratory arrest. For this child, bypass general noninvasive treatment and immediately begin assisted ventilation.

First, postion the patient to maintain an open airway. Then use suction. Suctioning is a basic technique to maintain an open airway. Children have tiny airways that are easily obstructed by secretions, vomitus, pus, blood, or foreign bodies. Children of different ages, with different clinical problems, need different types of suction devices and suctioning procedures. For a step-by-step explanation, see (Suctioning, Procedure 4).

If the patient is unresponsive, use an airway adjunct. Adjuncts may immediately improve the child's spontaneous ventilation. In addition, they may allow more effective bag-mask ventilation, reduce gastric inflation, and avert the need for endotracheal intubation. For a step-by-step explanation of this procedure, see (Airway Adjuncts, Procedure 5).

Then deliver assisted ventilation or **positive-pressure ventilation** using bag-mask. Bag-mask is usually the best method for providing oxygenation and ventilation during stabilization and transport. Use an age-appropriate rate of 30 breaths/min in infants and 20 breaths/min in older children. Saying the words, "Squeeze, release, release" will help time the ventilations to avoid a rate that is too rapid. Ensure that there is good chest rise. Good bag-mask technique will decrease the risk of gastric distention—a common complication leading to elevation of the **diaphragm**, decreased lung compliance, and increased risk of vomiting and aspiration of gastric contents. If a second rescuer is available, providing cricoid pressure using the Sellick maneuver

may help to further decrease gastric distension. With severe, lower airway obstruction, slower rates and longer expiratory times are indicated.

Bag-Mask Ventilation

Bag-mask ventilation is one of the prehospital professional's most useful skills in pediatric out-of-emergency department care. While the technique does not provide the definitive airway control that endotracheal intubation does, in most cases, bag-mask ventilation will be the best technique for providing oxygenation and ventilation during resuscitation and transport. For a step-by-step explanation of this procedure, see (Bag-Mask Ventilation, Procedure 8).

Minimize gastric distention during bag-mask ventilation with good bagging technique.

If the child does not respond to bag-mask ventilation, or if there is a long transport time with a critically ill or injured child who has an unstable airway, consider endotracheal intubation.

Case Study 3

A caregiver calls 9-1-1 because a 3-month-old girl has had three days of cough, runny nose and low-grade fever. The caregiver is concerned because the child seems to be working harder to breathe and is having a hard time taking feedings. On arrival, the child is found sitting on the caregiver's lap. She appears sleepy and does not make eye contact or respond to examination. She has audible wheezing and deep subcostal and intercostal retractions. There is nasal flaring. Her skin is mottled and she is diaphoretic. Respiratory rate is 70 breaths/minute and her heart rate is 180 beats/minute. Her breath sounds are tight with only fair air movement but you hear high-pitched, inspiratory and expiratory wheezes throughout. Pulse oximetry in room air is 74% with a pulse that corresponds to the patient's pulse on exam.

1. Is this child in respiratory distress or respiratory failure and what is the level of airway obstruction?
2. What are the first steps in the management of this child?

Management with Endotracheal Intubation

The indications for endotracheal intubation of a child in the out-of-emergency department setting are controversial. Potential advantages of intubation include definitive airway control, decreased risk of aspiration, and ease of assisted ventilation. Potential complications include transient hypoxia and hypercapnia due to prolonged intubation attempts, elevation of intracranial pressure, aspiration of stomach contents, and injury to the teeth, mouth, tongue, palate, larynx and soft tissues of the pharynx and neck. Failure of ventilation after intubation may be due to unrecognized misplacement of the tube (mainstem bronchus or esophageal intubation).

Dislodgment of the tube from the trachea during patient movement or transport is common and may be catastrophic. If an intubated patient fails to respond with improved color, oxygen saturation, heart rate, and appearance, the DOPE mnemonic may help to identify potential technical problems (**Table 3-7**).

Nasogastric/Orogastric Insertion

During positive-pressure ventilation, it is common to inflate the stomach as well as the lungs, with air. Gastric inflation with air slows downward movement of the diaphragm and decreases tidal volume, making ventila-

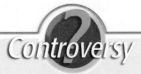

Controversy

The value of nasogastric and orogastric tubes is unknown. Avoid inserting a nasogastric or orogastric tube unless ventilation is impaired by a distended stomach.

Table 3-7	Troubleshooting the Endotracheal Tube: DOPE		
	Problem	**Assessment**	**Intervention**
Dislodgment	Esophageal intubation	End-tidal carbon dioxide monitor/detector reads no carbon dioxide or no color change Oxygen saturation < 90% Bradycardia Lack of chest rise with ventilation Auscultation of bubbling over the stomach	Extubate Bag-mask ventilation Reintubate
	Mainstem bronchus intubation	Asymmetric chest rise Asymmetric breath sounds	Pull tube back until breath sounds and chest rise are symmetric
	Accidental extubation	End-tidal carbon dioxide monitor/detector reads no carbon dioxide or no color change Oxygen saturation < 90% Bradycardia Lack of chest rise with ventilation Poor or absent air movement on auscultation	Bag-mask ventilation Reintubate
Obstruction	Tube blocked with blood, secretions, or kink	Decreased chest rise Decreased breath sounds bilaterally Oxygen saturation < 90% Increased resistance to bagging	Suction Extubate Bag-mask ventilation Reintubate
Pneumothorax	Tension pneumothorax, spontaneous or induced, compromises air exchange and may lead to decreased cardiac output	Asymmetric chest rise Asymmetric breath sounds Shock Oxygen saturation < 90% *Jugulovenous distention *Tracheal deviation	Needle thoracostomy
Equipment	Big air leak around tube Activated pop-off valve on resuscitator Oxygen tubing disconnected Oxygen tank empty		Check equipment "patient-to-tank"

* Not easily assessed in young children

tion more difficult and necessitating higher inspiratory pressures. In addition, inflation of the stomach with air increases the risk that the patient will vomit and aspirate. Gastric intubation with an NG or OG tube takes air from the stomach and helps positive-pressure ventilation. However, only use this technique if there is difficulty ventilating the patient. Insertion may be painful and frightening to the child and family. For a step-by-step explanation of this procedure, see

(Orogastric and Nasogastric Tube Insertion, Procedure 10).

Endotracheal Intubation
Successful endotracheal intubation allows optimal oxygenation and ventilation, provides a tube for medication delivery, and decreases the risk of aspiration and loss of airway control. A properly placed and secured endotracheal tube is a good tool for managing critical patients, but the procedure can take a long time, and there can be frequent and serious complications. For a step-by-step explanation of this procedure, see

(Endotracheal Intubation, Procedure 11).

Advanced Breathing Techniques
Rarely, standard bag-mask ventilation fails and ETI is difficult or impossible. Examples of such patients are children with massive head trauma and airway edema or hematoma of the mouth or upper airway, children with multisytem injuries and long transport times, or infants with significant congenital

or acquired airway abnormalities that cannot be ventilated. In such dire circumstances, some EMS systems allow prehospital professionals to perform advanced breathing techniques. These include use of the laryngeal mask airway (LMA), the gum elastic bougie, a lighted stylet, rapid sequence intubation (RSI) and needle cricothyrotomy. None of these techniques have been well evaluated in children in the out-of-hospital setting.

Table 3-8 summarizes the advantages and disadvantages of these advanced techniques. For a step-by-step explanation of the LMA, gum elastic bougie, lighted stylet, and RSI, see (Advanced Airway Techniques, Procedure 13).

(Needle Thoracostomy, Procedure 22) explains needle cricothyrotomy.

Confirmation of Endotracheal Tube Placement
Several products are currently available for confirming proper placement of the endotracheal tube. These include quantitative end-tidal carbon dioxide monitors or capnometers, which read out the blood carbon dioxide tension ($PACO_2$); colorimetric end-tidal carbon dioxide detectors that give a qualitative reading; and syringe and self-inflating bulb devices that distinguish endotracheal from esophageal intubation based on positive aspiration of air from the tube (not approved for children <5 years or 20 kg) (**Figure 3-19**).

The optimal method for tube confirmation in children in the out-of-hospital setting

Table 3-8	Advantages and Disadvantages of Rescue Breathing Techniques	
Technique	**Advantages**	**Disadvantages**
LMA	Simple insertion Good airway seal Adapts to bag-mask equipment	Does not prevent aspiration Few size choices
Gum elastic bougie	May facilitate ETT insertion	No equipment or data in infants and young children Prolonged attempts may worsen hypoxia
Lighted stylet	Does not require airway visualization	Poor information in children Unknown accuracy
Rapid sequence intubation	Paralyzes child and eliminates muscle resistance Improves visualization Allows mild hyperventilation	Drugs remove spontaneous breathing Drugs may decrease BP or RR **Succinylcholine** may cause high potassium
Cricothyrotomy	Provides tiny airway for life saving oxygenation/ventilation Bypasses obstruction	Technically difficult Bleeding Injury to other neck structures

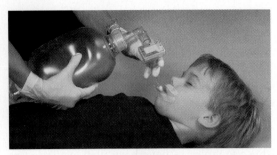

Figure 3-19 Using the carbon dioxide detector.

Tip

If an esophageal bulb or syringe is employed, cardiac arrest and low pulmonary blood flow should not affect the result.

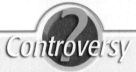

Controversy

The optimal method for tube confirmation in children in the out-of-emergency department setting is not known.

is not known. Because the child's airway is so short, even slight movement of the endotracheal tube can lead to extubation or main stem intubation. If capnometery shows no carbon dioxide, if the colorimetric detector fails to change color with ventilation, or if no air is aspirated into the esophageal bulb or syringe, these are indications that the endotracheal tube may not be in the trachea. In such cases, extubate the child, do bag-mask ventilation, and re-intubate after 1 to 2 minutes of oxygenation and ventilation.

The only exception to this approach is the patient in full cardiopulmonary arrest, where pulmonary circulation may be too low to generate detectable expired carbon dioxide. In this case, if the capnometer shows a negative end tidal carbon dioxide reading, or if the colorimetric device shows a yellow color (no carbon dioxide), observe for chest rise, auscultate bilaterally for air movement, and attempt to visualize the tube

passing through the vocal cords via direct laryngoscopy. If the endotracheal tube appears to be in proper position, leave the tube in place.

If an esophageal bulb or syringe is employed, cardiac arrest and low pulmonary blood flow should not affect the result. If air is aspirated, the tube is in the trachea. Hence, the esophageal bulb or syringe technique for confirmation of endotracheal tube placement may offer an advantage over the other two techniques in the setting of cardiac arrest and low pulmonary blood flow.

For a step-by-step explanation of these confirmation procedures, see Confirmation of Endotracheal Tube Placement, Procedure 12.

Summary of Management of Respiratory Failure

Respiratory failure or respiratory arrest can result from many different insults to the airway, mechanics of breathing, or gas exchange. Infection, trauma, and bronchospasm are important causes in children. Think respiratory failure when initial assessment reveals a child with altered appearance in the setting of significantly increased or decreased work of breathing. Bradycardia, poor air movement, and low oxygen saturation are key findings. In a child with respiratory failure or respiratory arrest, immediately begin assisted ventilation with a bag-mask device at an age-appropriate rate. Avoid gastric insufflation. Add specific treatment for airway obstruction, such as an inhaled bronchodilator, if indicated. Perform endotracheal intubation cautiously and be alert for the frequent "DOPE" complications in the intubated child who suddenly worsens or fails to respond. Always confirm proper placement of the endotracheal tube with capnometry, colorimetric carbon dioxide detection, or with an esophageal bulb or syringe. In some EMS systems, advanced breathing techniques are options in the child who cannot be ventilated by bag-mask ventilation or endotracheal intubation.

Initial Assessment: The Transport Decision—Stay or Go?

When a child has respiratory distress, begin general noninvasive treatment (position of comfort and oxygen) and consider specific treatment on scene. Never transport a child who is in respiratory failure without assisted ventilation. Also, never transport a child with a completely obstructed airway until after performing foreign body obstruction maneuvers. Immediate on scene care to support breathing will improve the outcomes of children with many respiratory emergencies. After opening the airway and providing assisted ventilation when necessary, or after simply giving general treatment, the prehospital professional must decide whether to stay on scene to assess further and treat specifically, or to go.

If the PAT and ABCDEs are normal and the child has no history of serious breathing problems, the child does not usually require urgent treatment or immediate transport. Take the time to get a focused history and physical exam and perform a detailed physical examination (trauma patient) on the scene if possible.

If the child has respiratory distress and signs of upper airway obstruction, transport is usually indicated after general noninvasive treatment. Consider specific treatment of suspected croup with cool mist and a dose of nebulized epinephrine on the way to the ED, if available. On the other hand, *if the child is an asthmatic and has lower airway obstruction with wheezing, begin specific treatment with a bronchodilator on scene, and then transport.*

For critical children, consider endotracheal intubation if the child is in respiratory failure and ventilation by bag-mask device is ineffective, or if an airway is difficult to maintain. However, endotracheal intubation increases scene time and delays the time to definitive care at the emergency department. There has been a high rate of complications documented in prehospital studies of endotracheal intubation in children. Intubation skills tend to extinguish rapidly because they are used infrequently. In most cases, bag-mask ventilation is probably a better option.

Additional Assessment

If the child has minimal respiratory distress and there are no immediate safety concerns for the child or prehospital professional, consider obtaining the focused history and physical exam and performing a detailed physical exam (trauma patient) on scene. Use the SAMPLE mnemonic to find important features of the complete respiratory history. **Table 3-9** gives examples of a focused history in a child with a breathing problem.

Do vigilant ongoing assessment of all children with respiratory distress or failure while on the way to the ED. Use the PAT to recall observational indicators of effective gas exchange, and watch respiratory rate, heart rate, and pulse oximetry. Be prepared to increase the level of respiratory support, or to correct complications of therapy if the child worsens or fails to respond.

Tip

When a child fails to respond to assisted ventilation with improvement in clinical status, quickly assess your equipment—from the oxygen tank to the patient—for mechanical failure.

Table 3-9	SAMPLE Components in a Child with Respiratory Distress
Component	**Explanation**
Signs/Symptoms	Onset and nature of shortness of breath Presence of hoarseness, stridor, or wheezing Presence and quality of cough, chest pain
Allergies	Known allergies Cigarette smoke exposure
Medications	Exact names and doses of ongoing drugs, including metered dose inhalers Recent use of steroids Timing and amount of last dose Timing and dose of analgesics/antipyretics
Past medical problems	History of asthma, chronic lung disease, or heart problems or prematurity Prior hospitalizations for breathing problems Prior intubations for breathing problems Immunizations
Last food or liquid	Timing of the child's last food or drink, including bottle or breastfeeding
Events leading to the injury or illness	Evidence of increased work of breathing Fever history

Chapter Review
Case Study Answers

Case Study ❶ page 51

This child is in respiratory distress but does not seem to have progressed to respiratory failure. She is exhibiting many of the signs and symptoms of upper airway obstruction. Her loud, harsh inspiratory breath sounds are consistent with stridor. This sound along with the supraclavicular and suprasternal retractions helps localize the obstruction to the upper airway. She has increased work of breathing, but does not show any signs of hypoxia or hypercapnia (carbon dioxide retention). Upper airway obstruction and stridor in a young child after a few days of an upper respiratory infection is most consistent with croup, a swelling in the trachea below the area of the vocal cords due to a viral infection. Other things that may cause upper airway obstruction include foreign bodies, bacterial infections (e.g., epiglottitis or retropharyngeal abscess) and airway edema due to allergic reactions.

Regardless of the cause, the management of children with upper airway obstruction is similar and is based on the severity of the symptoms. Keep this patient in a position of comfort, give humidified oxygen and transport to an emergency department for further care.

Advanced Life Support

Nebulized medications (e.g., epinephrine or racemic epinephrine), act as vasoconstrictors and decrease airway edema. These may be helpful en route to the emergency department.

The child should be closely monitored as her upper airway obstruction may progress and respiratory failure may develop.

Case Study ❷ page 63

This child is in respiratory failure. She has abnormal appearance (sleepy), poor color (pallor), and increased work of breathing (retractions, audible wheezing, flaring, tripod position). Her tachypnea, tachycardia, documented hypoxia, and poor air movement support this assessment. Her wheezing, and substernal and intercostal retractions localize her level of obstruction to the lower airway (within the thorax).

Further, she is being treated aggressively at home, with worsening symptoms despite steroids and utilization of her albuterol (salbutamol) MDI far more frequently than is recommended for patient self-administration. The fact that she was up all night indicates that she was in too much respiratory distress to recline or sleep.

Asthma is a chronic disease, involving inflammation of the small airways. Although bronchoconstriction, airway edema, and increased secretions all contribute to lower airway obstruction, the only part of this pathophysiology that can be reversed in the short time frame of a field response is bronchoconstriction.

General noninvasive treatment includes administration of high-flow oxygen, and position of comfort. Support ventilation with a bag-mask if her condition deteriorates. Positive-pressure ventilation will require high peak inspiratory pressures and may be associated with worse air trapping and barotrauma. If positive-pressure ventilation is required, it is important to use a very slow rate and allow for a long expiratory time to minimize air trapping.

Advanced Life Support

Specific treatment includes continuous high-dose nebulized albuterol (salbutamol), using 5–10 mg per dose, and "back-to-back" or continuous nebulizer treatments. Use ipratropium (0.5 mg) if available, with albuterol. Consider giving SQ epinephrine if she has little or no air movement (characterized by absent or faint breath sounds), does not respond to the first nebulizer treatment or if her condition worsens. If transport is long and assisted ventilation is required, consider endotracheal intubation.

Retained carbon dioxide may make patients so obtunded that the bag-mask is well tolerated. Also, the additional stimulation of intubation may make the patient struggle and gag. Intubation when the patient is struggling increases the risk of barotrauma and possible complications.

Case Study **3** page 69

Using the PAT, this child has an increased work of breathing, abnormal appearance, and poor circulation to the skin. She is in respiratory failure. Her wheezes and subcostal and intercostal retractions localize her airway obstruction to her lower airways. In the setting of preceding upper respiratory symptoms, fever, and progressive lower airway obstruction, the child probably has bronchiolitis. Open the child's airway and give high-flow oxygen. Do not delay transport because the child is not likely to have an easily reversible condition. This is unlike the child with asthma, who will likely benefit from a dose of a bronchodilator on scene, before transport.

En route, give continuous bronchodilators. Nebulized albuterol (salbutamol) or nebulized epinephrine may be given based on local protocol. Positive-pressure ventilation has a risk of complications in patients with lower airway obstruction and it may be wise to wait to see if bronchodilators lead to improvement in this patient.

During transport monitor the child's respiratory status closely. Any evidence of decreased respiratory effort or slowing of the respiratory rate should prompt initiation of positive-pressure ventilation with a relatively slow rate and a long expiratory time.

Suggested Readings

Textbooks

American Heart Association. *Textbook of Pediatric Advanced Life Support.* Dallas, TX, American Heart Association, 2002.

Gausche M: *Pediatric Airway Management for the Prehospital Professional.* Boston, MA, Jones and Bartlett Publishers, 2004.

Articles

Aijian P, Tsai A, Knopp R, et al. Endotracheal intubation of pediatric patients by paramedics. *Ann Emerg Med.* 1989; 18:489–494.

Bhende MS, Thompson AE, Orr RA. Utility of an end-tidal carbon dioxide detector during stabilization and transport of critically ill children. *Pediatrics.* 1992; 89:1042–1044.

Brownstein D, Shugerman R, Cummings P. Prehospital endotracheal intubation of children by paramedics. *Ann Emerg Med.* 1996; 28:34–39.

Gausche M, Lewis R, Stratton S, Haynes B, et al. Effect of out-of-emergency department pediatric tracheal intubation on survival and neurologic outcome: A controlled clinical trial. *JAMA.* 2000; 283:783–790.

Kellner JD, Ohlsson A, Gadomski AM, et al. Efficacy of bronchodilator therapy in bronchiolitis—a meta-analysis. *Arch Pediatr Adolesc Med.* 1996; 150:1166–1172.

Menon K, Sutcliffe T, Klassen T. A randomized trial comparing the efficacy of epinephrine with salbutamol in the treatment of acute bronchiolitis. *J Pediatr.* 1995; 126:1004–1007.

Qureshi F, Pestian J, Davis P, Zaritsky A. Effect of nebulized ipratropium on hospitalization rates of children with asthma. *N Engl J Med.* 1998; 339:1030–1035.

Sharieff GQ, Rodarte A, Wilton N, Bleyle D. The self-inflating bulb as an airway adjunct: Is it reliable in children weighing less than 20 kilograms? *Acad Emerg Med.* 2003; 10:303–308.

Cardiovascular Emergencies

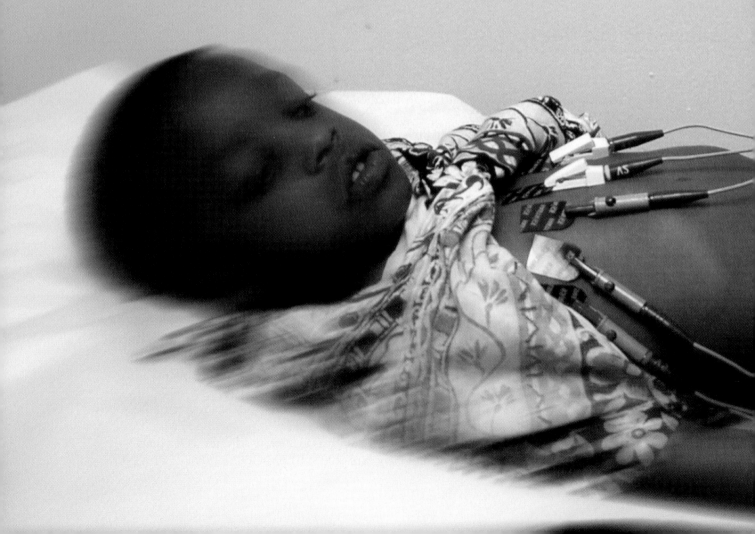

1 Describe how to assess circulation, using the PAT, ABCDEs, and additional assessment.

2 Explain the relationship between shock and blood pressure.

3 Differentiate between early (compensated) and late (decompensated) hypovolemic shock, and discuss appropriate management.

4 Explain when to treat tachycardia and bradycardia, and discuss management.

5 Order the steps in managing pediatric cardiac arrest due to asystole, pulseless electrical activity, ventricular fibrillation, and pulseless ventricular tachycardia.

6 Define indications in the use of the automated external defibrillators (AED) in pediatric patients.

7 Review key features in the management of drowning victims and the impact of hypothermia on outcome.

Case Study 1

A father calls 9-1-1 about an 18-month-old boy with a fever of 6 hours duration. On your arrival, the child is listless. He will not interact and cries inconsolably when held. There is a bluish rash of the face, trunk, and legs. There are no abnormal airway sounds. Breathing is rapid without retractions or flaring. The brachial pulse is faint, the skin is warm to touch, and capillary refill time is about 4 seconds. Respiratory rate is 60 breaths/min, and blood pressure is 60 mm Hg/palp. The cardiac monitor shows a heart rate of 190 beats/min.

1. What type of shock is present?
2. What differs in the management of this case from treatment of pure hypovolemic or cardiogenic shock?

Introduction

SERIOUS PEDIATRIC CARDIOVASCULAR problems are uncommon in the out-of-hospital setting. Cardiovascular emergencies may be the result of volume loss, vascular instability, cardiac failure, output obstruction, or a combination of any or all of these causes. Hypovolemia is the usual cause of abnormal circulation in children. Traumatic hemorrhage is a frequent etiology for *severe* hypovolemia in children, although sepsis and dehydration from gastroenteritis (vomiting and diarrhea) are other important etiologies as well, especially in infants and children under 3 years of age. *This is a different picture of circulatory emergencies than in adults, where primary cardiac disease such as dysrhythmia or congestive heart failure is the common reason for cardiovascular problems.* Such primary cardiac conditions are rare in children. Regardless of the type of cardiovascular emergency, early recognition and timely management can reduce the likelihood for serious morbidity or mortality.

Most circulatory problems in children arise from loss of intravascular fluid. The child's young, healthy cardiovascular system compensates for fluid loss by increasing heart rate and reducing blood flow to nonessential anatomic areas through the mechanism of peripheral vasoconstriction, or "clamping down." Vasoconstriction limits blood flow to less essential peripheral sites and preserves blood flow to the "core" organs such as the brain, heart, lungs, and kidneys. The physiologic process of restricting circulation to areas such as the skin and mucous membranes results in important physical signs of hypoperfusion.

Distributive shock is less common in children, and is usually due to sepsis. This type of shock primarily involves loss of vascular tone. Cardiogenic shock is unusual in pediatrics, except in children with congenital heart disease or acquired viral myocarditis. Cardiogenic shock results from congestive heart failure, with cardiac output insufficient to meet perfusion requirements. Obstructive shock is the rarest of all shock types in children. It is caused by pericardial tamponade or tension pneumothorax, secondary to injury to the chest.

Sometimes, identifying the type of shock is difficult, especially when the pathophysiology is mixed. For example, bacterial toxins or ingested poisons may have adverse effects on both vascular tone and myocardial function; sepsis may involve a volume deficit from third spacing (loss of plasma from the vascular space due to leaky blood vessels) as well as loss of vascular tone and myocardial depression. However, a careful history and physical assessment will usually identify the cause of shock and drive appropriate management. Shock from any cause, if unrecognized or inadequately treated, may advance to cardiac arrest. Once arrest has occurred, successful resuscitation is unlikely.

Prearrival Preparation

Based upon the dispatch information, prepare mentally for the assessment and management of a child with circulatory problems en route to the scene. Recall appropriate techniques for assessment, the role of vital signs, and the possible equipment, drug, and fluid requirements of the child. Consider when to stay and treat on scene and when to transport immediately.

Scene Size-up

Be sure that the scene is safe. Evaluate the environment and document potentially important features.

General Assessment: The PAT

Evaluating the Presenting Complaint

On arrival, determine the child's presenting complaint. Key questions include the onset of illness, presence of fever, frequency and amount of fluid losses (vomiting and diarrhea), and prior history of possible cardiovascular problems. Ask if the child has been injured. In children with mild circulatory compromise who are not in shock, obtain a more complete SAMPLE history (see **Table 4-1**) during the additional assessment.

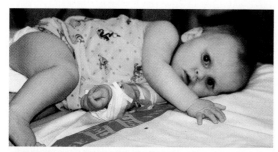

Figure 4-1 A child with decreased core circulation and too little blood and oxygen to the brain will have an abnormal appearance. This dehydrated child has listlessness, poor motor activity, and decreased interactiveness.

Assessment of Circulation

Using the PAT

The PAT is the first step in assessment of circulation, as outlined in Chapter 1. The PAT evaluates three characteristics: appearance, work of breathing, and circulation to skin. Knowing these characteristics helps to determine whether the child is sick or not sick, the type of physiologic abnormality, and the urgency for treatment. Circulatory problems affect each of these characteristics in identifiable patterns.

Appearance

First, assess the child's appearance. A child with decreased core circulation from any shock type may have signs of poor brain perfusion. The abnormality in the child's appearance will be variable, depending upon the type of perfusion problem, the degree of circulatory insufficiency, and the presence of associated problems such as fever, head trauma, or intoxication. Abnormal features in the appearance of a child with decreased core circulation include:

- Lethargy and/or listlessness
- Decreased motor activity
- Diminished interactiveness with caregivers, the prehospital professional, and the environment (**Figure 4-1**)
- Inconsolability
- Poor eye contact
- Weak cry

Sometimes the child in shock will be restless and inconsolable. *Appearance alone, however, is not a very accurate sign of circulatory problems.* An abnormal appearance may be caused by many different things, such as poor oxygenation/ventilation, head trauma, hypothermia, drugs, or fever as well as cardiovascular problems. Assessing appearance is a good way to tell if the child is ill, but not a good way to identify the physiologic problem. Assessment tools other than the PAT, such as the hands-on ABCDE assessment, will help distinguish the type of physiologic problem and the presence or absence of abnormal perfusion.

Work of Breathing

Next, assess the work of breathing. If circulation to vital organs is decreased, the child's respiratory rate will increase. "<u>Effortless tachypnea</u>," or a fast respiratory rate without increased work of breathing, is a common but nonspecific sign of shock. It reflects the child's attempt to blow off carbon dioxide and reduce the <u>metabolic acidosis</u> created by decreased perfusion to cells. Signs of increased work of breathing, such as abnormal positioning, retractions, flaring, or abnormal airway sounds such as grunting, stridor, or wheezing, are not usually present in a child with a pure circulatory problem. These signs reflect poor gas exchange and <u>hypoxia</u>, typically from a primary lung problem. While increased work of breathing is most commonly a function of respiratory disease, these signs may also occur with hypoxia and <u>pulmonary edema</u>, when cardiogenic shock results from <u>congestive heart failure</u>.

Circulation to Skin

After assessing appearance and work of breathing, assess circulation by looking at skin color. This will be difficult to interpret if the environmental temperature is low,

Tip

A child in shock may have tachypnea from metabolic acidosis, but will not usually have signs of increased work of breathing.

because <u>vasoconstriction</u>, as a reflexive effort to preserve heat, will falsely alter skin findings, especially in infants. Disrobe the child and look for mottling, pallor, and cyanosis, which reflect peripheral vasoconstriction or clamping down of nonessential skin perfusion to maintain essential core circulation. If a child has abnormal appearance and abnormal skin signs in a warm ambient environment, the child may be in compensated or decompensated shock.

Initial Assessment: The ABCDEs

After the PAT, perform the hands-on ABCDE assessment. After evaluating *Airway* and *Breathing*, as described in the previous chapters, assess the *"C"*: *Circulation*. There are four parts to the assessment of circulation:

1. Heart rate
2. Pulse quality
3. Skin temperature and capillary refill time
4. Blood pressure

Heart Rate

First, measure heart rate (HR) by feeling a pulse for 30 seconds, and then double the number. A normal heart rate is between 60 and 160 beats/min, depending on the child's age, as noted in Table 2-3. The radial or brachial areas are preferred sites to measure pulse rate in infants and children. The carotid pulse is acceptable in older children and adolescents, but it is hard to locate in infants. If a pulse is difficult to feel, determine heart rate by listening to the heart sounds directly with a stethoscope placed on the medial side of the child's left nipple. However, be aware that the presence of a "normal" heart rate by auscultation does not necessarily reflect adequate cardiac and perfusion.

Interpreting heart rate may be difficult, as explained in Chapter 1. Ranges of normal heart rates change inversely with advancing age. Also, many conditions can increase heart rate, ranging from serious physiologic problems to noxious stimuli that are rarely life-threatening. Stimuli that can cause <u>tachycardia</u> include

The carotid pulse is an acceptable site for measurement of pulse rate in older children and adolescents, but it is hard to locate in infants.

Bradycardia is always a critical sign in a young child, and reflects hypoxia or advanced shock.

pain, fever, fear, cold, and anger. Interpret heart rate in the context of overall signs of perfusion, age, presence or absence of noxious stimuli, and observed trends. While a single measurement of heart rate is usually of limited value in determining the degree of physiologic derangement, *a trend of mounting tachycardia, or a heart rate that is falling below the lower limits of normal, suggests a serious physiologic problem.* In addition, sustained tachycardia is a worrisome sign. Finally, be extremely vigilant when the child has <u>bradycardia</u>, as this may mean hypoxia or profound ischemia.

Pulse Quality

Presence of a strong central pulse (carotid, femoral, brachial in infants) with a strong peripheral pulse (<u>brachial</u> or <u>radial</u>, <u>pedal</u> in children) suggests a good blood pressure. A strong central pulse with a weak peripheral pulse indicates compensated shock. If a brachial pulse is not palpable, the child is probably hypotensive and in decompensated shock.

Skin Temperature and Capillary Refill Time

The next part of the hands-on cardiovascular assessment involves evaluating skin signs. Check skin temperature for warmth at the hands, feet, kneecaps, or forearms. Cool

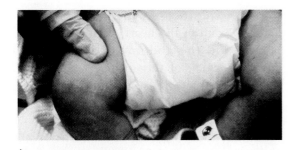

A

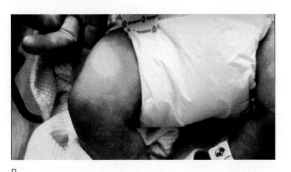

B

Figure 4-2 To determine capillary refill time, first depress the skin (A), and then count the seconds before color returns (B). Capillary refill time should be less than 2 to 3 seconds in a child who is not cold.

Tip

Practice capillary refill time and pulse quality on every child. This will help you to become comfortable with the technique and interpret key findings accurately.

hands and feet may be normal, but cool proximal extremities reflect poor perfusion and shunting of blood to the core. Determine capillary refill time (CRT) by pressing firmly on the skin. *Capillary refill time should be less than 2 to 3 seconds in a child who is not cold* (**Figure 4-2 A and B**). Again, inadequate core perfusion results in peripheral vasoconstriction, which will manifest as cool skin and delayed capillary refill time. While CRT is a good test of circulation in children, it must be interpreted in the context of overall signs of perfusion. The prehospital professional can become comfortable with the technique and interpretation of the key skin findings by practicing on every child.

Blip

CRT is a good test for circulation in children, but do not place heavy emphasis on this sign alone.

Tip

A normal minimal systolic blood pressure in a child over one year of age is 70 + (2 × years of age).

Blood Pressure

Last, consider taking a blood pressure. A high blood pressure value in a child is not clinically significant in the field, unless he has a history of hypertension, known renal disease, or acute head injury. On the other hand, a true low blood pressure value is significant and means late or decompensated shock. The challenges in the out-of-hospital setting are: knowing when to get a blood pressure reading; obtaining the blood pressure correctly; and interpreting it accurately.

Systolic blood pressure does not accurately reflect intravascular volume status until the acute volume loss is above 25% to 35% of normal circulating pediatric blood volume. *Therefore, a normal blood pressure does not mean the child has a normal blood volume or normal perfusion.* A normal minimal systolic blood pressure in a child over 1 year of age is 70 + (2 × years of age). Proper equipment, technique, and patience are required to obtain an accurate blood pressure in an infant or toddler. Because this can be a time-consuming process and may not contribute greatly to the clinical assessment of perfusion, in a child 3 years old or younger, attempt a blood pressure measurement only once or skip altogether. Inadequate perfusion will be better reflected in the other signs of perfusion described above (HR, pulse quality, CRT, and skin temperature).

In a child older than 3 years of age, make at least one blood pressure attempt in every patient. Use a cuff with a width that is

Table 4-1	SAMPLE Components in a Child with Cardiovascular Problems
Component	**Features**
Signs/Symptoms	Presence of vomiting or diarrhea
	Number of episodes of vomiting or diarrhea
	Vomiting blood or bile stools
	External hemorrhage
	Presence or absence of fever
	Rash
	Respiratory distress or shortness of breath (e.g., in cardiogenic shock with CHF)
Allergies	Known allergies
	History of anaphylaxis
Medications	Exact names and dosages of ongoing medications
	Use of laxatives or antidiarrheal medications
	Chronic diuretic therapy
	Potential exposure to other medications or drugs
	Timing and doses of analgesic/antipyretics
Past medical problems	History of heart problems
	History of prematurity
	Prior hospitalizations for cardiovascular problems
Last food or liquid	Timing of the child's last food or drink, including bottle or breastfeedings
Events leading to the injury or illness	Travel
	Trauma
	Fever history
	Symptoms in family members
	Potential toxic exposure

two-thirds the length of the upper arm. Applying too large a cuff will falsely decrease the blood pressure measurement, and too small a cuff will falsely increase it.

Additional Assessment

If the child is stable after the initial assessment, does not require immediate treatment, and if there are no immediate safety concerns for the child or prehospital professional, conduct the focused history and physical exam and the detailed physical exam (trauma patient) on scene. Use the SAMPLE mnemonic (**Table 4-1**) to recall important features of the focused cardiovascular history. Use age-appropriate approaches to gain the child's trust and speak directly to him. Ask the caregiver to add to the child's history. Obtain the history from the caregiver if the child is too young to speak or is unable to cooperate.

After the focused history, perform a focused exam of the heart, peripheral circulation, and the abdomen. Then, do an anatomic exam of the entire body, as outlined in Chapter 1. If the child has a traumatic injury, do a detailed physical exam as well, searching for other injuries.

Perform an ongoing assessment of all children with cardiovascular problems while on the way to the ED. The child's status may change during transport, so observe and document any physiologic trends. Use the PAT to monitor effective perfusion and watch respiratory rate, heart rate, blood pressure, and pulse oximetry. Keep a child who is in shock on a cardiac monitor. Be prepared to increase the level of respiratory and cardiovascular support if the child worsens or fails to respond to treatment.

Summary of Cardiovascular Assessment

The PAT provides a good first-line cardiovascular evaluation: abnormal appearance, normal work of breathing, and poor circulation to skin suggest a perfusion problem. Pallor, mottling, and cyanosis all indicate poor peripheral perfusion. The circulatory portion of the hands-on ABCDEs consists of evaluating heart rate, pulse quality, skin temperature, capillary refill time, and blood pressure. These physical features complement the PAT and will help identify the type and severity of circulatory compromise. Vital signs can sometimes be misleading and must be correctly obtained and interpreted for age. Trends in vital signs, or persistence in abnormal vital signs, such as tachycardia, are more accurate indicators of real physiologic problems than mild vital sign abnormalities on initial assessment.

Using the Assessment to Identify Shock

Shock is inadequate perfusion at the tissue level, with insufficient oxygen delivery to maintain normal cellular function. Oxygenation/ventilation, heart rate, intravascular volume,

Table 4-2	Summary of Different Types of Shock		
Shock Type	**Physiologic Insult**	**Common Causes**	**Treatment**
Hypovolemic	Volume loss	Hemorrhage Gastroenteritis (vomiting, diarrhea) Burns Prolonged poor fluid intake	Rapid transport IV fluid boluses
Distributive	Decreased vascular tone	Sepsis Anaphylaxis Drug overdose Spinal cord injury (neurogenic shock)	Rapid transport Fluid administration Epinephrine for anaphylaxis Dopamine for septic shock
Cardiogenic	Heart failure	Congenital heart disease Cardiomyopathy Dysrhythmia Drug overdose	Rapid transport Cautious crystalloid fluid administration, 10 mL/kg Consider a vasopressor like dopamine
Obstructive	Obstructed blood flow	Pericardial tamponade Pneumothorax	Rapid transport Needle thoracostomy Fluid administration

myocardial function, and vascular stability are all determinants of effective systemic cardiovascular function. If any one of these factors is impaired by illness or injury, the body will attempt to compensate and normalize perfusion through modification of other physiologic components. This is reflected in the clinical signs of decreased perfusion, such as tachycardia, vasoconstriction, and increased myocardial contraction.

There are four general classes of shock—hypovolemic, distributive, cardiogenic, and obstructive (**Table 4-2**)—reflecting impairment of the three major functional components of circulation: the blood volume, the vascular system, and the heart. Studies of hypovolemia—the most common type of pediatric shock—have allowed researchers to describe the clinical signs that characterize the progression of shock from a compensated state (adequate systolic blood pressure) to an uncompensated state (hypotension). However, the clinical signs characterizing the progression of distributive, cardiogenic, or obstructive shock are less well defined. This reflects the complex physiology of these other forms of shock.

Hypovolemic Shock

Hypovolemia (loss of fluid) is the most common cause of shock in children in the out-of-hospital setting. Bleeding from blunt injuries such as falls or vehicle collisions with the child as a pedestrian, bicyclist, or passenger is the most frequent cause of hypovolemia. Vomiting and diarrhea from gastroenteritis is a second common cause.

The signs and symptoms of hypovolemic shock vary with the amount, duration, and timing of fluid loss. As intravascular volume is further compromised by ongoing fluid losses (such as profuse diarrhea), the child may progress from compensated to decompensated shock.

Early (Compensated) Hypovolemic Shock

Children who lose bodily fluids through minor blood loss or dehydration from gastroenteritis usually show no clinically significant effects on circulation. However, if fluid losses are more than about 5% of body weight, the body compensates for decreased blood flow by predictable adjustments in cardiovascular physiology. This is compensated shock. Signs of compensated hypovolemic shock are tachycardia and peripheral vasoconstriction. Vasoconstriction causes the signs of abnormal circulation to skin: delayed capillary refill time, and decreased pulse strength, poor skin color (pallor or mottling), dry and cool skin temperature, delayed capillary refill time, and decreased pulse strength. A cold environment or hypothermia may cause vasoconstriction, which mimics poor perfusion. *Systolic blood pressure is normal in compensated shock.*

In the compensated stage of hypovolemic shock, appearance may be normal, or the child may appear slightly restless or less interactive. In a child with gastroenteritis the appearance may be abnormal because of fever, which can alter appearance regardless of the circulatory status.

Late (Decompensated) Hypovolemic Shock

In decompensated shock, perfusion is profoundly affected because compensatory mechanisms, increased heart rate and peripheral vasoconstriction, have failed to maintain sufficient circulation to core organs. The clinical signs are those of organ failure. While a child in decompensated shock may still be alert on AVPU, assessment of appearance will be abnormal because of inadequate brain perfusion. The child may be restless and agitated, or poorly responsive. Hypotension, or low blood pressure for age, develops when there is about a 25% loss of intravascular volume (blood volume). Other late signs are effortless tachypnea and extreme tachycardia. If not reversed, decompensated shock will lead to cardiac failure, with bradycardia and respiratory failure, and then to cardiac arrest.

While the course is less predictable, decreasing perfusion in children with distributive, cardiogenic, or obstructive shock will result in progressive changes in appearance, skin signs, and work of breathing. For example, a child with cardiogenic shock may present only with tachycardia and diminished peripheral perfusion, and then progress to respiratory distress and lethargy as cardiac output worsens and congestive heart failure develops. *In all shock types, hypotension is an ominous sign and represents decompensated shock.* Sometimes more than one type of shock can occur concurrently in the same patient, as previously described.

Tip

In all shock types, hypotension is an ominous sign and represents decompensated shock.

Distributive Shock

In pure distributive shock, the child has decreased vascular muscle tone (peripheral vasodilation) with a normal circulating blood volume. This loss of vascular tone creates a relative hypovolemia, and can be thought of as operating with a "less than full" tank. This change in the capacity of the vascular system and relative hypovolemia leads to hypoperfusion to vital organs. Patients with distributive shock may also have a component of hypovolemia. This would be the case in a patient with sepsis, who in addition to loss of vascular tone has "capillary leak" due to the effect of bacterial toxins. In this situation, hypovolemia is the result of "third spacing" of fluid from the vascular space into the surrounding tissues.

The most common cause of distributive shock is sepsis, especially in children under 2 to 3 years of age. Other causes of distributive shock are anaphylaxis, chemical intoxication with drugs that decrease vascular tone (e.g., beta blockers, barbiturates), or spinal cord injury (above T-6) with interruption of spinal sympathetic nerves to the muscle walls of peripheral arteries.

Special Features in Assessment of Distributive Shock

Signs of distributive shock reflect low peripheral vascular resistance (warm skin, decreased pulse quality, tachycardia, hypotension) and decreased organ perfusion (abnormal appearance). These signs may vary with the specific cause, as noted in the descriptions of the three major types of distributive shock. While the progression of physical signs in distributive shock is not as predictable as that in hypovolemic shock,

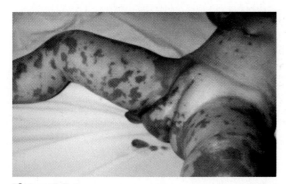

Figure 4-3 Purpura.

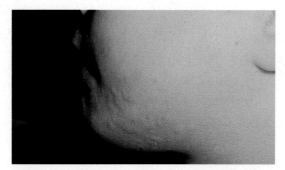

Figure 4-4 Hives suggest an allergic reaction and are usually present with anaphylaxis, the most extreme form of allergic reaction.

the late findings are indistinguishable from those of decompensated shock from any cause: abnormal appearance from poor brain perfusion and hypotension.

Major Types of Distributive Shock

Sepsis

Sepsis occurs when any type of infection, usually bacterial or viral, overwhelms the body's defense system and causes a generalized breakdown in core organ function. Distinctive signs of early septic shock are warm skin, tachycardia, and bounding pulses. A septic child's appearance will be abnormal and may include listlessness, lethargy, decreased interactiveness, restlessness, and poor consolability. Rash, fever, poor feeding, vomiting, diarrhea, and fussiness may also be present.

Ill children usually like to be held and cuddled. If a child with a fever does not want to be held but is more comfortable when left alone, the child may have para-doxical irritability. This may be a sign of meningitis where movement puts traction on the inflamed spinal cord.

Sometimes, a septic child has a petechial rash or purpura (non-blanching dark red or purple dots or splotches) (**Figure 4-3**). These skin lesions are the result of toxins that cause inflammation of the blood vessels and leakage of blood into the skin. Consider a child with shock in association with a rash and fever to be septic. He may require aggressive volume resuscitation in the field, and prehospital professionals should use strict infection control practices, including masks, to decrease their risk of infection.

Table 4-3	Drug Intoxications that May Cause Shock
Antihypertensives	Cyclic antidepressants
Beta blockers	Iron
Calcium antagonists	Opioids
Clonidine	Phenothiazines

Anaphylaxis

Anaphylaxis is a major allergic reaction that involves a generalized, multi-system response to an antigen (foreign protein). The airways and cardiovascular system are important sites of this often life-threatening reaction. The most common cause is an insect sting from a common bumblebee or fire ant. A child in anaphylactic shock will have hypoperfusion as well as additional signs such as stridor and/or wheezing, with increased work of breathing. The child will also have altered appearance with restlessness and agitation and sometimes a sense of impending doom. Hives, an intensely itchy skin rash, are usually present (**Figure 4-4**).

Shock from Drug Intoxication

There are numerous cardiovascular drugs that can cause loss of vascular tone and hypoperfusion when ingested. **Table 4-3** lists common agents. The mechanism usually involves direct depressant effect on the cardiovascular system.

Spinal Shock

Spinal shock is rare in children. It results from a mechanism of injury that involves the

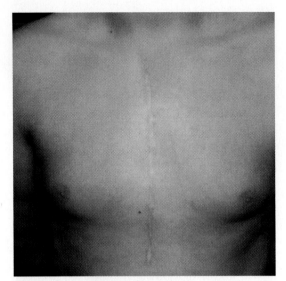

Figure 4-5 A midline sternal scar is an indicator of a cardiac history.

Table 4-4	Symptoms and Signs of Cardiogenic Shock

Possible historical findings in cardiogenic shock:

1. Preceding history of chest pain
2. Previous history of flu-like symptoms associated with weakness and fatigue
3. Difficulty feeding due to fatigue and sweating during feeding in the breast or bottle fed infant
4. No history of fever
5. No history of volume loss (e.g., diarrhea, vomiting, or blood loss)
6. Positive history of congenital heart disease
7. No history of asthma despite wheezing on exam
8. Persistent wheezing despite the administration of beta agonist (e.g., <u>albuterol</u> [salbutamol])
9. History of cyanosis
10. Recent history of exercise intolerance

Possible physical findings:

1. Tachypnea and/or grunting with clear lungs on exam
2. Unexplained dysrhythmias in the presence of a flu-like illness
3. Tachycardia disproportionate to the degree of fever
4. Persistent or worsening tachycardia despite fluid administration
5. Heart murmur, friction rub or gallop on exam
6. Presence of cyanosis that does not improve with the administration of oxygen
7. Crackles on lung exam
8. Peripheral edema/pitting edema
9. Hepatomegaly

back, neck, or both, and interrupts nervous system pathways. There is a loss of the autonomic nervous system's sympathetic control of circulation. The child will have motor paralysis and will be both hypotensive and bradycardic, with loss of the normal tachycardic response to actual or relative hypovolemia.

Cardiogenic Shock

<u>Cardiogenic shock</u> is uncommon in children, and is rarely diagnosed in the prehospital arena unless the child has a known cardiac history (**Figure 4-5**). In fact, the child's condition may be misdiagnosed as septic or hypovolemic shock, resulting in the administration of fluid boluses and <u>adrenergic agents</u>. The most likely cause is either congenital heart disease or cardiomyopathy from <u>myocarditis</u>. Myocarditis is a disease of the heart muscle, usually caused by a virus. A primary <u>dysrhythmia</u>, such as <u>supraventricular tachycardia (SVT)</u>, may also cause cardiogenic shock. Finally, overdose with a <u>cardiotonic</u> drug, such as a <u>calcium channel blocker</u> or beta blocker, is another possible etiology.

Special Features in Assessment of Cardiogenic Shock

A history from the caregiver will usually reveal that the child has had nonspecific symptoms such as loss of appetite, poor feeding, lethargy, irritability, and sweating over a period of days. There is often a history of congenital heart disease or the presence of a midline chest scar from heart surgery. **Table 4-4** summarizes the common symptoms and signs of cardiogenic shock.

Cardiogenic shock develops from left heart failure. Impaired left heart function causes decreased core organ perfusion. On physical assessment, the child may appear abnormal: sluggish, irritable, or agitated, and the skin color mottled or cyanotic. Heart rate is rapid; blood pressure may be high (early), normal, or low (late). The skin is cool and the child may be <u>diaphoretic</u> (not dry as with hypovolemic shock). Pulmonary edema causes increased work of breathing and inspiratory crackles or wheezing.

Increased right-sided cardiac pressures are also present in cardiogenic shock and result in liver enlargement (<u>hepatomegaly</u>). Hepatomegaly is an especially useful finding in infants and toddlers. Peripheral edema and <u>jugular venous distension</u> are rare in children.

Obstructive Shock

Several pathologic conditions may obstruct blood flow from the heart and cause shock. <u>Pericardial tamponade</u> and <u>tension pneumothorax</u> are two acute conditions that cause dramatic development of shock after penetrating injuries to the chest wall. <u>Hemopericardium</u> develops quickly after a gunshot or sharp object penetrates into a blood filled heart chamber, usually the right ventricle. The hole in the wall of the heart provides a route for blood to escape into the space between the two pericardial membranes. Because the membranes will not stretch easily, blood collects and collapses the right ventricle (tamponade). This interrupts venous return to the right heart and produces a profound drop in cardiac output.

Rarely, pericardial tamponade may develop after an infectious or inflammatory process in the chest. Cancer or chronic renal failure causes pericardial fluid accumulation. This type of fluid accumulation is slow and the membranes around the heart stretch. Therefore, obstructive shock rarely occurs.

Tension pneumothorax develops after a penetration into the pleural space. Sometimes blunt injury to the chest wall can also cause pneumothorax. Air and sometimes blood (hemothorax) collect in between the two membranes of the pleura. This causes a shift of the <u>mediastinum</u> and interrupts venous return to the right heart.

Special Features in Assessment of Obstructive Shock

Penetrating injuries to the chest wall are often deceptive. The appearance of the wound may be benign and seem superficial. Consider all gunshot wounds or stab wounds to the chest as major penetrations into the heart and/or pleura. Other types of penetrations from sticks or sharp objects may also cause severe internal injury. Be especially vigilant when the penetration has an entry site in the area between the two nipples and the

Tip

Be especially vigilant when the penetration has an entry site in the box between the two nipples and the clavicles, because this is a high risk location for cardiac injury.

clavicles, because this is a high risk location for cardiac injury. Blunt chest injury may also cause pneumothorax. Suspect this condition in a child with a significant blunt mechanism of injury and signs of obstructive shock.

The cardinal features of obstructive shock are signs of decreased circulation in an injured child with increased jugular venous distension. The increased jugular pressures reflect the obstruction to venous return to the right ventricle. Sometimes, however, blood loss into the chest (hemothorax) or other associated injuries may be associated with hemorrhage, so that jugular venous distension is not apparent.

General Noninvasive Treatment of Suspected Shock of All Types

Begin general noninvasive treatment of every child with suspected hypoperfusion after completing the PAT and initiating the hands-on ABCDEs. The general treatment is always the same: Allow the child to assume a position of comfort and supply oxygen, if tolerated. This will be the only management for most patients.

Positioning

Infants and toddlers may be most "comfortable" in their caregiver's arms or lap during assessment. If the initial assessment indicates that the child is physiologically unstable, place the child in a position of comfort that will decrease his anxiety and activity. This will usually be the supine position (**Figure 4-6**). *Putting a child in a head down position is not known to improve outcome.* A conscious child will not tolerate the shock position, and agitation will increase oxygen demand and complicate treatment.

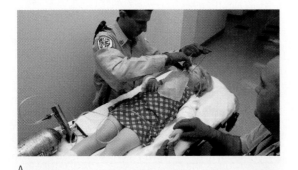

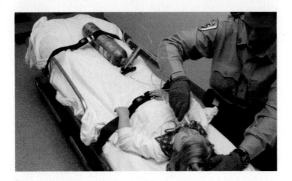

Figure 4-6 (A) Treat suspected hypovolemic shock with high-flow oxygen and supine positioning. (B) Keep the patient warm.

Do not place a conscious child in the shock position because it will not help and he will usually not tolerate it.

Oxygen

Treat all children who are unstable with high-flow oxygen. The prehospital professional must weigh the potential benefits of oxygen administration against the risk of agitating the child. "Blow-by" may be the only mechanism for delivering supplemental oxygen without upsetting the child and increasing their oxygen consumption.

Specific Treatment of Hypovolemia

After the initial assessment and beginning general supportive measures, provide additional specific treatment of shock. If the child has hypovolemic shock, consider how to stop the child's fluid losses and whether to attempt to replace them. In trauma patients, always look carefully for bleeding sites and assume there may be internal bleeding as well. Apply direct pressure to stop external bleeding. Consider appropriate immobilization and splinting of injured extremities, as described in Chapter 6.

If the child has severe fluid losses from vomiting and/or diarrhea, consider obtaining vascular access to give fluids. If the child has <u>decompensated</u> shock from illness, attempt an IV placement once in the field. Any further attempts should be made during transport to avoid a prolonged scene time. If the child is unconscious, consider an intraosseous (IO) needle insertion.

Advanced Life Support

Intravenous Access

Intravenous (IV) access makes it easier to give medications and provides a way to give fluid therapy in severe blood or fluid loss. IV delivery is the gold standard for giving medication, because it permits rapid drug and fluid treatment and allows titration of important drugs. See (**Intravenous Access, Procedure 15**).

IV Fluid Treatment of Early (Compensated) Hypovolemic Shock

If the child has mild–moderate volume losses as determined by HR, pulse quality, CRT, and skin temperature, and has a normal blood pressure, he is in compensated shock. Do not remain on scene to perform IV insertion and fluid administration. On the way to the hospital, consider obtaining vascular access and giving IV crystalloid fluid at 20 mL/kg boluses to stabilize the patient. Keep giving fluid boluses until the patient has a clinical response.

IV Fluid Treatment of Late (Decompensated) Shock

If the child has decompensated shock from illness, make one attempt on scene to establish vascular access. If the child is injured, delay all vascular access attempts until en route to the ED. With ongoing traumatic hemorrhage, in contrast, the value of establishing access and initiating volume resusci-

Tip

If the child has mild–moderate volume losses and has a normal blood pressure, the shock is compensated. Attempt an IV insertion en route to the ED, not on scene.

Tip

If the child is injured and has decompensated shock, delay all vascular access attempts until en route to the ED.

tation at the scene may be outweighed by continued blood loss. Once access is established during transport, give 20 mL/kg boluses of IV crystalloid fluid. Consider IO needle insertion, if vascular access cannot be obtained quickly and the child is unconscious. Repeat boluses (20 mL/kg up to 60 mL/kg) as needed to stabilize perfusion, based on ongoing reassessment of the PAT and vital signs.

IO Needle Insertion

Using an IO needle to give drugs or fluids is an excellent alternative to <u>cannulating</u> peripheral veins. The intraosseous space is highly vascularized and functions as a noncollapsible vein. Needle insertion into this space is quick, simple, effective, and is usually safe. Complications are infrequent and usually minor. See

Intraosseous Needle Insertion, Procedure 16 .

Specific Treatment of Distributive Shock

The primary difference between treatment of distributive and hypovolemic shock is the potential need for a <u>vasopressor agent</u> to improve vascular tone and heart muscle function when the child has distributive shock. Treat all shock conditions first with general noninvasive measures. Administer 100% high-flow oxygen and put the poorly responsive child with shock in a supine position.

Advanced Life Support

Treatment of Decompensated Distributive Shock

Attempt a vascular access on scene at least once. Deliver fluid boluses, up to 60 mL/kg of a crystalloid fluid solution in 20 mL/kg boluses on the way to the ED. If the child has lost protective airway reflexes or has refractory shock, support ventilation with bag-mask device or <u>endotracheal intubation</u>.

If cardiovascular instability (hypotension, markedly increased heart rate, and poor responsiveness) persists after volume therapy with 60 mL/kg of crystalloid fluid, try a vasopressor agent (<u>dopamine</u> or <u>epinephrine</u>). *Do not administer a vasopressor agent if you suspect untreated hypovolemia.*

Treatment of Anaphylaxis

A child with anaphylaxis requires special treatment with epinephrine and with a beta agonist if bronchospasm is present. Unlike a simple allergic reaction, anaphylaxis has dangerous cardiovascular effects (**Figure 4-7**).

Epinephrine is an excellent drug for treatment of anaphylaxis. It stimulates both the alpha- and beta-adrenergic receptors, leading to two important effects: (1) constriction of the blood vessels to help counter the vasodilation of anaphylaxis (alpha effect), and (2) opening up the airways to help

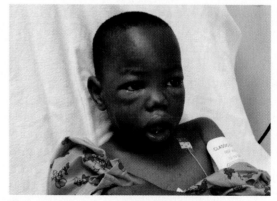

Figure 4-7 An allergic reaction, with edema of face, lips, and tongue.

reverse the bronchospasm of anaphylaxis (beta effect). For all children with allergic reactions associated with wheezing, administer epinephrine, 0.01 mg/kg (0.01 mL/kg) of 1:1000 solution (maximum 0.3 mg or 0.3 mL) subcutaneously (SQ). If a child has hypoperfusion with anaphylaxis, administer epinephrine by IV, using a maximum dose of 0.1 mg and a more dilute solution to decrease the possibility of an adverse drug reaction. Draw up 0.01 mg/kg (0.1 mL/kg) of the 1:10,000 epinephrine solution (maximum 0.1 mg or 1 mL of the epinephrine) and dilute the solution further with 10 mL of normal saline to reduce the epinephrine concentration to 1:100,000.

Treatment of Cardiogenic Shock

If cardiogenic shock is suspected by history and/or physical assessment, transport after general noninvasive treatment. On the way to the ED, consider vascular access. If the diagnosis of cardiogenic shock is uncertain, give a cautious fluid bolus of only 10 mL/kg of crystalloid fluid, and then reassess appearance, work of breathing, capillary refill time, heart rate, and blood pressure.

If there is no rhythm disturbance on the cardiac monitor, and the child remains poorly perfused after the initial fluid bolus, consider a vasopressor agent, either dopamine or epinephrine, if the transport time is long. Start vasopressors at low doses, based on per kilogram nomograms, and then titrate to achieve acceptable perfusion (improved appearance and skin circulation and decreased heart rate and respiratory rate). If the child is known to be in congestive heart failure with cardiogenic shock, avoid fluid boluses and consider vasopressor therapy as front-line treatment if perfusion is severely compromised.

The major difference between treatment of hypovolemic, distributive, and cardiogenic shock is the amount of fluid administration and consideration of a vasopressor.

Tip

Successful treatment of cardiogenic shock involves minimizing the volume of fluid administered and early consideration of a vasopressor.

Advanced Life Support

Treatment of Obstructive Shock

The additional option for treatment of obstructive shock from <u>pneumothorax</u> is needle <u>thoracostomy</u> to decrease air tension as explained in (Needle Thoracostomy, Procedure 22). This technique will not remove blood, but will place the pleural space at atmospheric pressure, and release air tension. Rapid transport is an essential feature of field management of chest injury.

Initial Assessment: Transport Decision

After completing the initial assessment and beginning general treatment when appropriate, the prehospital professional must decide whether to go or stay on scene. If the PAT and ABCDEs are normal and the child has no history of serious illness or injury mechanism, no anatomic abnormalities, and no pain, the child does not usually require urgent treatment or immediate transport. Take the time to get a focused history and physical exam and perform a detailed physical examination (trauma) on the scene if possible.

On the other hand, if the child has a serious mechanism of injury, a physiologic or anatomic abnormality, severe pain, or if the scene is not safe, transport immediately. With such patients, do the additional assessment and attempt specific treatment on the way to the hospital, if possible.

The transport decision is sometimes difficult in a child with a suspected cardiovascular problem who needs vascular access. If the child is in compensated shock and has a palpable brachial pulse or normal blood pressure, stabilize the spine (if the child is injured), manage the airway and breathing, control hemorrhage, and transport immediately. Attempt a vascular access for specific treatment on the way to the ED.

If the child is in decompensated shock, the prehospital professional has several options, depending on the clinical condition of the child, local EMS system regulations, comfort level, and the time to the nearest ED. If the child is injured, always transport immediately. If the child is ill with abnormal appearance and hypotension, consider attempting a vascular access once on scene, and then transporting without delay.

Summary of Shock States

There are four major classes of shock seen both in children and adults: hypovolemic, cardiogenic, distributive, and obstructive. Hypovolemic shock is most commonly the result of trauma and hemorrhage after injury. Vomiting and diarrhea with dehydration is most common medical cause of hypovolemia. Distributive shock may result from sepsis, anaphylaxis, drug intoxication, or

spinal injury. Always suspect sepsis in the infant or toddler who has fever and abnormal appearance. A petechial or purpuric skin rash is a red flag for sepsis. Cardiogenic shock is rare in children and difficult to identify in the field, unless the child has a known congenital cardiac problem. Obstructive shock will sometimes occur in conjunction with significant chest wall injury. Clinical findings may reflect more than one type of shock pathophysiology. Treatment of all shock types includes general noninvasive interventions, and then specific treatment based upon clinical findings. Consider rapid fluid boluses in children who are decompensated with abnormal appearance and hypotension. Vasopressor agents have a limited role in shock therapy in children.

Congenital Heart Disease

Children with congenital heart disease are at increased risk for the types of cardiovascular emergencies more commonly seen in the adult population, including dysrhythmias and congestive heart failure. These complications may present in infancy, or as late as the teenage years (**Table 4-5**). Advances in

Tip

If the child has a serious mechanism of injury, a physiologic or anatomic abnormality, severe pain, or if the scene is not safe, transport immediately.

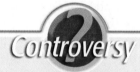

Controversy

The safety of vasopressor administration in the absence of infusion pumps is questionable. Mixing and infusing the small volumes necessary in young children cannot be easily achieved or monitored in ambulances.

Case Study 2

You are volunteering as a health professional at a local high school track meet when a 9-year-old boy collapses while running the 100-yard (meter) dash. You rush to his aid and find him apneic and pulseless. You immediately start CPR.

1. What should be the next step in your assessment/management of this child?
2. At what age is it appropriate to apply an AED to assess for ventricular fibrillation in a child?

Table 4-5	Congenital Heart Disease Causing Congestive Heart Failure at Different Times During Infancy
Age	**Type of Congenital Heart Disease**
Newborn	Hypoplastic left heart Pulmonic insufficiency Tricuspid insufficiency Third degree AV block SVT
First month	Aortic coarctation with patent ductus arteriosus Ventricular septal defect Total anomalous pulmonary venous return Tricuspid stresia Truncus arteriosus
First 6 months	Transposition of the great vessels Ventricular septal defect Patent ductus arteriosus
6–12 months	Ventricular septal defect Endocardial fibroelastosis Total anomalous pulmonary venous return

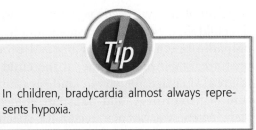

Tip

In children, bradycardia almost always represents hypoxia.

cardiovascular surgery have allowed the medical community to prolong the lives of children who just decades ago would have died in infancy. Many of these children are now living productive lives at home. Prehospital professionals must be prepared to treat "adult problems" in this younger population.

The initial assessment and management of any child experiencing a cardiovascular emergency is the same: airway, breathing, and circulation. However, in any child with a possible cardiac pathology, include a "quick look" at the cardiac rhythm. These children may have treatable cardiac dysrhythmias.

Dysrhythmias

Bradycardia

In children, bradycardia almost always reflects hypoxia, rather than a primary cardiac problem. It is a pre-arrest rhythm, and the prognosis is ominous if left untreated. Immediate delivery of high-flow oxygen and assisted ventilation are essential. Untreated bradycardia will quickly cause shock, hypotension, and death. In children with asthma or respiratory distress, bradycardia means profound hypoxia. Pulse oximetry, when avail-

able, will help determine the degree of hypoxia in the field.

Congenital heart block is an extremely rare cause of bradycardia in infancy and early childhood. Drug overdose (e.g., beta blockers, calcium channel blockers, digoxin) is another possible cause of bradycardia. Bradycardia may also result from <u>vagal</u> stimulation during medical procedures or gastric tube placement. However, while bradycardia that develops during <u>laryngoscopy</u> or suctioning may be the result of vagal stimulation, hypoxia may be the true cause. If bradycardia does occur in this setting, stop the procedure, administer supplemental oxygen and reassess the patient.

Bradycardia may also be a normal finding, especially in asymptomatic athletic adolescents. If bradycardia is an isolated finding, without signs of shock, in a well-perfused school-aged child or teen, no treatment is necessary in the field.

Assessment of the Child with Bradycardia

If the child has a heart rate below the normal range for age (see Table 2-3), evaluate carefully for signs of respiratory failure or shock. The PAT and ABCDEs, along with a brief history, will establish the likely cause, the severity of the problem, and the need for urgent treatment.

Treatment of Bradycardia

If the child is asymptomatic, consider no treatment, especially if the child is an adolescent, because slow heart rates are common in teenagers. If the child has bradycardia and an initial assessment demonstrates oxygenation, ventilation, or perfusion abnormalities, provide 100% oxygen and transport. If he does not respond to oxygen, begin assisted bag-mask ventilation. Check effectiveness of ventilation by observing for chest rise and an improvement in the PAT, heart rate, perfusion, and BP.

In rare situations, chest compressions for bradycardia are necessary. If the heart rate is below 60 beats per minute, *and* the child shows signs of poor systemic perfusion after oxygenation and assisted ventilation, begin chest compressions.

Drug Therapy for Symptomatic Bradycardia

Oxygenation and ventilation are the primary treatments for bradycardia. If the heart rate does not rise in response to assisted ventilation, in most cases administer epinephrine as the first-line drug at 1:10,000, 0.01 mg/kg IV or IO, or 0.1 mL/kg, every 3 to 5 minutes. Also administer <u>atropine</u>, 0.02 mg/kg IV or IO (minimum dose 0.1 mg) after epinephrine. Atropine will probably not help unless <u>atrioventricular heart block</u> or increased vagal tone (or poisoning by cholinergic drugs or agents such as organophosphates) is present. When the child has a known reason for cholinergic-mediated bradycardia, such as congenial heart block, give atropine first and monitor the response before administering epinephrine.

Before administering vasopressor drugs, always assess for mechanical problems with oxygen delivery and ventilation. Check for disconnected oxygen tubing, poor mask seal, airway obstruction, inadequate chest rise, endotracheal tube blockage, or <u>malposition</u>. Other causes of bradycardia from hypoxia or <u>ischemia</u> are pneumothorax, hypovolemia, <u>cardiomyopathy</u>, poisoning, or increased <u>intracranial</u> pressure.

When oxygenation, ventilation, and drug therapy for bradycardia fail, and the child remains in shock or cardiac arrest, consider electrical cardiac pacing of the heart.

Endotracheal Administration of Drugs

If neither IV nor IO access is available for giving drugs during resuscitation, the endo-

Be extremely careful with IV epinephrine and double check doses and preparation!

tracheal route is an alternative for at least four pediatric drugs: (LEAN) <u>lidocaine</u>, epinephrine, atropine, <u>naloxone</u>. While endotracheal drugs are probably not as effective as medications delivered by the IV or IO routes, endotracheal delivery is appropriate in the critical patient until IV or IO access is established. Use the technique for endotracheal drug delivery described in

Endotracheal Tube Drug Instillation, Procedure 19

. When administering epinephrine through an endotracheal tube to a child who has no vascular or IO access, give epinephrine at the higher concentration of 1:1000, and use the higher dose of 0.1 mg/kg (0.1 mL/kg). Note that this is the same total volume of epinephrine as the IV/IO dose, because the tenfold dose has ten times the concentration of 1:10,000.

Tachycardia

Tachycardia may be a nonspecific sign of fear, anxiety, pain, or fever and may not represent serious injury or illness. Tachycardia may also be a sign of a life-threatening problem such as hypoxia, cardiac abnormality, or hypovolemia. <u>Sinus tachycardia</u> is the most common dysrhythmia in children, and treatment is generally limited to fluid administration, supplemental oxygen, and transport.

Assessment of the Child with Tachycardia

Tachycardia must be assessed in conjunction with the PAT and ABCDEs. Always ask about a history of congenital heart disease and check for midline chest scars from cardiac surgery.

There are two characteristics in the child's rhythm strip to measure and use as a basis for treatment, along with the perfusion assessment: (1) the heart rate/min and (2) the width of the <u>QRS complex</u>. First, establish an accurate heart rate electronically from the rhythm strip. As in the assessment of bradycardia, interpret the heart rate based on knowledge of the normal range for age (see Table 2-3). Second, establish the width of the QRS from the rhythm strip. If the QRS complex is < 0.08 sec (< 2 standard boxes on the rhythm strip), consider the child to have a narrow complex tachycardia. If the width is > 0.08 sec (> 2 standard boxes on the rhythm strip), consider the child to have a wide complex tachycardia.

Table 4-6 distinguishes a narrow complex sinus tachycardia from narrow complex <u>supraventricular tachycardia</u> (SVT) and wide complex ventricular tachycardia (VT).

Specific Treatment of Tachycardia

If the child presents with tachycardia, determine the appropriate treatment by establishing perfusion status, and by assessing the rhythm strip for heart rate and QRS duration.

Narrow Complex Tachycardia If the child has a narrow QRS tachycardia (< 0.08 seconds), P waves are present, and the heart rate is variable and less than 220 beats/min in an infant or less than 180 beats/min in a child, the cause is usually sinus tachycardia (**Figure 4-8**) from non-cardiac conditions (e.g., hypoxia, hypovolemia, hyperthermia, metabolic abnormalities, toxins, fear, pain, or

serious trauma to the chest). No specific cardiac medical management of the sinus tachycardia is needed. Instead, treat with fluids, oxygen, splinting, analgesia, or sedation as indicated by the associated condition. If there is no change in heart rate after treatment, consider other etiologies, such as SVT.

Advanced Life Support

Specific Treatment of SVT If the QRS is less than 0.08 seconds, P waves are absent or abnormal, the rate is not variable and is greater than 220 beats/min in an infant or greater than 180 beats/min in a child, consider SVT as the likely etiology. If the child has no previous history of SVT, and the patient is stable, provide oxygen and transport to the ED. Delaying specific treatment for SVT until hospital arrival will permit the hospital staff to confirm SVT, and to run a continuous EKG while actively managing the dysrhythmia. A patient with a confirmed diagnosis of SVT may need long-term treatment with cardiac medications.

If the patient has a prior history of SVT, and is stable, consider a vagal maneuver

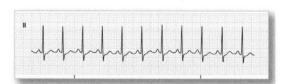

Figure 4-8 ECG of sinus tachycardia.

Table 4-6	Features of Sinus Tachycardia, SVT and VT					
	History	**Heart Rate**	**Respiratory Rate**	**QRS Interval**	**Assessment**	**Possible Treatments**
Sinus tachycardia	Fever Volume loss Hypoxia Pain Increased activity or exercise	< 220 beats/min (infant) < 180 beats/min (child)	Variable	Narrow < 0.08 sec	Hypovolemia Hypoxia Painful injury	Fluids Oxygen Splinting Analgesia/sedation
Supraventricular tachycardia	Congential heart disease Known SVT Nonspecific symptoms (e.g., poor feeding, fussiness)	> 220 beats/min (often 240–300 beats/min) < 180 beats/min (child)	Constant	Narrow < 0.08 sec	CHF may be present	Vagal maneuvers (ice to face) Adenosine Synchronized electrical countershock
Ventricular tachycardia	Serious systemic illness	> 150 beats/min	Variable	Wide > 0.08 sec	CHF may be present	Synchronized electrical countershock Lidocaine Amiodarone

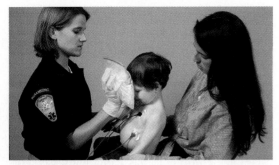

Figure 4-9 Placing a bag of ice on a child's face elicits the "diving reflex" and may convert SVT to sinus rhythm.

Prehospital personnel must be prepared to treat the adverse drug effects of all cardiac medications, even if the indication, dose, and route of delivery are correct.

first. Ice to the face (if available) evokes the "<u>diving reflex</u>" and is an effective management tool for SVT in infants and toddlers. Place crushed ice in a plastic bag, glove, or washcloth and apply firmly over the midface (cheeks and bridge of nose) for approximately 15 seconds, until the rhythm changes or the patient's condition dictates immediate cessation of the procedure (**Figure 4-9**). Do not occlude the nose (to allow breathing) and provide constant reassurance to the parent and child. Avoid ocular pressure (pressure on the eyeballs) as a method of vagal stimulation in a child. Only attempt a vagal maneuver once.

If the patient with narrow complex tachycardia has signs of poor perfusion and hemodynamic compromise (abnormal PAT, poor pulse quality, abnormal CRT and skin temperature, hypotension) and the heart rate does not convert to sinus rhythm after one attempt at vagal stimulation, give <u>adenosine</u> at 0.1 mg/kg up to a maximum first dose of 6 mg rapid IV or IO push and follow immediately with a 2 to 5 mL bolus of normal saline. Double the dose to 0.2 mg/kg, if the rhythm does not convert after the first dose of adenosine (maximum second dose = 12 mg). The IO administration of adenosine may be less effective than IV because of the slightly slower delivery of the drug bolus to the heart. Be prepared to treat the untoward effects of adenosine; it is a very potent cardiac drug. If given properly, it is usually effective in the treatment of SVT. Brief runs of bradycardia or even several seconds of asystole commonly occur with adenosine administration, but sustained or fatal dysrhythmias (e.g., asys-

tole, ventricular tachycardia, and ventricular fibrillation) are rare. Monitor the child closely and have resuscitative drugs as well as a <u>defibrillator</u> within reach.

If a child with suspected SVT is in shock or is unconscious, administer adenosine prior to electrical countershock if vascular access is possible within 90 seconds or three attempts. If there is no vascular access, and the child is unconscious, immediately administer synchronized electrical countershock at 0.5 to 1.0 joules(J)/kg as a starting electrical dose. If the initial shock is ineffective, double to 2 J/kg. If the child is in shock but still conscious and has vascular access, administer sedation if possible before delivering the electrical countershock. Do not delay electrical therapy for sedation. If electrical therapy fails to convert the child to sinus rhythm, consider using other anti-dysrhythmic drugs, such as <u>amiodarone</u> (5 mg/kg over 20–60 min) as per local EMS system guidelines. Do not give amiodarone and procainamide together.

Wide Complex Tachycardia If the patient is conscious, and has adequate perfusion, a heart rate of greater than 150 beats/min and a QRS interval of greater than 0.08 seconds, he is probably in stable <u>ventricular tachycardia</u> (VT). Sinus tachycardia with a conduction abnormality (bundle branch block) may look like VT, but usually occurs in a child with a history of heart disease or cardiac surgery. Likewise, SVT with aberrant conduction can result in a wide complex rhythm. In all such stable cases with wide complex tachycardias, provide oxygen and transport the patient to an appropriate ED, with close cardiac monitoring and equipment for electrical countershock immediately available.

If the child has VT, is conscious, but has signs of poor perfusion, administer lidocaine at 1 mg/kg IV. If lidocaine does not convert the rhythm to sinus and the child is still conscious, consider other anti-dysrhythmic drugs, such as amiodarone (5 mg/kg over 20–60 min) per local EMS system guidelines. Do not give amiodarone and procainamide together.

If the child has VT and shock, without pulses, or has pulses and poor perfusion but has not responded to anti-dysrhythmia drug treatment, immediately administer synchronized electrical countershock. If conscious, attempt to administer sedation before cardioversion. Use the same electrical charge as recommended for SVT, at 0.5 to 1 J/kg, increase to 2 J/kg if no response. After cardioversion, give an anti-dysrhythmia drug, either amiodarone, 5 mg/kg IV or IO over 20–60 min, or lidocaine, 1 mg/kg bolus IV or IO.

Most tachycardia in children is a response to non-cardiac stimuli (fever, fear, pain) and does not require dysrhythmia treatment.

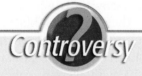

Ice to the face for SVT is a controversial field procedure. It has not been evaluated for efficacy or safety in the out-of-hospital setting, especially in children.

Automatic External Defibrillator (AED)

Cardiac arrest in children is usually the result of profound hypoxia or shock, which leads to asystole—the most frequent rhythm of pediatric cardiac arrest. Ventricular fibrillation (VF), however, does occur in pediatrics. The typical VF case is a child out of the infant age group who has had a witnessed collapse. Etiologies for VF arrest in children include myocarditis, an infection of the heart muscle, the "long QT syndrome," a congenital cardiac conduction problem, and idiopathic hypertrophic subaortic stenosis, an anatomic abnormality of the aortic valve. One other special circumstance for VF arrest is commotio cordis, which develops usually in a young athlete who is struck in the chest by a ball, stick, or other blunt object.

Perform rapid assessment for VF on all unresponsive children and administer defibrillation if VF is present on the cardiac monitor. Be especially vigilant for VF when the child is older and has suffered a witnessed collapse. There is no demonstrated benefit to defibrillation of asystole, and this procedure will only delay the key interventions of oxygenation, ventilation, and chest compressions.

The AED (**Figure 4-10**) allows early recognition of VF and rapid defibrillation. The American Heart Association currently recommends the use of an AED for treatment of VF in children of all ages, including younger children over 1 year of age. The US Food and Drug Administration has cleared several AEDs for use in children younger than 8 years of age. These devices have been shown to accurately identify VF and VT in young children and are also accurate in identifying pediatric rhythms that do not require defibrillation. When used with a designated pediatric pad-cable system, these AEDs deliver an energy dose that is smaller than that delivered with adult pads. AEDs may be used with CPR for treatment of prehospital cardiac arrest (victims who are unresponsive, with no breathing and no signs of circulation) in children 1 to 8 years of age.

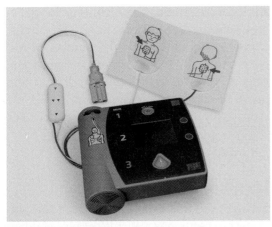

Figure 4-10 An AED.

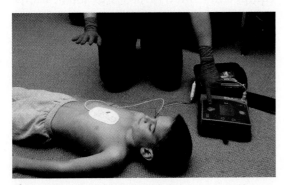

Figure 4-11 Using the AED with CPR in unresponsive children.

Use a pediatric AED or pediatric AED pads if available, but an adult AED can be used on a child. Perform 1 minute of CPR to ensure the problem is not respiratory in nature, before using the AED. Studies show that even school-age children with no prior experience or education in defibrillation can successfully operate an AED. **Figure 4-11** illustrates the recommended method of combining the AED with CPR in unresponsive children.

Summary of Dysrhythmias

Unlike adults, primary cardiac rhythm disturbances are rare in children. Bradycardia almost always reflects profound hypoxia and should be considered a pre-arrest rhythm. Tachycardia is most commonly a sinus rhythm, but may represent SVT or VT. While children can develop sinus

AEDs can be used on anyone. Preferably use a pediatric AED, but an adult AED can be used. Perform 1 minute of CPR on infants and children, to ensure the problem is not respiratory in nature, before using the AED.

tachycardia greater than 200 beats/min, do a careful evaluation for hypovolemia and hypoxia, and other treatable cause, and then treat the identified causes. Assume all rates over 220 beats/min in infants or over 180 beats/min in children, and all wide complex (QRS > 0.08 sec) tachycardias are primary cardiac dysrhythmias. The stable patient may need only general supportive care, regardless of cardiac rhythm. <u>Symptomatic ventricular dysrhythmias</u> may require drug therapy with lidocaine, amiodarone or proacainamide, and cardioversion or defibrillation. The AED is an important adjunct for prehospital professionals in unresponsive children with VF.

Cardiac Arrest

Causes

In contrast to adults, pediatric cardiac arrest is almost always a secondary event, the result of profound hypoxia or shock. Cardiac arrest in children usually follows a primary respiratory arrest, often from respiratory failure originating from common conditions such as pneumonia, bronchiolitis or asthma. <u>Myocardial infarction</u> and a <u>cardiac dysrhythmia</u>, frequent causes of cardiac arrest in adults, are extremely unusual in young children.

The primary age group for pediatric cardiac arrest is infancy, when <u>sudden infant death syndrome</u> (SIDS), infection, or inflicted injury precipitates respiratory failure. In toddlers and school-aged children, however, the causes of cardiac arrest change. In this older age group, the most likely causes

The only intervention associated with survival in pediatric asystolic cardiac arrest is time to airway and breathing support.

are hemorrhagic shock and blunt trauma from either vehicle-related injuries or falls.

Survival from cardiac arrest depends on several factors: time before the start of basic life support (BLS), time to advanced life support (ALS), and presenting rhythm. The shorter the "downtime" before BLS, the better the outcome. Among ALS interventions, the one that is associated with survival in pediatric asystolic arrest is time to airway and breathing support. As in adults, pediatric patients who present to EMS personnel in ventricular fibrillation are more likely to survive than children who present in asystole, as long as there is access to early defibrillation.

Assessment in Cardiac Arrest

A child in cardiac arrest is unresponsive, apneic, and pulseless. The cardiac monitor will show a cardiac arrest rhythm: asystole, pulseless electrical activity, VT or VF, or rarely SVT. Asystole is the most frequent rhythm. SVT and VT are rare causes of cardiac arrest.

Asystole reflects profound hypoxia and ischemia. Pulseless electrical activity may represent a variety of ischemic, hypoxic, hypothermic, and traumatic insults. Some pulseless electrical activity may arise from low-flow states with blood pressures too low to record in the out-of-hospital setting. VF occurs in children usually older than 2 years from a variety of conditions, including myocarditis, congenital anomalies, poisoning, electrocution, or hypoxia.

Chest Compressions

The American Heart Association recommends chest compressions as a key procedure in basic life support for pediatric and adult cardiac arrest. The technique for delivering chest compressions differs for adults, children, and infants, by the number of rescuers required, the placement of hands and fingers, rates of ventilation, and rates and depth of chest compressions. For a step-by-step explanation of this procedure, see

Cardiopulmonary Resuscitation, Procedure 17 .

Length-Based Drug Dosage

Treatment of infants and children in the out-of-hospital setting is difficult because children of different ages require different sizes of equipment, different doses of medications, and different amounts of fluids (**Figure 4-12**). Length is a good index for drug dosing and equipment sizing during resuscitations. From a measured patient length, either a computerized resuscitation software program or a color-coded tape can provide correct doses and equipment sizes. Computerized programs offer a wider range of drugs and additional safety features. The color-coded tape is easy to use but has limited drug information. For a step-by-step explanation of this procedure, see

Length-Based Equipment Sizing and Drug Dosing, Procedure 2 .

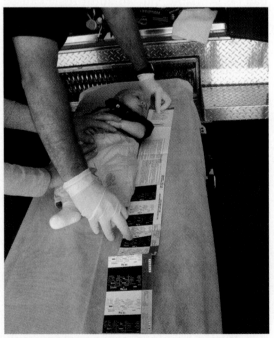

Figure 4-12 Resuscitation tape.

Presenting Cardiac Rhythm and Treatment

Priorities in the treatment of cardiac arrest are early airway management, oxygenation, and ventilation (usually via bag-mask or an endotracheal tube), chest compressions, and electrical countershock/defibrillation (if indicated). The presenting cardiac rhythm is a major determinant of the treatment of cardiac arrest. When the child is pulseless and apneic, the treatment of asystole and <u>pulseless electrical activity</u> (PEA) are the same.

Advanced Life Support

This includes multiple epinephrine doses at 0.01 mg/kg IV or IO, along with management of the airway, oxygenation and ventilation, and chest compressions.

In contrast, if the child has VT or VF as the presenting rhythm, the treatment includes electrical therapy and anti-dysrhythmia drugs. Perform initial defibrillation with 2 J/kg, then 4 J/kg, give epinephrine, repeat defibrillation at 4 J/kg, then administer drug treatment with: amiodarone, 5 mg/kg IV or IO; or lidocaine, 1 mg/kg bolus IV or IO. Use a pattern of CPR-drug-shock for sequencing interventions.

Survival from pediatric cardiac arrest requires good BLS care. IV or IO needle insertion and medication delivery are helpful but not primary determinants of survival. Endotracheal tube insertion offers no known benefit to survival. An important controversy is the role of "high dose" epinephrine. Many protocols allow administration of "high dose" or 0.1 mg/kg of epinephrine IV or IO after the initial 0.01 mg/kg dose, or for ET tube administration, if the "standard dose" is not successful in establishing a perfusing rhythm. This higher dose is unproven in humans and may be harmful in children.

The Transport Decision: Stay or Go

Deciding which pediatric cardiac arrest patients require hospital transport is another important controversy. Of all children in out-of-hospital cardiac arrest, only 3% to 5% will survive. Predictors of survival include type of presenting rhythm and early return of spontaneous circulation (<5 min) after BLS on scene. Survival from pulseless VT/VF is about 15%, versus about 3% for asystole. If children in cardiac arrest fail out-of-hospital resuscitation with BLS and ALS, they will not survive unless there is a special circumstance. Patients who are victims of hypothermia or drowning, or who have ingested massive amounts of sedative-hypnotic drugs (e.g., barbiturates) may have a greater chance of survival after prolonged resuscitation, and deserve extended treatment before death is declared.

In some cases, field resuscitation attempts can be stopped before transport if permitted by local EMS death-in-the-field policies. While survival in unwitnessed out-of-hospital cardiac arrest is rare, prehospital professionals may be uncomfortable in discontinuing resuscitative efforts in children. When resuscitation is terminated, skillful communication with the child's caregivers is critical (**Figure 4-13**), as explained in Chapter 11. *Never leave a family member on scene with the deceased child without appropriate supportive personnel.* A system to provide supportive care to the caregivers must be in place if EMS policy permits

Prehospital cardiac arrest treatment requires good BLS skills.

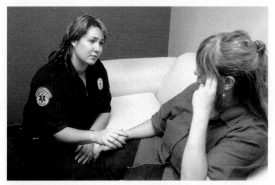

Figure 4-13 Skilled communication with the caregivers and family is imperative after the death of a child.

Never leave a family member on scene with the deceased child without appropriate supportive care.

discontinuation of resuscitative efforts in the field. These services might be provided by social services personnel, pastoral care, or grief counselors.

Cardiac arrest in children is associated with high provider stress. Critical incident stress debriefing may be helpful for prehospital professionals after such a tragedy.

Summary of Cardiac Arrest

Pediatric cardiac arrest is an uncommon event. Survival is unlikely, and asystole has the worst prognosis. VT/VF usually occurs in older children and has higher survival. Meticulous attention to airway, oxygenation, ventilation, chest compressions, and early defibrillation, when appropriate, will improve success. In all cases of pediatric cardiac arrest, grief counseling for the caregivers and critical incident stress debriefing for the prehospital professionals are extremely helpful.

Drowning

Drowning is suffocation after submersion in water. Drowning is the leading cause of unintentional death in children between the ages of 1 and 4 years, and the number two cause of death due to unintentional injury in children under 14 years (**Figure 4-14**). Unfortunately, drowning is not limited to the summer months. In warmer climates it occurs year-round, and in cooler climates it may occur due to submersion in lakes, buckets, hot tubs, and bathtubs.

Prevention

The best management for near-drowning is prevention. The installation of four-sided fencing prevents up to 90% of childhood

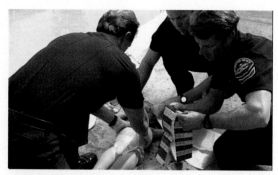

Figure 4-14 Drowning is the leading cause of unintentional death in children between the ages of 1 and 4 years.

residential swimming pool drownings and near-drownings. Eighty-five percent of boating-related drownings are preventable by wearing personal flotation devices.

Treatment

Early recognition of cardiac arrest and immediate bystander CPR has an important association with survival from severe submersion injuries. ALS care has an unproven benefit.

First remove the patient from the water and check for breathing and pulse. If the child is pulseless, open the airway and begin rescue breathing and chest compressions. Protect the cervical spine if there is potential head or neck trauma. Perform airway management, oxygenation, ventilation, and chest compression and follow protocols for drug therapy and electrical countershock depending upon presenting cardiac rhythm.

If the child has a pulse, open the airway and ensure appropriate oxygenation and ventilation, usually with a bag-mask device. Obtain IV or IO access and transport. Provide drug therapy, and rarely electrical countershock, as indicated for shock or dysrythmias.

Hypothermia

Hypothermia is an emergency resulting from exposure to cold temperatures. It most often occurs in association with submersion, but may be the result of prolonged exposure to cold ambient environment. When a child in cardiac arrest is also a cold water submersion victim, survival is improved even if the presenting rhythm is asystole.

Case Study **3**

You are dispatched to the location of an unresponsive 2-year-old boy recently removed from a swimming pool. Estimated downtime is unknown, but the parents are on scene and state that the child had been missing for over 30 minutes. The parents initiated CPR immediately. Upon arrival you find the child to be cool, blue, apneic, and pulseless.

1. What is the most important intervention for this patient to improve his chance for survival?
2. Should the child be actively re-warmed?

Treatment of Hypothermia

Remove clothing and prevent further heat loss by covering the head and body. If the patient is conscious, alert, and shivering, place warm packs in the axillae and groin, being careful not to cause burns. With profound hypothermia, aggressive rewarming in the field may do more harm than good. Not only may the hypother-

mic state be protective of brain function, but rapid rewarming can induce dysrhythmias. *In general, be extremely cautious using drug therapy if the child has suspected hypothermia.*

Do not rewarm frozen extremities until later in the hospital phase of the resuscitation because rewarming may worsen prognosis. Finally, do not pronounce the severely hypothermic patient dead in the field. Transport and continue resuscitation.

The hypothermic state is possibly protective of brain function. Rapid rewarming can introduce dysrhythmias unique to hypothermia.

If the child is unconscious, aggressive rewarming may do more harm than good.

Chapter Review

Case Study Answers

Case Study ❶ page 77

This child has septic or distributive shock. He has decompensated shock with hypotension. The rash is an ominous sign and aggressive treatment will be necessary to save the child's life. The appropriate first interventions are oxygen and bag-mask ventilation.

Attempt IV or IO access on scene once and give a 20 mL/kg crystalloid fluid bolus as fast as possible. Then transport and deliver 20 mL/kg fluid boluses to a maximum of 60 mL/kg while en route to the ED. Consider giving a vasopressor agent, either dopamine or epinephrine, if perfusion remains poor after fluid administration and the transport time is long. Endotracheal intubation may be necessary.

This case also requires universal precautions to protect the prehospital professionals as this child has a serious communicable disease. Direct specific questions about exposures and prophylactic treatment to your infection control personnel.

Case Study ❷ page 91

This cardiac arrest appears to reflect a primary cardiac event. While prompt CPR is imperative, so is a "quick look" at the cardiac rhythm. This child was in ventricular fibrillation due to a previously undiagnosed disorder known as "prolonged QT syndrome." Survivors from this disease often give a history of "blackouts" associated with exercise and stress. Other family members may also be affected by the same disorder. A look back at the family history can uncover unexplained deaths of relatives at young ages.

The initial treatment for children in ventricular fibrillation—as in adults—is rapid defibrillation. With the increasing availability of AEDs, many of these children will receive rapid recognition and defibrillation by bystanders. The AED is indicated this child.

Case Study ❸ page 101

After removal from the water, provide bag-mask ventilation with 100% oxygen. Rushing to intubate this child, before providing effective bag-mask ventilation with 100% oxygen, may result in worsened hypoxia and hypercarbia. Most drownings cause airway spasm with little or no water entering the lungs, so bag-mask may be effective. The best anatomic location for palpating a pulse in a 2-year-old child is over the brachial artery, which is located just proximal to the elbow and medially to the bicep muscle.

Rewarming severely hypothermic patients may do more harm than good. Not only may the hypothermic state be protective of brain function, but rapid rewarming can introduce dysrhythmias. In general, withhold drug therapy if the anticipated core temperature is below 30°C.

Suggested Readings

Textbooks

American Academy of Pediatrics and the American College of Emergency Physicians: *APLS: The Pediatric Emergency Medicine Resource,* 4th Edition. Sudbury, MA, Jones and Bartlett Publishers, 2004.

Articles

Han Y, Carcillo J, Dragotta, et al. Early reversal of pediatric-neonatal septic shock by community physicians is associated with improved outcome. *Pediatrics.* Oct 2003; 112(4):793–799.

Morris MC. Pediatric cardiopulmonary-cerebral resuscitation: An overview and future directions. *Crit Care Clin.* Jul 2003; 19(3):337–64.

Perondi M, Reis A, Paiva E. A comparison of high-dose and standard-dose epinephrine in children with cardiac arrest. *NEJM.* April 2004; 350(17):1722–1730.

Samson R, Berg R, Bingham R, et al. Use of automated external defibrillators for children: An update. An advisory statement from the pediatric advanced life support task force, international liaison committee on resuscitation. *Circulation.* 2003; 107:3250–3255.

Sirbaugh P, Pepe P, Shook J, et al. A prospective, population-based study of the demographics, epidemiology, management and outcome of out-of-hospital pediatric cardiopulmonary arrest. *Ann Emerg Med.* Feb 1999; 33(2):174–184.

Wenzel V, Krismer A, Arntz R, et al. A comparison of vasopressin and epinephrine for out-of-hospital cardiopulmonary resuscitation. *NEJM.* Jan 2004; 350(2):105–113.

Young K, Gausche-Hill M, McClung C, et al. A prospective population-based study of the epidemiology and outcome of out-of-hospital pediatric cardiopulmonary arrest. *Pediatrics.* Jul 2004; 114(1):157–64.

Young K, Seidel J. Pediatric Cardiopulmonary resuscitation: A collective review. *Ann Emerg Med.* 1999; 33(2):195–205.

5

Medical Emergencies

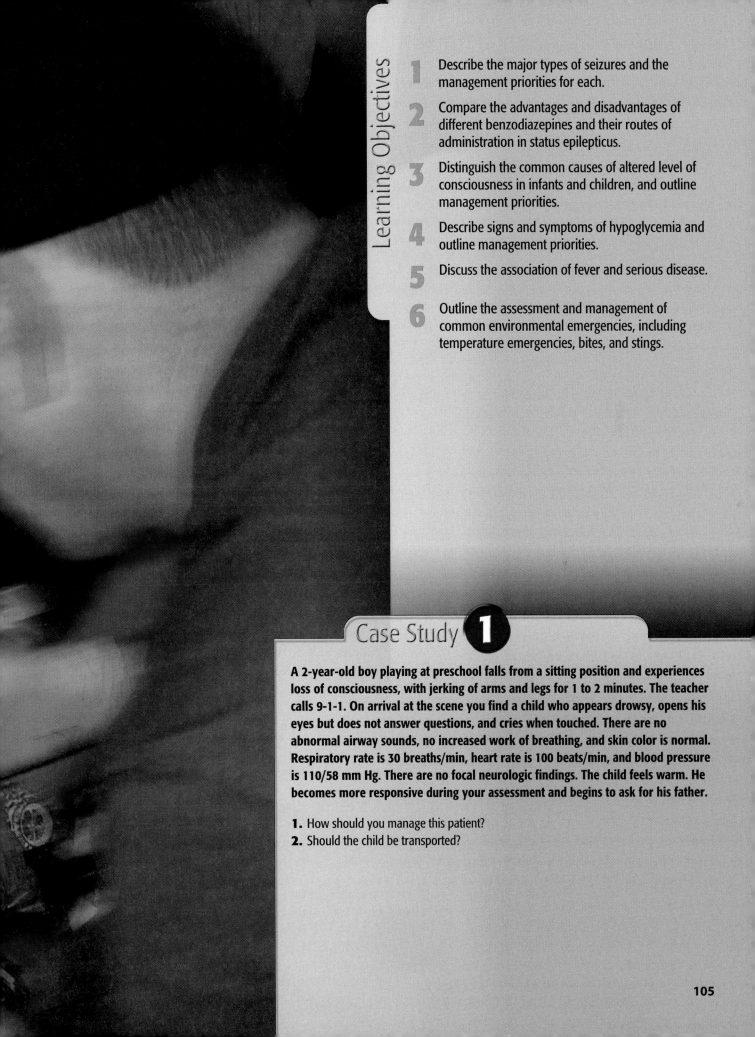

1. Describe the major types of seizures and the management priorities for each.

2. Compare the advantages and disadvantages of different benzodiazepines and their routes of administration in status epilepticus.

3. Distinguish the common causes of altered level of consciousness in infants and children, and outline management priorities.

4. Describe signs and symptoms of hypoglycemia and outline management priorities.

5. Discuss the association of fever and serious disease.

6. Outline the assessment and management of common environmental emergencies, including temperature emergencies, bites, and stings.

Case Study 1

A 2-year-old boy playing at preschool falls from a sitting position and experiences loss of consciousness, with jerking of arms and legs for 1 to 2 minutes. The teacher calls 9-1-1. On arrival at the scene you find a child who appears drowsy, opens his eyes but does not answer questions, and cries when touched. There are no abnormal airway sounds, no increased work of breathing, and skin color is normal. Respiratory rate is 30 breaths/min, heart rate is 100 beats/min, and blood pressure is 110/58 mm Hg. There are no focal neurologic findings. The child feels warm. He becomes more responsive during your assessment and begins to ask for his father.

1. How should you manage this patient?
2. Should the child be transported?

Introduction

APPROXIMATELY HALF OF all pediatric 9-1-1 calls are illness or "medical" complaints, and half are injury or "trauma" complaints. Calls involving children with pediatric medical complaints tend to be more serious as a whole, and the varied nature of these complaints makes this group especially challenging to assess and treat. This chapter reviews common out-of-hospital pediatric medical emergencies: seizures, altered level of consciousness (ALOC), fever, and environmental emergencies.

Respiratory illness and seizures are the two most common out-of-hospital pediatric medical emergencies. Fever is a common medical complaint, but is rarely an emergency in and of itself. Fever is a symptom of an underlying illness. The prehospital assessment of a febrile child must focus on identification of potentially treatable causes of fever. Fever may be associated with illnesses such as bronchiolitis, sepsis, or seizures in infant and preschool-aged children. All are conditions that have important prehospital treatments. ALOC is a less common characteristic of pediatric 9-1-1 patients, but it usually means the child has a serious or life-threatening medical emergency. Environmental emergencies occurring during childhood include heat- and cold-related emergencies, and envenomations by bites and stings. The young child is at increased risk for these environmental emergencies due to physiologic, behavioral, and developmental characteristics.

Accurately assessing a child with a medical illness requires an age-based approach to history taking and physical examination, as discussed in Chapters 1 and 2. Communicating with the child and family is essential. Effective communication is fundamental to good clinical care, establishment of trust, and development of comfortable interactions with the child.

Seizures

Seizures are caused by abnormal, sustained electrical discharges from a cluster of cerebral neurons. Seizures have varied physical manifestations, depending on the location of the abnormal electrical seizure activity in the brain and the age of the child. Seizures in infants, whose central nervous system (CNS) is immature, can be very subtle, consisting only of abnormal gaze, sucking motions, or "bicycling." In older children, with a more mature CNS, seizures are usually more obvious, and typically manifest as repetitive muscular contractions (tonic-clonic activity) and unresponsiveness. These "generalized" seizures are the most common type in children. "Partial" or "focal" seizures, in which consciousness is maintained during a state of localized motor jerking, are a second type, but are less common. About 5% of all children will have at least one seizure by 6 years of age. Over half of those children will never have another seizure.

The term epilepsy refers to a chronic disorder that causes recurrent seizures over time, with or without a known underlying cause. While caregivers of children with epilepsy may be very calm at the scene of a 9-1-1 call, those who are witnessing a first time seizure are usually very frightened, may fear that the child is dying, and may have initiated CPR efforts.

Febrile Seizures

The most frequent type of seizure in childhood is the febrile seizure. By definition, a simple febrile seizure is a generalized, tonic-clonic seizure of less than 15 minutes duration that occurs in a febrile child between 6 months and 3 years of age with no underlying neurological abnormalities. "Simple" febrile seizures do not cause brain injury, even if the child has repeat febrile seizures. The vast majority of simple febrile seizures will have stopped spontaneously before the arrival of prehospital professionals. Complex febrile seizures last longer than 15 minutes, may be focal rather than generalized, and may be associated with baseline developmental or neurologic abnormalities. This type of seizure has a higher association with serious illness and requires more evaluation in the hospital. While the diagnosis of febrile seizure is usually correct in a young, febrile postictal child whose level of consciousness is improving and who looks well in the field, other serious causes of fever and seizures, such as meningitis, must be ruled out in the hospital. A child who has a seizure and a fever may not necessarily have had a febrile seizure, and requires physician evaluation to exclude a serious disease. *A prehospital professional cannot make a diagnosis of a febrile seizure.*

A prehospital professional cannot make a diagnosis of a febrile seizure.

Afebrile Seizures

While childhood seizures are frequently associated with fever, there are many other possible causes of seizures that do not have fever. These include trauma (including child abuse), hypoxia, hypoglycemia, infection, ingestion, CNS bleeding, metabolic disorders, and congenital neurologic problems. A common group of children with afebrile seizures are those with known epilepsy who have not received therapeutic doses of their anticonvulsant medication, and experience "breakthrough" seizures.

A seizure with a fever is not the same as a febrile seizure.

Status Epilepticus

The classic definition of status epilepticus is either: (1) a series of two or more seizures without recovery of consciousness, with the child unable to carry on verbal communication between the seizures, or (2) a continuous seizure more than 20 minutes long. A newer "operational" definition of status was developed in the late 1990s by a group of neurologists specializing in seizure management. Based on data indicating that the majority of

seizures stop spontaneously in less than five minutes, they redefined the term "status epilepticus" and set a threshold for initiating pharmacological treatment as a seizure lasting longer than 5 minutes. Accordingly, consider any child who is actively seizing on arrival of the prehospital professional to be in status epilepticus, and treat with drug therapy to stop the seizure. Such patients inevitably have been seizing for at least 15 minutes, given the average response times in most EMS systems.

Status epilepticus may occur as the child's first seizure. The age of the child in status epilepticus helps forecast the likely cause of the seizure. Children under 3 years of age tend to have acute, sometimes progressive causes of status epilepticus, such as hypoxia, infection, or toxic ingestion. Children over 3 years of age who present with status epilepticus tend to have chronic, static causes (e.g., epilepsy and inadequate anticonvulsant treatment). Therefore, be especially vigilant in care of infants and young children with status epilepticus if they do not have a history of fever or epilepsy.

Status epilepticus is a medical emergency. Early treatment in the field is key because the longer the duration of the seizure, the harder it is to stop pharmacologically. Stopping the seizure will also facilitate airway management and support of oxygenation and ventilation, as well as transport. However, the risk of long-term neurological injury is most closely associated with the underlying *cause*, rather than with the *duration*, of the seizure. For example, a child who has a 20-minute complex febrile seizure is unlikely to sustain brain injury, while a child with meningitis who has a seizure of the same duration is at high risk for long-term neurological problems.

During status epilepticus, the risk of brain injury is most closely related to the cause of the seizure, not the length of the seizure.

Table 5-1	Classification of Seizures
Type	**Description**
Generalized	
Tonic-clonic (*grand mal*)	Trunk rigidity and loss of consciousness, with sudden jerking of both arms and/or both legs; may be only tonic (muscle contraction; rigidity), or clonic (muscle relaxation; jerking)
Absence (*petit mal*)	Brief loss of awareness without any abnormal body movements; the child may appear to be staring or may blink his eyes repetitively
Partial (focal)	
Simple	Focal motor jerking, without loss of consciousness; may be sensory, autonomic, or psychic; may progress to complex seizure activity
Complex	Focal motor jerking, with loss of consciousness; sometimes there is secondary generalization to a tonic-clonic seizure
Neonatal	
Subtle	Chewing motions, excessive salivation, blinking, eye deviation, swallowing, swimming arms, pedaling legs, apnea, or color change
Tonic	Rigid posturing of trunk and extremities, may have fixed eye deviation
Focal–clonic	Rhythmic twitching of muscle groups, particularly the extremities and face
Multifocal	Similar to clonic with multiple muscle groups involved
Myoclonic	Brief focal or generalized jerks of extremities or parts of the body with distal muscle groups, may occur as a single jerk or series of repetitive jerks

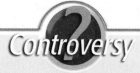

When to treat a seizure is a matter of debate. Although most seizures will stop spontaneously and do not need any treatment, some untreated children will go on to the dangerous condition of status epilepticus. The best practical approach is to treat if the child is seizing upon arrival.

Do not treat absence or simple partial seizures because they will not cause brain injury.

Classification of Seizures

The type of abnormal motor activity and the age of the child are factors important to classify seizures, as shown in **Table 5-1**. The main distinction is whether the seizure involves the entire body (generalized) or only one part of the body (partial). A generalized seizure usually involves abnormal muscle jerking (grand mal seizure), but may have only loss of attention and eye blinking (absence or petit mal seizure). When the child has had a partial seizure, establish whether consciousness and verbal interaction is preserved (simple partial seizure) or impaired (complex partial seizure). <u>Simple partial seizures</u> can progress to <u>complex partial seizures</u> or to <u>generalized seizures</u>. When a partial seizure evolves to a generalized seizure, it is called "secondary generalization". <u>Neonatal seizures</u> tend to be more subtle, because tonic-clonic activity may not occur during the first month of life.

Complications

Seizures may cause hypoxia from airway obstruction, aspiration, or inadequate respiratory drive. Good prehospital management will minimize these complications. A second concern is brain injury from prolonged seizure activity in a child with a serious underlying condition such as infection, intoxication, or hemorrhage. Support of airway and breathing, control of seizure activity, and rapid transport to a facility with pediatric intensive care capability are the best strategies for minimizing morbidity in this population of critically ill children.

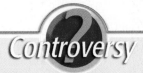

Table 5-2	Initial Airway Management in Seizing Children

Position the head to open the airway.

Clear the mouth with suction.

Consider the <u>lateral decubitus position</u> if the child is actively vomiting and suction is inadequate to control the airway (**Figure 5-1**).

Provide 100% oxygen by nonrebreathing mask or blow-by.

Consider a nasopharyngeal airway.

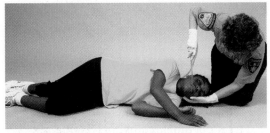

Figure 5-1 Position the head to open the airway, place the child in the lateral decubitus position, and clear the mouth of vomitus with suction.

Assessment and Treatment of the Actively Seizing Child

If a child is actively seizing when the prehospital professional arrives, there are several essential steps:

1. *Open the airway.*
   Managing the airway is the most important initial action (**Table 5-2**).

Advanced Life Support

Without the use of neuromuscular blockade agents, successful endotracheal intubation during a seizure is extremely difficult, and complication rates are high. *Do not attempt to intubate a seizing child.* If the airway is not maintainable, attempt to stop the seizure through the administration of anticonvulsant medications. Once the seizure is stopped, perform airway management as needed.

Consider spinal stabilization as part of airway management in a post-traumatic seizure, although it will not be very effective until the seizure activity has stopped.

2. *Breathing.*
   All seizures are associated with some degree of hypoventilation. Attempt to gently assist ventilation if the child is cyanotic, or has a measured oxygen saturation less than 90% on supplemental oxygen. Be aware, however, that it is difficult to obtain an accurate pulse oximetry reading in a child who is having an active grand mal seizure. Again, stopping the seizure is the key to successful ventilation. Opening the airway, coordinating positive-pressure ventilations with the patient's spontaneous respiratory effort, and expanding a rigid chest wall are technically difficult procedures during a generalized seizure. Often the result of assisted ventilation is stomach inflation with air. Consider a nasogastric tube to decompress the stomach if bag-mask ventilation visibly distends the abdomen.

3. *Circulation.*
   Unless a child has seizures associated with sepsis or trauma, fluid resuscitation in the field or in transport is not necessary. Signs of poor perfusion are most likely associated with prolonged seizure activity, hypoxia, and metabolic acidosis. Once again, treating the seizure will address these problems.

Table 5-4	Benzodiazepine Administration During Seizures			
Generic Name	**Initial Dose**	**Route**	**Pros**	**Cons**
Diazepam	0.1 mg/kg	IV, IO	Rapid onset Inexpensive No refrigeration	Sedating Respiratory depression Short duration of action for seizure control (15 min)
Diazepam	0.5 mg/kg	PR	Rapid onset No IV required	Sedating Respiratory depression
Lorazepam	0.05–0.1 mg/kg	IV, IM, IO	Rapid onset Long duration of action for seizure control (12–24 hours)	Store away from heat and extreme temperature
Midazolam	0.05–0.15 mg/kg	IV, IM, IO	Rapid onset	Medium duration of action for seizure control (30–120 min)

4. *Disability.*
Check the bedside glucose level and treat documented hypoglycemia, as described in **Table 5-3**.

While most seizures will have stopped before the arrival of prehospital professionals, the child who is still actively seizing will usually benefit from pharmacologic treatment. Consider options for anticonvulsant administration, in terms of medications approved in the EMS system and available routes of administration. The goal is to stop the seizure, while minimizing medication side effects.

Benzodiazepine drugs are excellent first-line anticonvulsants. Common drugs in this class are **diazepam**, **midazolam**, and **lorazepam**. **Table 5-4** provides doses and routes of administration.

While each of the benzodiazepines has the same mechanism of action, differences in specific agent and route of administration lead to significant clinical differences in the time to peak effect, and the duration of action.

Lorazepam

Of the benzodiazepines, lorazepam, 0.05–0.1 mg/kg probably has the best pharmacologic profile for prehospital seizure management. It has a rapid onset of action, can be given IV, IO, IM, or PR, and has a long half-life. The drug may be given IM, but usually try the IV mode of administration

Table 5-3	Dextrose Administration Guidelines During Seizures

Indications
- Infant and child with glucose level < 60 mg%
- Newborn with glucose level < 40 mg%

Treatment
- Newly born: Give $D_{10}W$, 2 mL/kg IV or IO
- Neonate: Give $D_{10}W$, 5 mL/kg IV or IO bolus (1 part $D_{50}W$, 4 parts sterile water or normal saline)
- Child < 2 years old: Give $D_{25}W$, 2 mL/kg IV or IO bolus (1 part $D_{50}W$, 1 part sterile water or normal saline)
- Child > 2 years old: Give $D_{50}W$, 1 mL/kg IV or IO bolus

first. If no vascular access is possible, then administer the drug deep IM in a large muscle mass. There is little experience with out-of-hospital PR lorazepam administration in children, and drug doses are not well established. In general, this drug has not been widely used by prehospital professionals due to the manufacturer's recommendation regarding refrigeration. Lorazepam may be stocked un-refrigerated on prehospital ALS units if it is replaced every 30 days.

Diazepam

Diazepam is a time-honored drug for status epilepticus. IV diazepam, at 0.1 mg/kg, is an effective treatment for status epilepticus or prolonged seizures, but rapid IV administration may cause **respiratory depression**. Do not give diazepam IM because it is not well absorbed and is irritating to muscle tissue.

Table 5-5	Second-Line Anticonvulsant Drug Administration			
Generic Name	**Initial Dose**	**Route**	**Rate of Infusion**	**Maximum Rate of Infusion**
Phenytoin	20 mg/kg	IV, IO	1 mg/kg/min	50 mg/min
Fosphenytoin	20 mg/kg (phenytoin equivalents)	IV, IO, IM	3 mg (PE)/kg/min	150 mg (PE)/min
Phenobarbital	20 mg/kg	IV, IO	1 mg/kg/min	50 mg/min

Sublingual and intranasal administrations have been described, although there is little out-of-hospital experience.

The requirement for cannulating a peripheral vein in a seizing child often slows down delivery of essential ALS drugs, especially in infants and toddlers. *The rectum is an effective alternative route for emergency diazepam administration.* Rectal (PR) diazepam is effective, causes less respiratory depression and is easy to administer. Use a higher dose of 0.5 mg/kg. Rates of respiratory depression associated with PR diazepam are lower than for IV diazepam. However, onset of action is longer, with time to clinical effect in the range of 5 minutes. For a step-by-step explanation of the rectal diazepam administration procedure, see

Rectal Aministration of
Benzodiazepines, Procedure 20.

Diazepam begins to work quickly but its anticonvulsant action does not last long, a serious limitation in long field or transport times. Another dose of diazepam (or another anticonvulsant medication, if available) may be necessary within 10 to 20 minutes if the drug is given. Consider half the normal dose of diazepam, if the child is on phenobarbital or has received other benzodiazepines in the previous few hours, to minimize the risk of respiratory depression.

Midazolam

IM midazolam is another benzodiazepine that can be given to a patient without IV access. The dose is 0.05–0.15 mg/kg IM. While onset of action is delayed when compared to IV diazepam, the time to cessation of seizure activity may be less, because IM administration is usually much faster than IV. Midazolam works IV and IO, and may also work intranasally and sublingually to stop seizures, but the nasal and sublingual

administration procedures and doses have not yet been well studied.

When administering any benzodiazepine, watch closely for respiratory depression, a common side effect of this class of drugs, and be prepared to provide bag-mask ventilatory support. Even in the case of apnea following benzodiazepine administration, a bag-mask device will usually suffice, as the respiratory depressant effects of the drugs are transitory. Endotracheal intubation is rarely necessary.

If the seizure does not stop after two doses of a benzodiazepine, further doses are unlikely to terminate the seizure. Consider a second drug if the local EMS system permits. Common choices for second-line anticonvulsants include phenytoin, fosphenytoin, and phenobarbital, the dosing and administration of which are described in **Table 5-5**.

Phenobarbital is preferred as the first line drug in neonates. Phenytoin is probably the best second line drug in neonates, infants, and children. Give phenytoin in normal saline at a rate no faster than 50 mg/min. Place the child on a cardiac monitor and watch carefully for bradycardia and hypotension—the most common serious complications of IV or IO phenytoin. Complications are caused by the diluent, or mixing solution, propylene glycol. Fosphenytoin, a recent "prodrug" or metabolic precursor to phenytoin is another second line option. While fosphenytoin can be administered more quickly than phenytoin IV or IO and can also be given IM, it then takes about 15 minutes to metabolize to phenytoin, the active metabolite. *Hence, the total time it takes to get an effective drug level in the blood and brain to stop the seizure is approximately the same with phenytoin and fosphenytoin.* A disadvantage of fospheytoin is that the drug is much more expensive than phenytoin.

Tip

Always give oxygen to a child who is having a seizure or who is postictal.

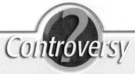

Controversy

Both lorazepam and midazolam may be effective when given sublingually or intranasally. However, the exact doses, and the relative effectiveness and safety of benzodiazepines given by this route are unknown.

Transport

After providing airway and breathing support and administering a benzodiazepine, wait a few minutes for the seizure to stop and initiate transport. Some EMS regions allow second-line anticonvulsant medications in transport. Perform the focused history and physical exam and the detailed physical exam (trauma patients), if possible, on the way to the hospital. During transport, do ongoing assessment using continuous cardiac monitoring and pulse oximetry, if available. If a patient has not stopped seizing after administration of several doses of a benzodiazepine and a second-line drug (e.g., phenytoin and phenobarbital), the risk for a prolonged seizure is high. Consider options in terms of transport destination because this subset of children is likely to require intensive care.

Assessment of the Postictal Child

Usually the child's seizure is already over when the prehospital professional arrives. This "postictal" state is characterized by abnormal appearance with sleepiness, confusion, irritability, and decreased interactiveness that may last from minutes to hours.

If the child is physiologically stable, perform a complete assessment in the field,

Table 5-6	Worrisome Circumstances with the Postictal Child
Post-traumatic seizure	
Post-ingestion seizure	
Seizure and sustained hypoxia	
Seizure in a neonate (< 4 weeks of age)	
First seizure in a child > 6 years	
More than one seizure	
Seizure time > 5 min	
Low glucose level	

including the focused history and physical exam and the detailed physical exam (trauma patients). Some examples of a stable postictal patient are the child with a previous diagnosis of epilepsy who experiences a brief grand mal seizure, or the child under 3 years of age with fever and a possible febrile seizure. Most children who have had a brief seizure will show improvement in level of alertness, muscle tone, and interactiveness within 15 to 30 minutes. Failure to "wake up" over a 30 to 60 minute period following the seizure may reflect a serious underlying problem and trigger early transport with completion of the assessment en route to the hospital. **Table 5-6** lists some of the conditions that might lead to a prolonged postictal state that require urgent treatment in the ED. If the child has had a seizure after closed head injury, always stabilize the <u>cervical</u> spine, as discussed in Chapter 6.

If the postictal patient has a previous diagnosis of epilepsy, include the name and dosage of anticonvulsant medications and when the last dose was given in the focused history. Inquire when the last blood levels were obtained and whether the levels were adequate. Determine the duration of the seizure and ask for a description of the motor activity, including where it started, how it progressed, and how long the child was unconscious. From this information, determine the type of seizure (e.g., generalized or partial, or partial with secondary generalization). Ask carefully about head trauma. Consider the possibility of an ingestion or overdose.

Calm parents' fears about the seizure, but do not diagnose or provide them uncertain information about the cause of the seizure or chance of recurrence.

Attempt to allay the caregiver's fears. If the child has had her first seizure, the caregiver may be extremely frightened.

Summary of Seizures

Seizures are common in children, and frightened caregivers frequently call 9-1-1 to assist in managing this problem. Usually the seizure has stopped before ambulance arrival, in which case the tasks include only assessment of the postictal child and transport to the hospital with no treatment.

Sometimes the child is seizing on arrival and requires medical management. The treatment includes opening and clearing the airway, giving oxygen, then administering a benzodiazepine medication, usually diazepam or lorazepam. Rectal diazepam stops most seizures in children. Effective alternatives are IV or IM lorazepam or midazolam or IV diazepam. The benzodiazepine medications often cause temporary respiratory depression, which requires bag-mask ventilation support without endotracheal intubation, in most cases. If treatment with a benzodiazepine is unsuccessful, second line drugs such as phenobarbital, phenytoin, and fosphenytoin are good options, based on local EMS protocol.

Table 5-7	AEIOU TIPPS: Possible Causes of Altered Level of Consciousness
Alcohol	
Epilepsy, endocrine, electrolytes	
Insulin	
Opiates and other drugs	
Uremia	
Trauma, temperature	
Infection	
Psychogenic	
Poison	
Shock, stroke, space-occupying lesion, subarachnoid hemorrhage	

Altered Level of Consciousness

ALOC is an abnormal neurologic state in which the child is less alert and interactive than is age-appropriate. The term ALOC refers to a range of abnormal appearances, from irritability to total unresponsiveness. Sometimes, the concern of the caretaker is vague, and the complaint is simply that his child is "not acting right." Understanding normal developmental or age-related changes in behavior, and listening carefully to the caregiver's opinion about alterations from an individual's norm are key features in the assessment. A mnemonic AEIOU TIPPS recalls many of the severe causes of ALOC (**Table 5-7**). The

Case Study **2**

You respond to a call about an unresponsive child. The caregiver states that the 3-year-old boy could not be awakened from his nap. The child is "sleeping" on your arrival, with no abnormal airway sounds or retractions. He is pale. Respiratory rate is 20 breaths/min, cardiac monitor shows a narrow complex with a rate of 160 beats/min, and blood pressure is 80/60 mm Hg. Pupils are small and slow to constrict to light and the child withdraws to pain. There is no sign of trauma. The caregiver states that the child was playful and appeared healthy prior to his nap.

1. What are the immediate treatment priorities for this child?
2. What additional history may be helpful?

mnemonic is the five vowels in the alphabet [AEIOU], followed by tips [TIPPS], and reflects the major causes of ALOC.

Assessment

Use the PAT and the disability component of the hands-on ABCDEs to quickly assess neurologic status. These two parts of the initial assessment work in concert to evaluate both <u>cortical</u> and <u>brain stem functions</u>, as described in Chapter 1. There is a difference between "abnormal appearance" and ALOC. Abnormal appearance is a more subtle measure of brain function and is evaluated using the TICLS mnemonic (Table 1-1). ALOC is a more severe signal of mental status alteration and is evaluated with the AVPU scale. While ALOC is always associated with an abnormal appearance, some children with more subtle abnormalities in appearance would not have ALOC using the AVPU. For example, a child who is irritable or listless and has abnormal appearance on the PAT, may be "alert" on the AVPU scale of disability during the ABCDE hands-on evaluation.

The AVPU system is a quick way to determine level of consciousness and to assess *major* changes in level of consciousness during transport. A child with sepsis or brain hemorrhage from inflicted injury, for example, has a serious degree of brain dysfunction and may score "verbal" or lower on the AVPU.

Finally, observe <u>motor activity</u> and check the pupils. In the assessment of motor activity, watch for purposeful and symmetric movement of extremities, <u>ataxia</u>, seizures, <u>posturing</u>, or <u>flaccidity</u> (<u>hypotonia</u>). In the assessment of pupils, check size (small or large), equality, and response to light. Pupils may have abnormal size or reactivity in the presence of drugs, ongoing seizures, hypoxia, or impending <u>brain stem herniation</u>.

Look for a Medical Alert Bracelet and ask about important medical history that may account for the child's ALOC, such as diabetes or a seizure disorder (**Figure 5-2**).

Management

Regardless of the cause of ALOC, focus on the ABCs.

1. *Open the airway.*
   In the poorly responsive patient with compromised airway reflexes, suction the mouth to relieve potential obstruction from secretions or vomitus. If there is no <u>gag reflex</u> or if the patient is totally unresponsive, position the head and insert an oropharyngeal or nasopharyngeal airway. Keep the spine stabilized if there is a suspicion of head or neck injury.

2. *Ensure adequate breathing.*
   Patients with altered levels of consciousness may have inadequate breathing despite spontaneous respiratory effort, based on inadequate respiratory rate or inadequate tidal volume. Administer 100% oxygen by nonrebreathing mask. Start bag-mask ventilation with 100% oxygen if the patient is cyanotic, has oxygen saturation less than 90% on 100% oxygen by nonrebreathing mask, is breathing at a rate too slow for age, or has shallow or irregular respiratory effort.

There are many causes of altered level of consciousness, but management must focus on the ABCs.

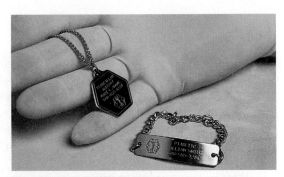

Figure 5-2 In a child with altered level of consciousness, look for a bracelet with his medical history.

There is a difference between abnormal appearance and ALOC. Abnormal appearance is a more subtle measure of brain function and is evaluated using the TICLS mnemonic. ALOC is a more severe signal of mental status alteration and is evaluated with the AVPU.

Advanced Life Support

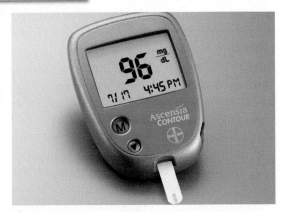

Figure 5-3 Perform a bedside blood glucose test.

Consider endotracheal intubation to protect the airway and to avoid aspiration. Ventilate the patient with suspected brain injury but do not hyperventilate the patient (see Chapter 3). Place the patient on a cardiac monitor and a pulse oximeter.

3. *Safeguard circulation.*
Establish vascular access and obtain blood for <u>serum glucose</u> measurement. Always start isotonic fluids at a To-Keep-Open (TKO) rate, unless the child is in shock. Reassess the child's level of consciousness.

4. *Perform a bedside blood glucose test* (**Figure 5-3**).
Administer glucose only to children with documented hypoglycemia. Neurological outcome in patients with diffuse brain injury is worse when the child also has hyperglycemia. If a bedside glucose test shows hypoglycemia (<40 mg% in a newborn, <60 mg% in a child), give an IV glucose

bolus or IM glucagon as outlined in **Table 5-3**. Administer <u>oral glucose</u> to a child with diabetes and hypoglycemia who is conscious and has a gag reflex.

5. *In the child with ALOC and depressed respirations, consider naloxone administration.*
The <u>naloxone</u> dose is 0.1 mg/kg, with maximum doses up to 2 mg. Naloxone may be given by a variety of routes: IV, IM, IO, SQ, or ET tube. Caution must be exercised when giving naloxone to a depressed newly born of a <u>narcotic</u>-addicted mother, because it may induce acute withdrawal symptoms and seizures. Instead of giving naloxone, consider supporting ventilation and transporting the newborn to the hospital. Outside of the newly born, narcotic overdose is an unlikely cause of ALOC in children, but is an important consideration in teenagers. Constricted pupils are a universal finding in pure opiate overdoses.

Hypoglycemia

Hypoglycemia is defined as a serum glucose concentration of less than 40 mg% in a newly born, or less than 60 mg% in a child. The most frequent scenario for out-of-hospital hypoglycemia is a child with known diabetes who uses too much insulin, exerts herself excessively, or delays a meal (<u>transient</u> hypoglycemia). Hypoglycemia is also seen in children with sepsis. *Check a bedside glucose in any acutely ill appearing child, especially in the presence of abnormal appearance or ALOC.* Other causes of hypoglycemia in children are poor food intake in the face of an acute illness, especially in infants and toddlers with limited glycogen reserves.

Assessment

Signs and symptoms of hypoglycemia can be hard to detect, especially in younger infants who have mild hypoglycemia. The changing signs and symptoms are noted in **Table 5-8**. Depending on the blood sugar level, signs and

Table 5-8	Signs and Symptoms of Hypoglycemia	
Mild	**Moderate**	**Severe**
Hunger, irritability, weakness, agitation, tachypnea, tachycardia	Anxiety, blurred vision, stomach ache, headache, dizziness, sweating, pallor, tremors, confusion	Seizure, coma

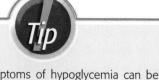

Signs and symptoms of hypoglycemia can be nonspecific.

symptoms may range from mild to profound. Tachycardia, tachypnea, sweating, agitation and tremor all reflect increased catecholamine release as the body responds to inadequate sugar supplies to support cellular metabolism. When blood sugar is dangerously low, seizures, coma, and death can occur.

Management

Diabetes Mellitus

Children with Type 1 (insulin-dependent diabetes mellitus, IDDM) <u>diabetes mellitus</u> are often well aware of the symptoms and signs of hypoglycemia, based on past experiences with insulin. If a diabetic patient is physiologically stable and cooperative but is hypoglycemic by blood sugar testing, allow her to attempt oral glucose replacement. Give 0.5 to 1.0 g/kg of sugar. There are 20 g of glucose in 13 ounces of cola or orange soda and in 12 ounces of orange juice or apple juice.

There is an increasing prevalence of Type 2 diabetes (non-insulin-dependent diabetes mellitus, NIDDM) in childhood. Such children are usually adolescents, often with associated obesity. The child may be on oral hypoglycemic agents, rather than insulin. Hypoglycemia is an occasional complication of this type of drug therapy as well and can be more difficult to stabilize. Give the child oral glucose replacement if signs and symptoms of hypoglycemia occur and the child is physiologically stable and cooperative, or treat with IV <u>dextrose</u> or glucagons if the child has ALOC.

Treatment of Hypoglycemia

Treat hypoglycemia if the child has ALOC and a measured serum glucose of less than 40 mg% in a newborn or less than 60 mg% in a child, as outlined in **Table 5-3**. Children have different tolerances to hypoglycemia,

so a child may be alert and cooperative with a blood sugar level between 40 to 50 mg%. A child in this condition can take oral glucose or breastfeed.

For the physiologically unstable patient with hypoglycemia and ALOC, give IV or IO dextrose immediately. Recheck the serum glucose if scene time or transport is prolonged, and repeat glucose doses as needed. Infuse dextrose as a slow push, and avoid infiltration, because the concentrated solution is quite irritating to skin tissues.

If there is no IV access, give glucagon. Repeat in 20 minutes as needed. Glucagon will stimulate a transient increase of the blood glucose level as long as there are liver stores of glycogen (long chains of stored glucose molecules).

Transport

After giving IV or IO dextrose or IM glucagon, reassess. Watch for a return to normal appearance and behavior. If the child with ALOC does not return to normal in a few minutes, transport immediately and conduct additional assessment on the way to the ED. If the child returns to normal, consider doing additional assessment on scene.

Additional Assessment

Do a focused history when possible. Ask key questions, such as:

- How quickly did the symptoms progress?
- Does the patient have diabetes or any other known illness?
- If the patient is a diabetic, has there been a recent change in medication or meals?
- Is the child on insulin or an oral hypoglycemia drug?
- Is this the first episode? If not, how often does this happen?

- Is it possible that the child was exposed to drugs or alcohol?
- If the patient is a newborn, has the mother received prenatal care?
- Has the mother had any medical problems with the pregnancy?
- Is the mother a diabetic?
- What is the newborn being fed and how often?
- How many caregivers are giving medications? Are they doubling up doses?

After the focused history, perform a physical exam. Reassess. If the child has diabetes and received too much __insulin__, and if there are no physiologic or anatomic abnormalities on reassessment, consider contacting medical oversight. In some EMS systems, the child with Type 1 diabetes may be left at the scene with management directed by the primary care physician in consultation with the caregiver. However, the circumstances with Type 2 diabetes are somewhat different, because the oral drugs that are taken for this condition have a longer duration of action than most insulin, and the child may need ongoing administration of glucose to maintain blood sugar. *Do not leave Type 2 diabetic patients on oral agents, who have experienced hypoglycemia on the scene.* Transport such patients to the emergency department.

Summary of Altered Level of Consciousness and Hypoglycemia

There are many causes of ALOC in children. The caregiver may be the best judge of ALOC, especially in the infant or toddler where developmental assessment is more challenging. Appearance and the AVPU scale work in concert to help assess ALOC. Address the ABCs first and especially consider reversible causes such as hypoglycemia. In some EMS systems, the child with Type 1 diabetes who has had a hypoglycemic event may be left at the scene with management directed by the primary care physician in

Do not leave Type 2 diabetic patients on oral agents, who have experienced hypoglycemia, on the scene.

Fever <106°F by itself does not cause brain damage.

consultation with the caregiver. Do not leave a Type 2 diabetic patient who has experienced hypoglycemia on the scene.

Fever

Fever is a sign of infection or inflammation, rather than a problem itself. Children can run high fevers in response to either bacterial or viral infections. High fever (>40°C or 104°F) can be due to minor illness such as a cold or serious problems such as pneumonia, meningitis, or sepsis. Fever leads to an increase in basal metabolic rate, causing a more rapid respiratory rate, increased cardiac output, higher oxygen consumption, and a greater need for fluids and calories. The ill child frequently is not interested in eating or drinking and with the increased metabolic demands of fever may be at risk for volume depletion and hypoglycemia. Body temperature less than 106°F is not in and of itself harmful, but is a common cause of concern to caregivers who fear brain damage as a result of fever.

Determine the presence of fever by history and field evaluation. Knowing the temperature, however, usually does not change field management.

Assessment

The initial assessment will help determine the severity of the child's illness and the urgency for treatment. If the initial assessment is normal, take a focused history and perform a detailed physical exam (trauma). Ask about important signs and symptoms of infection such as chills, <u>malaise</u>, poor feeding, <u>lethargy</u>, vomiting, diarrhea, abdominal pain, stiff neck, headache, and irritability.

Ask about exposure to known childhood communicable diseases. Many childhood illnesses begin with a fever before any other symptoms are present. Determine if the child has any significant medical history, because children that may be immune deficient (e.g., patients with <u>sickle cell disease</u>, cancer, human immunodeficiency virus [HIV], or post-organ transplantation) have a higher risk of serious infection as the cause of fever.

Febrile respiratory infections are very common in children, and are characterized by fever, tachycardia, tachypnea, nasal congestion, cough, and respiratory distress. Fever may make a child with a minor illness appear sicker than he really is, and parents will often report a marked improvement in symptoms after administration of <u>antipyretics</u> like <u>acetaminophen</u> or <u>ibuprofen</u>. After the focused history, if the child has no physiologic abnormalities, do a focused examination to look for possible sources of infection.

While the height of fever is not reflective of the degree of illness, certain findings suggest a serious underlying illness, and must prompt rapid transport. These include a <u>bulging fontanelle</u> (if <18 months of age, palpate with the child sitting up), nuchal rigidity (stiff neck), <u>paradoxical irritability</u> (an infant who is crankier when picked up and held than when left alone) (**Figure 5-4**),

seizures, prolonged capillary refill time, or a petechial or purpuric rash (**Figure 5-5**).

Age and Fever

In addition to signs and symptoms, the age of a child is important in assessing the significance of fever. A fever in an infant less than 4-weeks-old may be the only indication of serious infection, but the degree of temperature may be lower in comparison to the severity of illness or in comparison to older children with the same problem. The symptoms of serious bacterial infection in a young infant may be nonspecific, such as fussiness, poor feeding, and sleepiness. Because these very young infants have an immature immune system and are difficult to assess because of their limited range of behaviors and activities, any infant less than four weeks old with fever >38°C (100.4°F) will require blood, urine, and spinal fluid cultures as well as <u>antibiotics</u> in the ED. In the first few days of life, only <u>jaundice</u> may be a sign of serious bacterial infection.

Management

Management of fever in the child who has a normal initial assessment includes:

1. *Prevent transmission of disease to the prehospital professional.*
   Use standard precautions for infection control.
2. *Treat for shock.*
   See Chapter 4 for details on the signs and treatment of shock.
3. *In a febrile child who is older than 3 months, consider administration of*

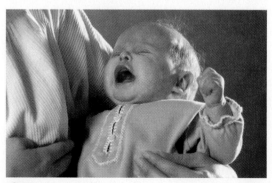

Figure 5-4 An infant suffering from paradoxical irritability.

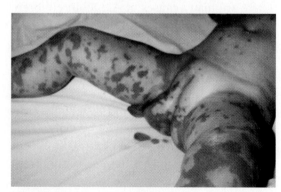

Figure 5-5 Purpuric rash in a child with meningococcemia.

antipyretics if none have been administered in the past 4 hours. Give acetaminophen at a dose of 10–15 mg/kg orally or rectally. Another option for the alert pediatric patient is ibuprofen at 5–10 mg/kg orally if awake. Consider the pediatric patient's level of consciousness or recent vomiting before administering anything by mouth. Avoid <u>aspirin</u> in a febrile child. Parents may need explanation that over-bundling a febrile child retains heat and may increase fever.

4. Cool the feverish child by undressing her, but avoid hypothermia.
   Do not use cold water, fans, ice, or alcohol baths to lower temperature.
5. Transport with ongoing reassessment for deterioration.
6. Explain to the caregiver that fever alone is not dangerous to the child.

Summary of Fever

Fever is a response to any type of infection. It is rarely a problem in and of itself. The age of the child and other associated signs and symptoms are important in determining probability of serious illness. In most cases, simple cooling measures and transport are the primary actions for the prehospital professional.

Communicable Diseases

Many communicable diseases are common during childhood. While most are viral in origin, and mild in terms of severity, infectious diseases on occasion cause significant compromise in the pediatric patient, resulting in the need for prehospital transport.

Never use ice, cold water, fans, or alcohol baths to cool a feverish child.

Gastroenteritis

<u>Gastroenteritis</u> is an inflammation of the gastrointestinal tract that presents as vomiting and diarrhea in the pediatric patient. This infectious illness can result in volume depletion, particularly in younger children. Causes of gastroenteritis are often viral, but can be due to bacteria or parasites. Beware that signs and symptoms most commonly associated with gastroenteritis such as fever, abdominal pain, or vomiting can also herald more serious abdominal emergencies like appendicitis and bowel obstruction. The diagnosis of "gastroenteritis" requires exclusion of more serious causes, and this determination is not possible in the field.

Assessment

Focus the assessment of a child with presumed gastroenteritis on the child's state of hydration.

The focused history should include questions regarding:

- The onset and frequency of vomiting and/or diarrhea
- Amount of oral intake
- Number of wet diapers in the past eight hours
- Last urination or wet diaper

The physical exam should include attention to:

- Presence or absence of fever
- Level of consciousness
- Hydration of mucous membranes: moist or dry
- Presence or absence of tears
- Extremity warmth and pulse quality
- Abdominal tenderness or distention

Always check a bedside glucose in a child with a history of vomiting, diarrhea, and poor oral intake.

Management

Management of the pediatric patient with presumed gastroenteritis depends on the degree of dehydration. Prevention of disease transmission to the prehospital professional is an additional component of care.

1. *Use standard precautions to reduce the likelihood of disease transmission.* Gastroenteritis, whether bacterial, viral, or parasitic in origin, is transmitted by the fecal–oral route. Ingestion of even a few pathogenic organisms can lead to disease in some cases. Some organisms can survive on exam instruments and surfaces for hours, so special care of clothes and instruments as well as careful hand washing are essential.

2. *Provide supplemental oxygen and airway management for the unstable pediatric patient.*

Advanced Life Support

3. *Provide fluid replacement for severe clinical dehydration.* Establish vascular access, IV or IO, and initiate fluid replacement using crystalloid fluid at 20 mL/kg initial bolus if the child has severe clinical dehydration as evidenced by elevated HR, poor pulses, delayed capillary refill time, cool extremities, and abnormal coloration. Repeat the bolus until perfusion is stabilized.

4. *Treat documented hypoglycemia.*
5. *Reassess vital signs.*
6. *Transport.* Transport decisions will depend on the degree of dehydration and local resources. A child with mild-to-moderate dehydration and ongoing vomiting and diarrhea may require transport alone without treatment. Sometimes provide oral fluids in the field to children with dehydration, if permitted by the EMS system. The child with signs of severe dehydration or shock will benefit from immediate fluid replacement before hospital transport.

| Sepsis and Meningitis

Sepsis implies an overwhelming, life-threatening bacterial blood stream infection.

Some children with sepsis will also have meningitis, resulting from infection and inflammation of the meninges, the membranes that cover the brain and spinal cord. Other children will present with sepsis or meningitis alone. The causative agent of meningitis may be viral or bacterial. While children with viral or aseptic meningitis may appear quite ill, the infection is not often life-threatening. On the other hand, bacterial meningitis is rapidly progressive, with death sometimes following the onset of symptoms within hours to days. While fever is always present, except occasionally in the neonatal period, other symptoms may vary from stiff neck and headache to impending brain stem herniation.

Infants in the first year of life are at highest risk for sepsis and bacterial meningitis, and the organisms vary with age. Since the introduction of the *Hemophilus influenza* vaccine in the late 1980s, this previously common cause of childhood illness has almost disappeared. Bacterial sepsis and meningitis in the first month of age is most commonly caused by bacteria acquired from the maternal vaginal area during delivery. These include *Escherichia coli, Group B streptococcus,* and *Listeria Monocytogenes.*

Outside of the youngest age group, community acquired infection is the source of sepsis and meningitis, with common bacterial causes in immune-competent children including *Streptococcus pneumoniae* (also the most common cause of bacterial ear infections, sinusitis, and pneumonia in children) and *Neiserria meningidites* (meningococcus). The pneumococcal vaccine recently available throughout the United States is significantly reducing the incidence of childhood bacteremia and sepsis from the pneumococcal organism. Hemophilus influenzae meningitis has also decreased significantly due to widespread vaccine use. The enteroviruses are also common causes of viral meningitis, especially during summer and fall months.

Meningococcal sepsis or meningitis is a life-threatening emergency that presents acutely with high fever, ALOC, and a characteristic petechial rash or purpura. The presence of such a rash should always trigger rapid transport by the highest level of provider to the highest level of care available, as these children can deteriorate very quickly, requiring aggressive life support.

Assessment

In a physiologically unstable child with presumed sepsis or meningitis, limit the scene assessment. Perform the focused history and physical exam during transport, if possible.

The focused history should include:

- Known exposure to illness
- Perinatal history for infants <1 month of age
- Onset of symptoms and rapidity of progression
- Presence or absence of fever
- Associated symptoms/signs such as irritability, vomiting, nuchal rigidity, rash (petechiae or purpura)
- Immunization history

The physical exam should include attention to:

- Fever
- Level of consciousness
- Adequacy of perfusion
- Nuchal rigidity
- Presence of a rash (petechiae or purpura)
- Photophobia

Because children with sepsis and meningitis are in a hypermetabolic state, they can develop hypoglycemia. Check a bedside glucose on any patient with presumed sepsis or meningitis.

Management

Management of the pediatric patient with sepsis or meningitis must include infection control precautions. Interventions will vary based on the patient's clinical presentation.

1. *Prevent disease transmission.*
The prehospital professional should use standard and respiratory precautions, including gowns, gloves, and masks to avoid contact with patient secretions.

2. *Provide supplemental oxygen.*
Unstable patients may need assisted ventilation or airway management.

> **Advanced Life Support**

3. *Establish vascular access.*
4. *For inadequate perfusion, initiate fluid replacement.*
For the pediatric patient with inadequate perfusion, initiate fluid replacement using crystalloid fluid at 20 mL/kg initial bolus. Because of the effects of bacterial toxins on the blood vessels, children with sepsis may develop distributive shock requiring aggressive fluid resuscitation with as much as 60 cc/kg of crystalloid fluid.

5. *Treat hypoglycemia.*
6. *Reassess vital signs frequently.*
Use continuous cardiorespiratory monitoring and pulse oximetry, if available. Anticipate deterioration in transport.
7. *Transport.*
Since these children are at risk for rapid deterioration and may need ALS intervention, transport by the highest level of service available. Children with sepsis or meningitis generally require intensive care. Consider this when determining a transport destination.

Environmental Emergencies

Common pediatric environmental emergencies include temperature-related problems, bites, and stings. Each of these emergencies can range from mild to severe. Match the intensity of intervention to the severity of the illness or injury.

Heat-Related Emergencies

Heat-related emergencies in the pediatric population occur most commonly when young children are left in a closed car, or older children who are not heat-acclimated participate in sports during periods of high environmental temperatures and do not hydrate adequately (hyperthermia). Because of the difficulty of obtaining temperature readings in the field, the assessment of such

Table 5-9	Typical Clinical Presentation of Heat-Related Emergencies
Clinical Presentation	**Signs and Symptoms**
Heat cramps	Normal level of consciousness Slightly elevated body temperature Painful muscle spasms
Heat exhaustion	Mild ALOC Tachycardia, tachypnea, hypotension Core temperature 100.4°–104.0°F (38°–40°C) Fatigue Headache Diaphoresis
Heat stroke	Severe ALOC; confusion to coma Tachycardia, hypotension Core temperature >104.0°F (40°C) Flushed, dry skin Nausea and vomiting

patients often occurs without the benefit of an objective temperature.

Physiologic considerations in infants and toddlers with heat-related emergencies include: immature thermoregulatory systems, greater body surface area to mass ratio, and a lesser ability to dissipate heat (**Table 5-9**).

Assessment

The focused history should include:

- Environmental temperature
- Activities and events prior to symptom development
- Pre-existing medical conditions

Management

The management of heat-related illness depends on the severity of symptoms, especially the patient's level of consciousness and cardiovascular status.

Heat Cramps
- Cool environment
- Remove excess clothing
- Oral rehydration with an electrolyte containing solution
- Establish vascular access with normal saline at TKO rate

Heat Exhaustion
- Cool environment
- Cool mist or light sponging with tepid water and allow moisture to evaporate

Early recognition and frequent reassessment of a heat-related emergency is important, as the patient's temperature may continue to rise despite initial management techniques.

- Establish vascular access and initiate fluid replacement with crystalloid fluid at 20 mL/kg for treatment of shock

Heat Stroke
- Airway management, intubate if indicated
- Establish vascular access and fluid replacement with crystalloid fluid at 20 mL/kg
- Cool mist or light sponging with tepid water and allow moisture to evaporate
- Aggressive cooling measures: wet sheets, ice bags to axilla, groin, and neck
- Frequent re-measurement of core temperature
- Avoid shivering
- Treat for shock

Summary of Heat-Related Emergencies

Rapid recognition of heat-related emergencies is essential to effective management. Reassess vital signs frequently to evaluate the patient's response to treatment.

Cold-Related Emergencies

<u>Hypothermia</u> is a core temperature of less than 95°F (35°C). Infants and toddlers are at especially high risk for hypothermia, due to their greater body surface area to mass ratio, decreased body fat, increased permeability of thin skin, and limited ability to shiver and produce heat. Extended exposure to a cold environment and immersion in cold water are the two most common causes of hypothermia in young children. Children with severe illness or injury may also develop hypothermia. Finally, infants and young children may become hypothermic while being

exposed for medical evaluation, especially in cold environments. The presence of hypothermia may complicate resuscitation, regardless of the underlying condition.

Assessment

Focused history should include:

- Recent illness or injury
- Circumstances of exposure

The physical exam should include special attention to:

- Airway and breathing. Because hypothermia leads to a slowing of metabolism, the child may hypoventilate, with slow or shallow respirations

Circulation

Bradycardia and hypotension may be present due to hypothermia itself, or to a concurrent hypoxic insult. Hypothermia may also lead to cardiac dysrhythmias. Skin is often pale and cool.

Disability

Mental status may range from confusion to coma, depending on the degree of hypothermia. Again, hypoxia may be the underlying cause of ALOC, especially in submersion victims, so ensure the adequacy of oxygenation and ventilation.

Core Body Temperature

Obtain core body temperature, when possible, with a thermometer that registers below 94°F.

Determine degree of hypothermia:

- Mild: 93°F to 95°F (35°C–36°C)
- Moderate: 86°F to 93°F (30°C–34°C)
- Severe: < 86°F (< 30°C)

Loss of the compensatory mechanism of shivering to generate heat is characteristic of moderate to severe hypothermia.

Management

Management of the patient with hypothermia will depend on the core temperature.

1. *Support airway, breathing, and circulation as indicated.*

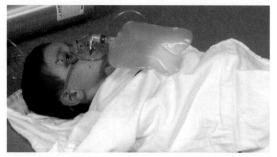

Figure 5-6 Provide warmed, humidified oxygen.

2. *Prevent heat loss.*
   In every hypothermic patient, prevention of further heat loss is key. Remove wet clothing, dry the skin, and cover the patient once the exam is completed. Apply a hat or head wrap because a high proportion of heat is lost through the head.

3. *Rewarm.*
   External rewarming is appropriate for mild-to-moderate hypothermia. In the case of severe hypothermia, external rewarming may shunt cold blood to the core, leading to further complications. Core rewarming in the ED is the appropriate therapy for these patients.

   a. Mild hypothermia: apply warm blankets, increase ambient temperature of the ambulance— prehospital professionals should be uncomfortably warm!

   b. Moderate hypothermia: warm blankets, heat packs to axilla and groin.

   Advanced Life Support

   c. Severe hypothermia: cautious movement, warmed, humidified oxygen (**Figure 5-6**), warmed IV solution, rapid transport to a definitive care facility for core rewarming.

Summary of Cold-Related Emergencies

Pediatric patients' physiologic and developmental characteristics place them at risk for the development of cold-related emergencies.

Tip

Use caution when rewarming the severely hypothermic pediatric patient in the prehospital environment, as cold acidemic blood from the periphery could lead to further deterioration. Focus instead on preventing further heat loss and supporting the ABCs.

Accurate assessment of the degree of hypothermia is essential to effective management of children in the prehospital environment.

Bites and Stings

Bites and stings typically result in a puncture type wound or laceration. The majority of these injuries will be minor. However, some stings, such as from the bumblebee or fire ant, may produce a severe allergic, or **anaphylactic reaction**. Some bites, such as from a rattlesnake or spider, can cause life-threatening **envenomations** or bleeding problems. Bites and stings may pose a greater risk to the pediatric patient because of their smaller body weight and higher metabolic rate.

Assessment

Focused history should include:

- Time and type of bite or sting
- Activities since the injury
- Known allergies to bites or stings
- Immunization history

The physical exam should include special attention to:

- Clinical presentation will vary depending on the type of bite, the presence or absence of envenomation, and the time since the bite occurred.
- Assess airway, breathing, and circulation; respiratory distress and **anaphylaxis** may be the initial signs of a bite envenomation.
- Inspect for type, anatomic location, and number of punctures or wounds.
- Assess for swelling, discoloration, and pain at or around the site.

Management: Bites

Management will depend on the type of insect, snake, or animal involved in the envenomation.

General Management

- Support airway, breathing and circulation, establish vascular access.
- Treat anaphylaxis if present (see Chapter 4).

Local Management

- Stop bleeding, perform wound care.
- If an envenomation is suspected, consider cool compresses or an ice pack to the affected area to reduce spread of venom.
- Minimize the activity level of the pediatric patient. Most venom is transported through the lymphatic system and increased physical activity will increase the rate of spread throughout the body.
- Immobilize an affected extremity at the level of the heart.

Tip

Abnormal behavior may be the first clue that the pediatric patient has been bitten or stung. A thorough inspection of the patient's skin, particularly around the waist, distal extremities, axillae, and neck may reveal the location of the bite or sting.

- Transport rapidly to evaluate for possible <u>antivenin</u> administration and for definitive care.
- Remove any clothing or jewelry on the affected area or limb.

Management: Stings

General Management

- Support airway, breathing and circulation, establish vascular access.
- Treat anaphylaxis if present (see Chapter 4).

Local Management

- Apply cold compresses.
- Consider medications based on clinical presentation: <u>diphenhydramine hydrochloride</u>.

Summary of Bites and Stings

Insect bites are common in children, and may result in complications ranging from mild local reaction to life-threatening anaphylaxis. Other types of envenomations, such as snake or scorpion stings, are more regionally specific. Early recognition of the nature of the injury is important. Field treatment of anaphylaxis may be life-saving. Prompt transport to a definitive care facility is key if antivenin treatment is needed.

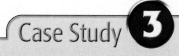

Case Study 3

A 6-year-old boy with a known allergy to bee stings has been playing outside in the garden. The caregiver calls 9-1-1 when the child develops noisy breathing. On arrival at the scene the PAT reveals a pale, irritable child, with audible stridor, and supraclavicular retractions. Respiratory rate is 32 breaths/min, heart rate is 140 beats/min, and blood pressure is 90 mm Hg/palpable. His skin is covered in pink welts.

1. What are the possible causes of respiratory distress in this child?
2. What are the immediate management priorities?

Chapter Review

Case Study Answers

Case Study **1** page 105

The child is physiologically stable, and can be further assessed on the scene. As you manage the child, allay the caregiver's fears. Use the opportunity to provide the caregiver with education regarding seizures and fever. Take a focused history. The story suggests a possible febrile seizure.

Transport all children with a history of seizure activity to the hospital because it is impossible to "diagnose" a febrile seizure in the field. There are many causes of seizures, including serious infections such as meningitis.

Limit field treatment to simple cooling methods if the child is still febrile. Do not sponge or bathe the child in cold water or alcohol to lower temperature; these methods can lead to shivering and actually can increase the core temperature. Reassess the patient frequently and be prepared for repeat seizures.

Advanced Life Support

If multiple seizures occur or a seizure lasts longer than 5 minutes, treat with a benzodiazepine; rectal or IV diazepam, IV or IM lorazepam, or IM midazolam. While brief seizures do not require pharmacologic treatment, prompt treatment of seizures lasting longer than 5 minutes will have the greatest success in terms of seizure cessation. Continuous, careful monitoring during transport is especially important if drug therapy has been given, since administration of benzodiazepines and phenobarbital can result in apnea or respiratory depression.

Case Study **2** page 113

Open and manage the airway with positioning. Administer 100% oxygen by nonrebreathing mask. If there is no trauma, place the patient in the sniffing position and use the jaw thrust maneuver to maintain the airway. If respirations are shallow or irregular, or if oxygen saturation is less than 90% on supplemental oxygen, assist ventilation with appropriate-sized bag-mask device. Insert an oropharyngeal or nasopharyngeal airway as needed to maintain a patent airway.

Advanced Life Support

Use a length-based resuscitation tape or computer software program, as described in Length-Based Equipment Sizing and Drug Dosing, Procedure 2, to determine drug doses. Rapidly assess the serum glucose. If the glucose level is less than 60 mg%, establish an IV and give $D_{25}W$ 2 mL/kg by IV bolus. If there is no IV access, give glucagon IM 1.0 mg. If bedside glucose determination is normal consider other causes of ALOC and consider administering naloxone 0.1 mg/kg (maximum 2 mg).

Case Study **3** page 125

A previously healthy child playing outdoors with an acute onset of respiratory distress should be assessed for bites and stings. This child's prior history of **hymenoptera** (bumblebee) allergy, the presence of hives in addition to respiratory distress and the sudden onset of symptoms all suggest anaphylaxis.

Provide supplemental oxygen and give inhaled bronchodilators for wheezing. Administer epinephrine SC.

Advanced Life Support

Establish vascular access and give IV diphenhydramine.

Even if the child shows marked improvement with these treatments, transport urgently, as symptoms may recur as the medication effect wears off. Monitor carefully during transport.

Suggested Readings

Textbooks

American Academy of Orthopaedic Surgeons: *Emergency Care and Transportation of the Sick and Injured,* 9th Edition. Sudbury, MA, Jones and Bartlett Publishers, 2005.

American Academy of Pediatrics and the American College of Emergency Physicians: *APLS: The Pediatric Emergency Medicine Resource,* 4th Edition. Sudbury, MA, Jones and Bartlett Publishers, 2004.

Baram T, Shinnar S: *Febrile Seizures.* San Diego, Academic Press, 2002.

Barkin R: *Pediatric Emergency Medicine,* 2nd Edition. St Louis, Mosby-Year Book, 1997.

Bledsoe B, Porter R, Cherry R: *Essentials of Paramedic Care,* New Jersey, Prentice Hall, 2003.

Hazinski M, Zaritsky A, Nadkarni V, et al: *PALS Provider Manual,* American Heart Association, 2002.

Articles

Freedman S, Powell E. Pediatric seizures and their management in the emergency department. *Clinical Pediatric Emergency Medicine.* Sep 2003; 4(3).

Reuter D. Common emergent pediatric neurologic problems. *Emerg Med Clin North Am.* Feb 2002; 20(1):155–76.

Warden CR. Evaluation and management of febrile seizures in the out-of-hospital and emergency department settings. *Ann Emerg Med.* Feb 2003; 41(2):215–22.

Trauma

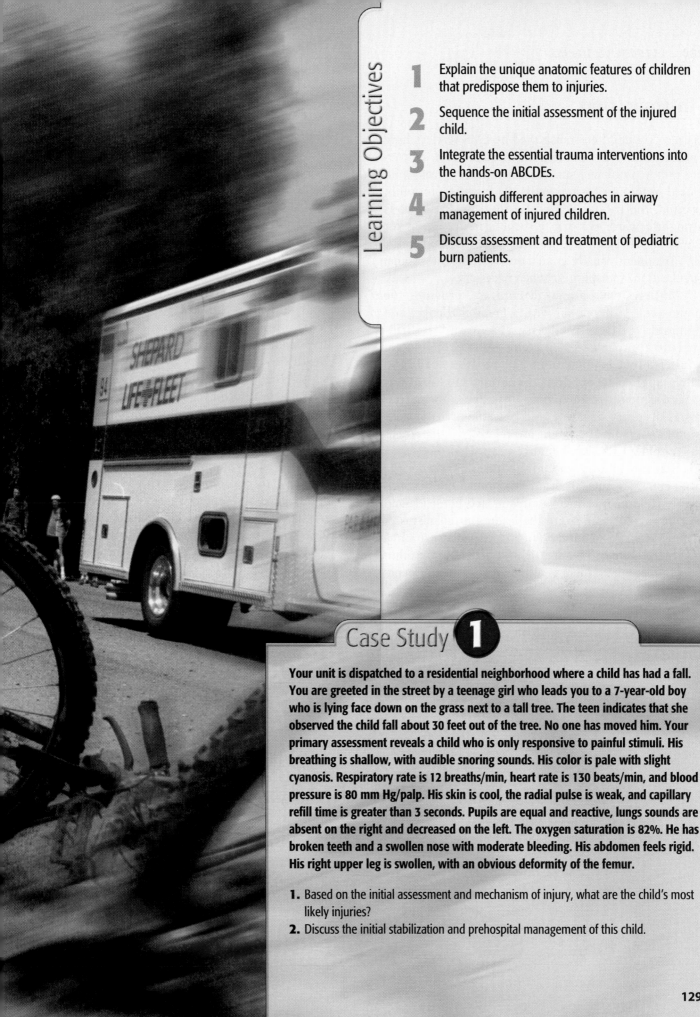

Learning Objectives

1 Explain the unique anatomic features of children that predispose them to injuries.

2 Sequence the initial assessment of the injured child.

3 Integrate the essential trauma interventions into the hands-on ABCDEs.

4 Distinguish different approaches in airway management of injured children.

5 Discuss assessment and treatment of pediatric burn patients.

Case Study 1

Your unit is dispatched to a residential neighborhood where a child has had a fall. You are greeted in the street by a teenage girl who leads you to a 7-year-old boy who is lying face down on the grass next to a tall tree. The teen indicates that she observed the child fall about 30 feet out of the tree. No one has moved him. Your primary assessment reveals a child who is only responsive to painful stimuli. His breathing is shallow, with audible snoring sounds. His color is pale with slight cyanosis. Respiratory rate is 12 breaths/min, heart rate is 130 beats/min, and blood pressure is 80 mm Hg/palp. His skin is cool, the radial pulse is weak, and capillary refill time is greater than 3 seconds. Pupils are equal and reactive, lungs sounds are absent on the right and decreased on the left. The oxygen saturation is 82%. He has broken teeth and a swollen nose with moderate bleeding. His abdomen feels rigid. His right upper leg is swollen, with an obvious deformity of the femur.

1. Based on the initial assessment and mechanism of injury, what are the child's most likely injuries?
2. Discuss the initial stabilization and prehospital management of this child.

Introduction

HALF OF THE children transported by EMS services have an acute injury. Fortunately, the most common injuries are minor problems, such as lacerations, burns, mild closed head injuries, and extremity fractures. In minor trauma, the role of the prehospital professional is straightforward: perform a scene size-up, assess for physiologic or anatomic problems, and transport to the ED. Treatment usually entails only wound care, spinal stabilization, and splinting when necessary.

Multisystem trauma, in contrast, provides the prehospital professional with a great challenge, and demands a disciplined assessment and a child-specific approach to treatment. Most principles of adult trauma management can be effectively and safely applied to children. Important modifications in assessment are related to differences in mechanisms of injury, anatomy, and physiologic responses. Modifications in treatment are related to differences in equipment sizes and emergency procedures.

Between infancy and adulthood, injuries are the most common cause of death. Intentional injuries, primarily child maltreatment in infants and homicide and suicide in adolescents, are the leading mechanisms of traumatic death. About 80% to 90% of pediatric trauma involves a blunt mechanism. This differs from the adult population, where there is a higher incidence of pene-trating injuries. Handgun injuries, however, are on the rise in children and are now the most common cause of penetrating injuries in adolescents.

Most injuries are preventable. Child restraint devices in automobiles, bicycle helmets, swimming pool fences, and window barriers have significantly reduced the incidence of blunt injuries and drownings. Stricter building codes have reduced the incidence of burns, although burns continue to be a leading cause of death in children under 12 years of age. Pediatric trauma challenges the prehospital professional to manage not just the injury and related physiologic abnormalities, but also to treat the child's pain and communicate with the injured child and the "injured family."

Death or serious injury of a child from trauma causes tremendous emotional stress on prehospital professionals, who may project feelings and fears about their own children's vulnerability onto the situation. This common provider response may lead to difficulty in maintaining an appropriate emotional distance, and it may compromise objective performance. Experience and education in the care of ill and injured children will help the prehospital professional have a greater sense of confidence, competency, and control in these stressful situations. Critical incident stress management may be valuable to the prehospital professional after treating a seriously injured child.

Fatal Injury Mechanisms

Table 6-1 summarizes the most frequent fatal mechanisms of injury in children and adolescents. Vehicular trauma (including automobile occupant, pedestrian, all-terrain vehicles [ATV], and bicyclist injuries) is the most common cause of death in all age groups. Drowning is the second leading cause. House fire is a significant cause of death, especially in the eastern United States. Falls are common, but rarely cause major injury unless the length of the fall is greater than the child's height and the stopping surface is unyielding, such as concrete.

Table 6-1	Leading Mechanisms of Injury-Related Death
Preschoolers/ Children	**School-aged**
Vehicular trauma	Vehicular trauma
Drowning	Drowning
Fires	Abuse
Abuse	Fires
Falls	Gunshot wounds

Unique Anatomic Features of Children: Effect on Injury Patterns

Head

Head injury is the most common cause of serious trauma in children. Even in multisystem trauma, the severity of <u>traumatic brain injury (TBI)</u> usually defines the

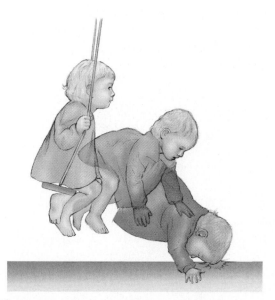

Figure 6-1 A disproportionately large head size in children explains their tendency to fall "head first," leading to a high rate of traumatic brain injury.

patient's medical and functional outcome. Many of the essential interventions in managing pediatric trauma are directed at preserving brain function.

Until early school age (5-years-old), the child's head is disproportionately large in relationship to overall body mass and surface area, when compared to adults. Because of this anatomic feature, in a fall or in an acceleration-deceleration event such as a motor vehicle crash, the head functions like the heavy end of a lawn dart, becoming the lead point (**Figure 6-1**). Consequently, the head and brain are more commonly injured in blunt trauma in children than adults.

Spinal Column

As a group, children do not suffer many vertebral fractures or dislocations. When vertebral fractures do occur, the event typically involves a high-energy mechanism (e.g., motor vehicle crash or diving incident) with axial loading of the spine or extreme flexion or extension. Traumatic spinal cord injury, or disruption of the central nerve pathways, is also rare in children. Spinal cord injury does occur without vertebral injury, however, when the cord is injured and there are no vertebral fractures.

It is difficult to find a cervical collar that really fits an infant or toddler. When a properly sized collar is not available, stabilize the child's spine on a long board with padding to prevent movement.

The most common cervical spine injuries in children occur at the level of the high cervical spine. Weaker neck muscles and spinal ligaments, in conjunction with a "heavy" head, create greater vulnerability to acceleration-deceleration forces common in motor vehicle crashes and falls. In reality, most children with high cervical injury are in full arrest on the scene and die despite all medical interventions.

The most common lower spine injuries occur in the mid to lower thoracic spine. Mechanisms include direct blows, falls, or spinal compression during a motor vehicle crash from improper seat belt use. The use of booster seats in vehicles may reduce these types of injuries by allowing proper fitting of the seat belt.

Chest

The ribs of the child are more pliable and compressible than those of the adult as they are comprised mainly of cartilage. For this reason, rib fractures and flail chest are uncommon in younger children, even with high energy transfers. On the other hand, this bony compressibility in conjunction with a chest wall that is poorly protected by fat or muscle, leads to transfer of energy

Injuries cause almost half the deaths among children from 1 to 4 years of age, and outrank all other causes of death combined among older children and adolescents.

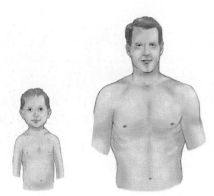

Figure 6-2 The child's chest wall is not well muscularized, so it lacks the soft tissue protection from injury that is present in adolescents and adults.

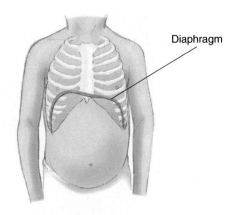

A

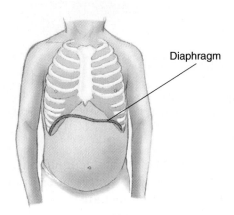

B

Figure 6-3 The diaphragm can rise as high as the nipple line during full expiration (A) and can flatten to the level of the lowest ribs during full inspiration (B). Therefore, injuries to the abdominal organs may occur after chest trauma.

on impact directly to the lungs and heart (**Figure 6-2**). Serious injuries of the thoracic organs can be present with or without external signs of injury, such as <u>abrasions</u>, bruises, or tenderness.

<u>Pulmonary contusion</u>, or bruising of the lung tissue itself, is the most common form of serious lung injury in children. You may suspect this condition in a child who sustains blunt chest trauma and has hypoxia or respiratory distress; however, pulmonary contusions can only be diagnosed by x-ray, which makes the distinction between pulmonary contusion and pneumothorax impossible in the field.

If a child has a blunt injury mechanism, be careful about placing a needle in the pleural space because a contusion is more likely than pneumothorax. In contrast, a child with hypoxia and respiratory distress after a penetrating injury probably does have a pneumothorax, and needle decompression is indicated.

The diaphragm of a child can rise as high as the nipple line during full expiration. When there is blunt or penetrating trauma to the chest below the nipple line or below the scapula, internal injury may include both chest and abdominal organs (**Figure 6-3 A and B**).

Penetrating chest trauma may cause serious problems in oxygenation and ventilation. When the chest wall, back, or high abdomen is penetrated, look for <u>tension pneumothorax</u> and <u>sucking chest wounds</u>. These injuries are unusual in children but, if present, require specific immedi-

Tip

Since the child's chest wall is smaller, thinner, and less muscular than an adult's, lung sounds may be transmitted throughout the chest cavity, making it difficult to appreciate asymmetric breath sounds. Listening along the lateral sides of the chest wall under the axillas (armpits) may improve the ability to distinguish sound variability between the right and left lungs.

ate life-saving treatment in the field. <u>Needle decompression</u> may save the life of a child with a tension pneumothorax. The procedure is similar for a child and adult, the major difference being the size of the catheter. The procedure is illustrated in

Needle Thoracostomy, Procedure 22.

If there is penetration of the chest wall below the nipples, or below the scapula, anticipate abdominal injury as well as tension pneumothorax.

Remember that young children rely heavily on their diaphragm to breathe. Do not restrict the abdomen when stabilizing the patient's spine.

Abdomen

The <u>abdomen</u> is often the site of serious blood loss in pediatric patients and is the most common site of injury causing shock. The solid organs of the upper abdominal cavity are the liver, <u>spleen</u>, and kidneys. These organs are disproportionately larger and more exposed than in adults and are poorly protected by the child's softer ribs and relatively undeveloped abdominal muscles (**Figure 6-4**). The spleen, located in the left upper quadrant, is one of the most commonly injured abdominal organs. Injuries to the hollow organs of the abdomen—the stomach, small bowel, and bladder—are less common than solid organ injuries. Although <u>pelvic fractures</u> are uncommon in children, they become more frequent in adolescents, who have adult anatomy.

Assume that every child with a serious trauma has a life-threatening abdominal injury. Many children with abdominal injury have no localizing signs and may not complain of pain. Fear, young age, or other distracting injuries may hide signs and symptoms. When present, signs include growing abdominal distention or rigidity, tenderness, abdominal wall contusions or abrasions, and hemodynamic instability. <u>Serial examinations</u> in timed intervals (5–10 minutes) may improve the accuracy of abdominal assessment.

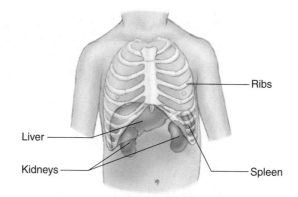

Figure 6-4 The solid organs of the upper abdominal cavity are disproportionately large and more exposed in children than in adults. They are poorly protected by the thin chest wall and undeveloped abdominal muscles.

The abdomen is the most frequent site of injury causing shock. Serial examinations greatly improve the accuracy of assessment of abdominal injury.

Never overlook the possibility of solid organ injury when there has been blunt injury, because fear, young age, or other distracting injuries may mask signs and symptoms.

Extremities

Children's bones are more flexible and their muscles are not as well developed as those of adults. They are especially vulnerable to fractures at the weak, cartilaginous growth plates at the ends of the bones (**Figure 6-5**). Fractures that disrupt the <u>periosteum</u> on only one side of the bone (often called <u>greenstick fractures</u>) are common, as are "<u>buckle fractures</u>" in which the pliant bone is compressed with <u>axial loading</u>. These fractures may be present in the absence of significant swelling, bruising, or deformity. *Suspect a fracture whenever there is point tenderness or limited range of motion, especially around a joint.*

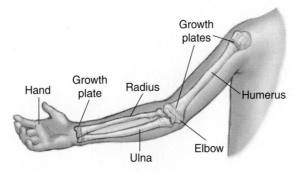

Figure 6-5 The physeal (growth) plates at the ends of children's bones are easily fractured.

The most serious complications of extremity injuries are <u>neurovascular</u> problems and blood loss into the soft tissues at the fracture site. Blood loss may be severe in long-bone fractures (e.g., fractures of the femur) or in pelvic fractures. The symptom usually associated with serious extremity injuries is pain.

Advanced Life Support

Pain is frequently underestimated and undertreated in children! Consider analgesia for pain management in children with isolated extremity fractures. <u>Morphine</u> sulfate is the medication of choice. Repeat with half doses as needed for pain control. Be extremely careful with morphine administration in children with a serious injury mechanism or signs of compensated or decompensated shock. Morphine can rapidly drop the child's blood pressure and critical perfusion when it is administered to a hypovolemic patient. Always be alert for signs of respiratory depression, especially if multiple doses of a narcotic are administered.

Suspect an extremity fracture whenever findings include point tenderness or limited range of motion.

Injuries to the <u>**physeal plate**</u> or growth plate of a long bone can be permanently damaging to the limb.

Skin

The skin provides temperature regulation. Children have more skin surface area in relation to their overall size and weight than do adults. Because of this, heat loss from the skin is rapid. Even without injuries such as burns that damage the skin, injured children are at increased risk for hypothermia, which can in turn compromise core organ function. The signs and symptoms of hypothermia can mimic those of hypovolemia and shock. To avoid hypothermia, especially in a preschool-aged child, prevent heat loss by ensuring that the child is dry and covered, and limiting time that the undressed child is exposed for assessment and procedures. Turn up the heat in the ambulance! For the temperature to be warm enough for an infant who is disrobed, it must be uncomfortably hot for an adult.

Mechanism of Injury: Effect on Injury Patterns

The different mechanisms of injury in children in combination with their unique anatomic features lead to predictable patterns of injury. Head injury due to blunt trauma is very common in children. While there are many cases of minor closed head injuries associated with play that do not have neurological consequences, high energy impacts are often associated with TBI. Because of a child's small size, high energy blunt impacts can lead to <u>multisystem trauma</u>, including the head, chest, abdomen, and long bones.

Table 6-2 lists the common mechanisms of pediatric injury and the associated patterns of injury. **Figure 6-6 A–D** illustrates several typical injury sequences in children.

Table 6-2	Common Mechanisms and Associated Patterns of Pediatric Injury*	
Mechanism of Injury	**Associated Patterns of Injury**	
Motor vehicle crash (child is passenger)	Unrestrained	Multiple trauma, head and neck injuries, scalp and facial lacerations
	Air bag	Head and neck, facial and eye injuries
	Restrained	Chest and abdominal injuries, cervical and lower-spine fractures
Motor vehicle crash (child is pedestrian)	Low speed	Lower-extremity fractures
	High speed	Chest and abdominal injuries, head and neck injuries, lower-extremity fractures
Fall from a height	Low	Upper-extremity fractures
	Medium	Head and neck injuries, upper- and lower-extremity fractures
	High	Chest and abdominal injuries, head and neck injuries, upper- and lower-extremity fractures
Fall from a bicycle	Without helmet	Head and neck injuries, scalp and facial lacerations, upper-extremity fractures
	With helmet	Upper-extremity fractures
	Hitting handlebar	Internal abdominal injuries

*Adapted from *Teaching Resource for Instructors in Prehospital Pediatrics (TRIPP),* 1998 Version 2.0, Center for Pediatric Emergency Medicine (CPEM), New York, NY.

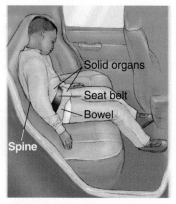

Figure 6-6 A A restrained child in a motor vehicle crash may have a lap belt injury involving the solid organs, the bowel, and the spine.

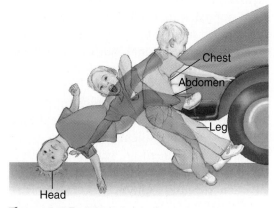

Figure 6-6 B Children frequently sustain multisystem injuries involving the head, chest, abdomen, and long bones.

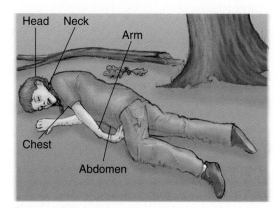

Figure 6-6 C A fall from height frequently involves injuries to the head and neck, chest, abdomen, and the extremities.

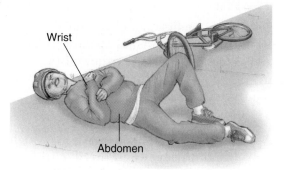

Figure 6-6 D A fall over the handlebars of a bike may result in injuries to the abdomen and extremities.

Assessment of the Injured Child

The initial steps in assessing the injured child follow the generic approach for all children outlined in Chapters 1 and 2. This includes pre-arrival mental preparation based on dispatch information and a scene size-up on arrival. Always use <u>universal precautions</u> or personal protective measures and equipment to prevent potentially harmful or infectious exposures to bodily fluids.

The on-scene trauma evaluation includes: (1) general assessment using the PAT; (2) the initial assessment with the hands-on ABCDEs, then (3) additional assessment consisting of a focused history and physical exam and a detailed physical exam (trauma). A child with multisystem injuries needs a prioritized, efficient on scene approach to assessment and treatment, and rapid transport to the ED. Typically, the prehospital professional will get no further than the initial assessment of a child with multisystem trauma, since the recognition and management of life-threatening physiologic problems will be the focus of field care. The anatomical problems identified in the additional assessment are generally not life-threatening, and can be treated in the hospital when the child is physiologically stable.

The General Assessment

The PAT

The PAT is the first part of the initial assessment of trauma as well as medical patients, and allows rapid determination of the type of physiologic disturbance, severity of injury, and urgency of treatment.

Appearance

Appearance reflects brain function, which may be abnormal in injured children because of <u>primary brain injury</u> (caused by direct trauma to the brain tissue itself) or <u>secondary brain injury</u> (caused by an indirect insult to the brain tissue by hypoxia or ischemia). The most likely causes of abnor-

There are many potential causes of abnormal appearance in a pediatric trauma patient, including closed head injury; hypoxia; hemorrhage; and pain from fractures, burns, and soft-tissue injuries.

mal appearance in a pediatric trauma patient are: closed head injury; hypoxia; hemorrhage; and pain from fractures, burns, and <u>soft-tissue injuries</u>.

Toxins may also cause an abnormal appearance, but are uncommon causes of poor responsiveness in the preschool and school-aged trauma patient. However, toxins—most often recreational drugs—are an important contributor to trauma in the adolescent, who may incur injuries due to high risk behaviors while "under the influence." **Table 6-3** lists common causes of abnormal appearance in injured children.

Table 6-3	Common Causes of Abnormal Appearance in Injured Children
Category of Injury	**Examples**

Primary brain injuries	Closed head injury
	    Brain edema
	    Concussion
	    Contusion
	    Intracranial hematoma
	    Intracranial hemorrhage
	    Penetrating brain injuries

Secondary brain injuries	Hemorrhage with hypoperfusion/shock due to:
	    Solid organ abdominal injury
	    Hemothorax
	    Pelvic fracture
	Hypoxia due to:
	    Aspiration of gastric contents
	    Failure of central respiratory drive
	    Pulmonary contusion
	    Smoke inhalation
	    Tension pneumothorax

Pain	Burns Fractures Soft-tissue injuries
Toxins	Alcohol Recreational drugs Carbon monoxide

Table 6-4	Injury Causes of Increased Work of Breathing in Injured Children
Cause	**Examples**
Airway injuries	Hematomas or lacerations of the tongue, mouth, or neck Smoke and hot gas inhalation Penetrations into the upper airway
Chest injuries	Pulmonary contusion Sucking chest wound Tension pneumothorax/hemothorax
Abdominal injuries	Diaphragmatic injury Solid or hollow viscus injury with pain and "splinting"

Work of Breathing

Work of breathing is increased by injuries that affect the airway, lungs, or pleura. **Table 6-4** summarizes the causes of increased work of breathing in pediatric trauma patients. Effortless tachypnea, or a rapid respiratory rate in the absence of increased work of breathing, may be seen in a child with traumatic shock. This is a reflexive mechanism to compensate for <u>metabolic acidosis</u> caused by <u>hypoperfusion</u> by "blowing-off" carbon dioxide.

Listen for abnormal airway sounds, such as stridor or change of speech, which may reflect tracheal injury or obstruction. Wheezing reflects lower airway irritation and bronchospasm. This may occur from inhalation of vaporized toxins, as in a house fire. Grunting indicates decreased gas exchange at the level of the alveoli, and may be seen with pulmonary contusion. After listening, look for retractions and nasal flaring to further assess for hypoxia.

Circulation to Skin

Circulation to skin reflects the blood flow to the skin and mucous membranes. If skin color and skin temperature are abnormal in an injured child who is not in a cold environment, it suggests hypovolemia and poor perfusion. Hemorrhage from abdominal solid organ injury is the most common cause of hypoperfusion and shock in pediatric trauma patients. An isolated closed

head injury cannot account for signs of hypoperfusion or shock in children outside of infancy, since the closed space of the skull cannot accommodate a significant volume of blood. However, infants can lose large volumes of blood based on intracranial bleeding, because the plates of their skull (sutures) are not yet fused, and the skull can expand under pressure. *Because of their large surface to volume ratio, children are at higher risk than adults to develop hypovolemia and shock.*

Figure 6-7 and **Figure 6-8** show the PAT findings for the two most common patterns of major pediatric trauma: closed head injury and multisystem injury.

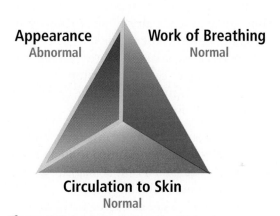

Figure 6-7 A patient with closed head injury has an abnormal appearance, but normal work of breathing and normal circulation to skin.

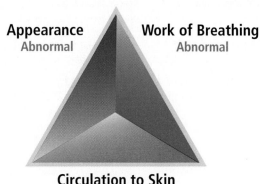

Figure 6-8 A patient with multiple system injury has an abnormal appearance, abnormal work of breathing, and abnormal circulation to skin.

The Initial Assessment

Hands-on ABCDEs

The ABCDEs are the hands-on initial assessment. The trauma ABCDEs have a special focus on spinal precautions and control of blood loss.

The pediatric assessment, including the PAT and ABCDEs, does not require any specialized equipment. Potentially life-threatening problems should be treated as they are identified in the ABCDE sequence. **Table 6-5** lists the key features of the pediatric trauma ABCDEs and interventions specific to the trauma patient.

Airway

Airway is always the first priority. Trauma victims are at risk for airway obstruction from bleeding, <u>emesis</u>, edema, or foreign objects. TBI may cause loss of protective airway reflexes or impair central respiratory drive.

Consider spinal injury in a child with any of the following:

- A mechanism of injury involving high velocity forces transmitted to the head or spine (e.g., fall from a height, ejection from a motor vehicle)
- Physical evidence of trauma to the head or spine (e.g., scalp hematoma, tenderness to palpation of the cervical spine)

Tip

Adult equipment must be adapted to properly immobilize a child. Use of pediatric immobilization devices can speed the process, but is not necessary to achieve full spinal stabilization.

- Altered level of consciousness (ALOC)
- Neck or back pain
- Weakness or numbness

If the child has any of these findings, stabilize the entire spine while managing the airway. While great care must be taken to prevent further injury in the unlikely event of an unstable spine injury, these concerns must not take precedence over appropriate management of the child's airway. *An injured child is far more likely to die from untreated hypoxia or shock than spinal trauma.*

Actions If airway obstruction is present, use a modified jaw thrust maneuver combined with manual spinal in-line stabilization (**Figure 6-9**) to establish and maintain airway patency. Insert an <u>airway adjunct</u> if unable to maintain an open airway and the child has no gag reflex. Use suction to clear any fluid or Magill forceps to remove foreign bodies from the mouth, nose, or upper airway. Be prepared to turn the child on his side and suction if he vomits, to prevent aspiration of stomach contents. Quickly but carefully

Table 6-5	Pediatric Trauma ABCDEs
Element of Assessment	**Special Interventions**
Airway	Modified jaw thrust maneuver while maintaining cervical spine stabilization Consider airway adjunct
Breathing	Needle thoracostomy Dressing to sucking chest wound
Circulation	External hemorrhage control Splinting of fractured extremity
Disability	Elevated intracranial pressure management (head midline, head of backboard up, assisted ventilation to maintain normal CO_2 levels)
Exposure	Prevent heat loss

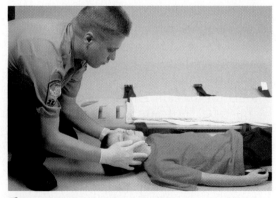

Figure 6-9 If airway obstruction is suspected in a child with possible spine injuries, use the modified jaw thrust maneuver combined with manual spinal in-line stabilization.

Never let concern for spinal injury compromise appropriate management of the child's airway.

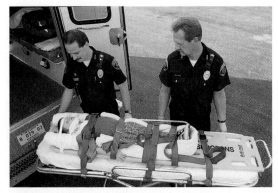

Figure 6-10 Spinal stabilization must secure the body so that there is no spinal movement.

logroll the patient if vomiting occurs before he is secured to a spine board. Once the spine is fully stabilized, the entire backboard can be turned, if necessary to protect the child from aspiration.

Spinal Stabilization The spinal column is made of 33 articulating bones, the vertebrae, and its structure changes significantly during childhood growth. The incidence and type of spinal injuries will depend on the age of the child and the mechanism of injury, which in turn is influenced by the child's developmental level and activity. Cervical spine trauma can lead to <u>quadriplegia</u>, the most devastating type of spinal injury. Always perform complete spinal stabilization including stabilization of the thoracic and lumbar areas (**Figure 6-10**). Spinal cord injuries and life-long paralysis may follow thoracic or lumbar trauma. For a step-by-step explanation of this procedure see

(Spinal Stabilization, Procedure 21).

Breathing

Breathing is the second priority in the ABCDEs. Injuries to the airway, chest wall, lungs, or abdomen as well as gastric distention due to air swallowing may compromise oxy-genation and ventilation. Head and cervical spine injuries will sometimes depress central respiratory drive or diminish protective airway reflexes. Pulmonary aspiration of gastric contents is a common and potentially serious complication of head injuries that results in hypoxia and increased work of breathing.

Look for soft-tissue or penetrating injuries of the chest or back. Watch for the adequacy and symmetry for chest rise, and then listen with a stethoscope to assess air entry and equality of breath sounds. Feel the chest wall for <u>crepitus</u>, pain, or instability. Apply a pulse oximeter to assess for hypoxia, as pallor and cyanosis can be late findings. A normal pulse oximetry reading does not, however, rule out respiratory distress. A child with profound tachypnea or increased work of breathing may need assisted ventilation regardless of the reading on the oximeter, if he exhausts his compensatory mechanisms.

Actions If breathing is inadequate, position the child and assist ventilation. Pull the jaw

Case Study **2**

You are dispatched to a local recreation field where a 4-year-old boy was struck in the head by a baseball that was hit into the stands. The child has a large hematoma on his forehead and is crying inconsolably in his father's arms. The child did not lose consciousness but is not making eye contact with you or his dad. Other than his altered appearance, the PAT is normal and the hands-on ABCDEs reveals normal vital signs and no other apparent injuries. The child becomes increasingly somnolent during your assessment, and is difficult to arouse.

1. What is the child's greatest threat to life?
2. What interventions are required?

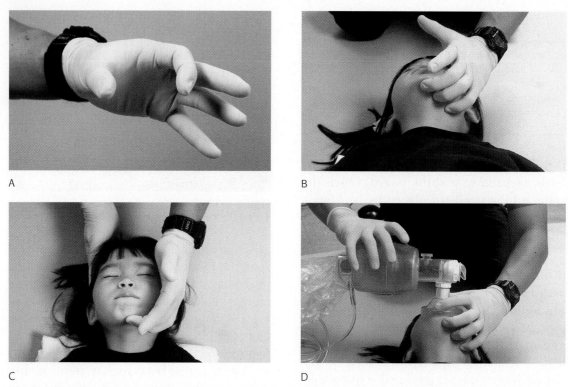

Figure 6-11 The E-C clamp technique will facilitate proper hand placement for good mask-to-face seal. (A) Hand displaying E-C shape. (B) Fingers resting on bony ridge of jaw. (C) Fingers positioned to hold mask. (D) Bag-mask ventilation in place.

into the mask. Pushing the mask onto the face to make a seal may cause cervical spine flexion. The E-C clamp technique (**Figure 6-11 A–D**) will help with proper hand placement for good mask-to-face seal. Consider inserting an airway adjunct to help maintain an open airway, although an oral airway will not be tolerated by a child with an intact gag reflex.

Give 100% oxygen or bag-mask ventilation. Use a properly fitted oxygen mask. Provide assisted ventilation with a bag-mask device if the child's respiratory effort is inadequate or if he has deteriorating cardiopulmonary or mental status. Use the "squeeze-release-release" timing technique, as the tendency is to bag too fast. Allow a brief pause between each breath to minimize the chance of gastric distention. *Only hyperventilate children who are experiencing brain stem herniation.* Be extremely careful, because hyperventilation may decrease perfusion to the brain. The pupillary reactions can help guide rate of ventilation in a child with suspected brain stem herniation, as outlined in **Table 6-6.** In each breath, provide only enough tidal volume to just achieve chest rise.

Table 6-6	Using Pupils to Guide Ventilation Rates in Closed Head Injury
Patient Category	**Rate of Ventilation**
Pupils equal	Normal for age[a]
Both pupils fixed and dilated	Above normal rate,[b] until pupils constrict
Pupils asymmetric	Above normal rate,[b] until pupil constricts
Child posturing	Above normal rate,[b] until posturing stops

[a]30 breaths/min for infants; 20 breaths/min for toddlers and children
[b]35 breaths/min for infants; 25 breaths/min for toddlers and children

Treating penetrating chest injuries, sucking chest wounds, impaled objects, and tension pneumothorax in pediatrics is the same as in adults. Cover sucking chest wounds with an <u>occlusive dressing</u>, such as a petrolatum gauze, taped on three sides (**Figure 6-12**) or a specially designed bandage/seal for sucking chest wounds. This technique will allow trapped air to escape while helping to prevent the entrance of air and development of tension pneumothorax. *Do not remove impaled objects.* Instead, stabilize them in place.

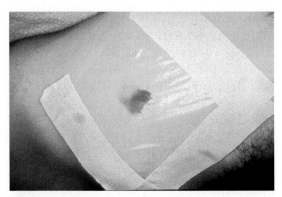

Figure 6-12 Management of a sucking chest wound. Cover sucking chest wounds with an occlusive dressing such as a petrolatum gauze taped on three sides.

Tip

Pulmonary aspiration of gastric contents is a common and potentially serious complication of head injuries.

Tip

If a patient with penetrating chest trauma also has respiratory distress, hypoxia, and hypoperfusion, perform needle decompression to treat possible tension pneumothorax.

Advanced Life Support

Management of Tension Pneumothorax If a patient with penetrating chest trauma also has respiratory distress, hypoxia, and hypoperfusion, perform **needle decompression** to treat possible tension pneumothorax.

Needle decompression may also be necessary in the child with blunt chest injury if the child has serious blunt chest-wall injury and respiratory distress, especially if he worsens with assisted ventilation. In this situation, when there is a closed pneumothorax, positive pressure ventilation quickly increases the air pressure in the **pleural space**, creating a dangerous level of "tension." Tension pneumothorax not only compromises ventilation of the affected lung,

but impairs venous return to the heart. This can lead to shock unresponsive to fluid resuscitation. Needle decompression of the pneumothorax will improve oxygenation, ventilation, and perfusion. For a step-by-step explanation of this procedure, see Needle Thoracostomy, Procedure 22.

Management of Gastric Distention with a Nasogastric/Orogastric Tube Assisted ventilation or prolonged crying can cause air swallowing and gastric distention. Nasogastric (NG) or orogastric (OG) tube placement may improve ventilation by decreasing the upward pressure on the diaphragm caused by the distended stomach, and reduce the risk of vomiting. If possible, insert an NG tube after endotracheal intubation of a comatose patient, because positive pressure ventilation can cause gastric inflation even in an intubated child. **Contraindications** for NG insertion include midfacial trauma and suspected **basilar skull fracture** (raccoon's eyes, Battle's sign, or suspected CSF rhinorrhea or otorrhea) because of the risk of passing the tube through the disrupted cribiform plate into the cranial vault. In these cases, perform OG insertion. Weigh the benefits of **gastric decompression** against the possible complications of vomiting and aspiration during passage of the tube or tube misplacement into the trachea. For a step-by-step explanation of this procedure, see Orogastric and Nasogastric Tube Insertion, Procedure 10.

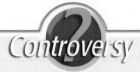

Controversy

Studies suggest that rapid administration of crystalloid fluids to adult patients with internal bleeding due to penetrating trauma may worsen outcome. These studies have not been confirmed in children, who usually sustain blunt trauma. In the absence of data to change practice, provide aggressive volume resuscitation of the pediatric trauma patient with signs of shock.

Frequently reassess heart rate, preferably with an electronic monitor. Tachycardia may be a response to pain, fear, cold, or anxiety, but a trend of rising heart rate suggests ongoing blood loss.

Circulation

Multisystem pediatric trauma more often involves respiratory failure than shock. Sometimes, however, shock develops because of external or internal bleeding, pneumothorax, spinal injury, or pump failure due to cardiac contusion or **tamponade**. The combination of the PAT and the hands-on ABCDEs allow ongoing perfusion evaluation. Measure heart rate continuously with a cardiac monitor, or with frequent pulse checks. Tachycardia may be due to pain, fear, cold, or anxiety, but a trend of rising heart rate suggests ongoing blood loss. Blood pressure measurement is not a good indicator of hypovolemia, since a child can be in compensated shock with a normal blood pressure. Blood pressure is mainly useful if it is low. When there is frank hypotension, assume the child is in decompensated shock. If it is significantly higher than normal in a child with possible TBI, consider possible **intracranial hypertension**.

Because of the technical challenges of obtaining a reliable blood pressure (due mainly to having the proper cuff size) and because skin signs, capillary refill time, and pulse quality are good signs of perfusion, make only one attempt at obtaining a blood pressure in children over 3 years of age. Make sure the blood pressure cuff size is correct, or the measurement will be inaccurate. In children *under* 3 years of age, taking the time on scene to get a blood pressure is of limited value.

Advanced Life Support

Controversies in Volume Resuscitation of the Pediatric Trauma Patient The indications, technique, and rate of volume resuscitation for perfusion support of the pediatric trauma patient are controversial. Recent studies suggest that rapid use of crystalloid fluids may worsen outcome in adult patients with internal bleeding from penetrating injury. In this circumstance, **volume resuscitation** increases perfusion, which in turn increases the rate of bleeding. Dislodgment of a clot may also be a factor as well as progressive dilution of red cells with crystalloid, which may further decrease oxygen carrying capacity. However, shock in most pediatric patients is due to blunt trauma, not penetrating major vessel injury. The applicability of the adult research in penetrating injury on volume resuscitation in pediatric blunt trauma victims is unknown. Treat traumatic shock in children with isotonic fluids. However, a child with ongoing hemorrhage is likely to lose more blood during prolonged attempts to establish vascular access at the scene than can be replaced during transport with crystalloid. Therefore, crystalloid treatment is detrimental if transport is delayed. Infuse enough fluids to maintain core perfusion. Reassess fluid status frequently, and stop hemorrhages if possible.

Do not use **military anti-shock trousers (MAST)** in children. The leg compartments may cause ischemia to the lower extremities and the abdominal compartment may compromise ventilation by impairing diaphragmatic movement. In adults, MAST do not appear to improve outcome from multiple trauma. No controlled studies in children are available at this time.

Actions Stop any visible external bleeding with direct pressure on the wound. Use sterile gauze compresses, and use gloves and personal protective equipment. Splint any extremities with obvious deformity. Apply oxygen and place the child in a supine position for transport.

Begin transport when the airway is properly secured, ventilation is adequate, and the child's spine is fully stabilized.

Volume Resuscitation If the child has signs of shock or significant ongoing blood loss, obtain vascular access and start volume resuscitation on the way to the ED. Look first for peripheral IV sites in the upper extremities or external jugular vein. Attempt to secure two lines. Insert an IO needle if IV access is problematic *and* the child has signs of decompensated shock.

In a poorly perfused patient, administer 20 cc/kg of crystalloid fluid as quickly as possible. Use a pressurized system or the pull-push method, with an in-line, three-way stopcock and a large syringe to maximize the infusion rate (**Figure 6-13 A and B**). Repeat 20 mL/kg boluses as needed to improve appearance and stabilize vital signs.

Never delay transport in an effort to establish vascular access. Only about one-third of crystalloid remains in the vessels after administration, and crystalloid has no useful oxygen-carrying capacity. The benefits of crystalloid administration are outweighed by the risks of ongoing hemorrhage with prolonged scene time.

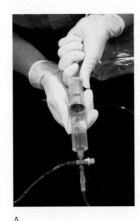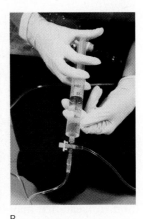

A   B

Figure 6-13 Infuse boluses using a pressurized system or the pull-push method with an in-line, three-way stopcock and a large syringe. (A) Pull fluid bolus into syringe after turning stopcock off to patient. (B) Push fluid bolus into patient after turning stopcock off to IV bag.

Military anti-shock trousers (MAST) have not been proven to be useful, and may be dangerous in children. They may cause ischemia to the lower extremities or limit ventilation.

Disability

Disability in the context of trauma care relates to TBI or spinal cord trauma. Injuries may be open or closed. Children may have primary or secondary brain injuries, or both.

Primary brain injury is the direct result of the traumatic insult and may include brain hemorrhage, cerebral edema (brain swelling), or diffuse <u>axonal shearing</u>. Increased intracranial pressure may develop quickly

after primary brain injury. Untreated, the downward spiral of increased intracranial pressure can lead to <u>brain stem herniation</u>, cardiopulmonary arrest, and <u>brain death</u>. By the time that the prehospital professional reaches the scene, any damage incurred from the primary brain injury is complete.

Secondary brain injury results from central nervous system hypoxia and/or ischemia. The prehospital professional has a key role in preventing secondary brain injury. Hypoxia may be the result of airway or chest injury, or of compromised central respiratory drive due to the primary brain injury. Brain ischemia may result from hemorrhage, usually in the abdomen or chest. Ensuring adequate oxygenation, ventilation, and perfusion is the key to preventing secondary brain injury.

A 9-1-1 call sometimes involves an infant with altered level of consciousness, apnea, or seizures with no report of preceding trauma. Assessment of these infants may not reveal any physical exam findings suggestive of head trauma or TBI, despite the fact that they have sustained severe traumatic brain injury. This is a typical scenario in <u>shaken baby syndrome</u>, where the infant is forcibly shaken by a caregiver, sometimes with impact of the baby's head against a fixed object. This mechanism involves severe acceleration-deceleration forces to the infant's brain and consequent <u>diffuse axonal injury</u> and/or intracranial hemorrhage. Shaken baby syndrome is further discussed in Chapter 12.

Assess the injured child's degree of neurologic disability with the AVPU scale (see Table 1-9). Disability, as categorized in the AVPU scale, is not the same as "abnormal appearance" in the PAT. An injured child may have an abnormal appearance for many reasons other than brain or spinal cord injury, such as pain, fear, shock, hypoxia, or intoxication. Appearance may be quite abnormal in a child who is "alert" on the AVPU scale. Appearance is a more subtle indicator of overall physiologic function in children than AVPU. The AVPU scale is more helpful in categorizing children with severe neurologic insults, including critical primary or secondary brain injuries.

Some EMS systems use a Pediatric Glasgow Coma Scale (PGCS) to assess neurological injury (**Table 6-7**). Neither the AVPU score nor the PGCS have been validated in young children. Though both systems attempt to objectively assess neurologic function, the AVPU is less complex and easier to remember. When using the PGCS, pay special attention to the motor component of the score, which has the highest value in predicting neurologic outcome from TBI.

After evaluating the level of consciousness with AVPU or the PGCS, note abnormal positioning and seizures, and check for pupil size, symmetry, and <u>reactivity</u>. The pupils provide important information about brainstem function and the papillary exam will help determine the need for hyperventilation in comatose patients.

Actions In pediatric trauma patients with AVPU scores of P or U, provide assisted ventilation to maintain good oxygenation and adequate ventilation. Hypoxia is an important cause of secondary brain injury in these children with TBI. Hypoxia may be associated with increased intracranial pressure, a situation that may occur rapidly and sometimes deceptively in a child with a primary brain injury.

Children with TBI require careful oxygenation/ventilation, but the rate of ventilation is controversial. While hyperventilation was widely recommended in the past

Table 6-7	Pediatric Glasgow Coma Scale	
Score	**Child**	**Infant**
Eyes		
4	Opens eyes spontaneously	Opens eyes spontaneously
3	Opens eyes to speech	Opens eyes to speech
2	Opens eyes to pain	Opens eyes to pain
1	No response	No response
_____ = Score (Eyes)		
Motor		
6	Obeys commands	Spontaneous movements
5	Localizes	Withdraws to touch
4	Withdraws	Withdraws to pain
3	Flexion	Flexion (decorticate)
2	Extension	Extension (decerebrate)
1	No response	No response
_____ = Score (Motor)		
Verbal		
5	Oriented	Coos and babbles
4	Confused	Irritable cry
3	Inappropriate words	Cries to pain
2	Incomprehensible words	Moans to pain
1	No response	No response
_____ = Score (Verbal)		
_____ = Total Score (Eyes, Motor, Verbal) Scores will range from 3 to 15		

Source: James HE, Anas NG, and Perkin RM. *Brain Insults in Infants and Children.* Orlando, FL: Grune & Stratton; 1985. Reprinted with permission.

as a way of rapidly decreasing intracranial pressure, extreme hyperventilation can itself cause decreased brain perfusion and secondary brain injury. In addition, there are no data that demonstrate improved neurological outcomes for patients who have been hyperventilated. Reserve hyperventilation for victims of TBI who have signs of impending brain stem herniation, and use appropriate breathing rates and tidal volumes, as outlined in **Table 6-6.**

If the patient with TBI has <u>impending herniation syndrome</u>, use mild hyperventilation. Consider this intervention if the child has a severe neurologic disability, as defined by a rating of P or U on the AVPU scale, a score of less than 9 on the PGCS; and a fixed and <u>dilated</u> pupil, <u>asymmetric</u> pupils, or <u>posturing</u>

(<u>decerebrate</u> or <u>decorticate</u>). Ventilate at a rate that is 5 breaths/min more than recommended for age. The rate, for example, is 35 breaths/min in an infant less than 1-year-old, or 25 breaths/min in a child older than 1 year. When the pupils constrict or the posturing stops, resume the normal ventilation rate for age.

Advanced Life Support

Management of Elevated Intracranial Pressure If the child has ALOC (not alert on AVPU or <15 on the PGCS), anticipate elevated intracranial pressure. Take a graded approach to intracranial pressure management, always balancing risks and benefits of treatment.

- Support the patient's head in a midline position to facilitate jugular venous return to the heart.
- If the patient is not in shock, elevate the backboard. Ensure adequate oxygenation and ventilation.
- Consider hyperventilation only in patients with signs of impending herniation syndrome.
- If there is head injury and hypovolemia, administer fluid to maintain brain perfusion. The injured brain hates ischemia!
- <u>Mannitol</u> may be useful to acutely decrease intracranial pressure in the child with asymmetric pupils or posturing, but

must be used with caution in a child with associated injuries who is at risk for hemorrhagic shock.

Exposure

Exposure is the last step in the initial assessment. Good exposure allows full assessment of the child's entire anatomy, including the extremities. Quickly examine the back during the spinal stabilization procedure for soft-tissue or penetrating injuries. Assess circulation and neurologic function <u>distal</u> to obvious or suspected extremity injuries. Although not usually life-threatening, complicated extremity injuries (such as open fractures of the humerus or femur) may cause significant blood loss and pain. Remember to cover the patient after the exam to prevent heat loss and hypothermia.

Summary

The assessment of the injured child requires knowledge of anatomic and functional differences that lead to pediatric-specific patterns of injury. The child's airway is small and easily obstructed, the lungs are vulnerable to contusion, and the solid organs and long bones are poorly protected. The prehospital professional's primary role in multisystem trauma is to ensure an open airway, assist ventilation, and minimize secondary brain injury. Treatment goals are to avoid hypoxia and hypotension. Short time on scene and rapid transport to the ED are over-riding priorities for all children who are physiologically unstable or have concerning mechanisms of injury. Vascular access and volume resuscitation are secondary tasks to be considered on the way to the hospital.

Use assisted ventilation to maintain oxygenation and to avoid carbon dioxide retention in pediatric trauma patients with AVPU scale scores of P or U.

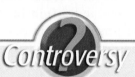

The rate of ventilation in comatose patients is controversial. No one has studied enough children with serious closed head injury to know at what point the benefit of hyperventilation and reduction of cerebral blood flow to decrease intracranial pressure outweighs the associated risk of brain ischemia.

In the out-of-hospital environment, endotracheal intubation is not always the optimal airway management tool.

Special Airway Considerations in Pediatric Trauma

Children with severe head injuries with neurologic disability and impending herniation often require field interventions to:

- Protect the airway and prevent aspiration
- Improve or control ventilation
- Improve or control oxygenation

Optimal airway management balances the potential risks of the procedure against the potential benefits to the patient. While endotracheal intubation has long been considered the best method for airway

Do not attempt blind nasotracheal intubation in children.

management in a critically injured patient, the procedural risks are significant. These risks may include prolonged scene time, worsened hypoxia, vomiting and aspiration, elevation of intracranial pressure during laryngoscopy, or a misplaced tube. The decision to support ventilation using a bag-mask device versus an endotracheal tube is a complex one, and must take into consideration the following factors:

- Risk of increasing intracranial pressure (by increasing the child's combativeness or inducing gagging during intubation procedure)
- Ability to access the airway
- Length of on scene and transport times
- Personnel availability and experience
- Ability to perform rapid sequence intubation (RSI)

Table 6-8 lists the factors that the prehospital professional must consider to choose the optimal airway management approach for each patient.

Table 6-8	Factors Influencing Optimal Airway Management Decisions
Factors Favoring BLS (Bag-mask ventilation)	
Combativeness, strong gag reflex	
Presence of **trismus** (spasm of jaw muscles)	
Short on scene and transport times	
Factors Favoring ALS (endotracheal intubation)	
Inability to ventilate with a bag-mask device	
Unresponsive child	
Absent gag reflex	
Apnea, poor muscle tone	
Long extrication or transport times	
Limited personnel to assist during transport	
Availability of RSI	

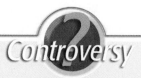

Rapid sequence intubation for pediatric endotracheal intubation, with sedatives and paralyzing drugs, is standard practice in many EDs and in a limited number of EMS regions. Its effectiveness and safety in the field are controversial.

Advanced Airway Management of the Pediatric Trauma Patient

If a severely injured child needs endotracheal intubation, the preferred path is orotracheal, with manual neutral stabilization of the cervical spine see

Orogastric and Nasogastric Tube Insertion, Procedure 10 .

Although blind nasotracheal intubation may cause less cervical spine motion in the adult than the orotracheal technique, the procedure is not applicable to children because of the anterior location of the <u>larynx</u> and the increased risk of <u>adenoidal</u> bleeding. *Do not attempt blind nasotracheal intubation in any child younger than 8 years of age.*

RSI for pediatric endotracheal intubation, with sedatives and paralyzing drugs, is standard practice in many EDs and in a limited number of EMS regions. Its effectiveness, safety, and feasibility are controversial. Further study is required to determine its safety and effectiveness as a tool for out-of-hospital pediatric airway management. See

Advanced Airway Techniques, Procedure 13 for a

detailed explanation of this procedure.

The Initial Assessment

The Transport Decision: Stay or Go?

After the initial assessment and initiation of life support, consider the timing for transport. *Immediately transport every pediatric trauma patient who has any abnormal physiologic or anatomic findings, severe pain, or a serious*

mechanism of injury. Stable trauma patients with apparently minor injuries may undergo further evaluation and treatment on scene. If the scene size-up suggests circumstances that could be dangerous to the child or prehospital professional, transport immediately. Potentially dangerous conditions that would warrant immediate transport and completion of assessment in the ambulance include proximity to fire or hazardous materials, threatened violence, angry bystanders or caregivers, and suspected child maltreatment.

Additional Assessment

The additional assessment consists of the focused history and physical exam and the detailed physical exam (trauma patient). This part of the assessment is directed at *anatomical* problems. Perform the focused history and physical exam, and the detailed physical exam in the field only if the patient is physiologically normal and the conditions are safe. Otherwise, address these components of the assessment in the ambulance while on the way to the ED. In physiologically unstable patients, defer the additional assessment altogether.

When obtaining the focused history, use the SAMPLE template, as outlined in Chapter 1. Focus only on points likely to affect initial trauma assessment and interventions. **Table 6-9** provides a SAMPLE template oriented to pediatric trauma patients.

The focused physical exam includes a careful look at the anatomy in the suspected areas of injury. This may involve a conscientious examination by exploration and palpation of the head and scalp for a child with closed head injury, observation and palpation of the back and axillae in a child with a penetrating chest injury, or inspection and palpation of the neck in a child with a strangulation injury.

The detailed physical exam (trauma) is a head-to-toe sequence or (in infants, toddlers, and preschool-aged children) toe-to-head, then front-to-back complete physical examination of the patient. This exam uses the traditional assessment tools of observation, palpation, and auscultation as outlined in Chapter 1. The detailed physical exam

Table 6-9	SAMPLE History in Pediatric Trauma
Component	**Explanation**
Signs/symptoms	Time of event Nature of symptoms or pain Age-appropriate signs of distress
Allergies	Known drug reactions or other allergies
Medications	Chronic medications—timing and dose of last dose Timing and dose of <u>analgesic</u>/antipyretics
Past medical problems	Prior surgeries Immunizations
Last food or liquid	Time of the child's last food or drink, including bottle or breastfeeding
Events leading to the injury	Key events leading to the current incident Mechanism of injury Hazards at the scene

(trauma) tends to be redundant in young children with small anatomy, and has greater utility in older children or children with multiple injuries.

Once the child is on the way to the ED, perform ongoing reassessments, especially with patients with abnormal physiology. This includes serial evaluations of the PAT, ABCDEs, pulse oximetry, vital signs, heart rate and rhythm on the cardiac monitor, anatomic problems, and response to treatment. Be sure to monitor and treat pain, if possible. When the child arrives in the ED, diagnostic testing with blood tests and imaging studies may assist with continued assessment.

Summary

After the initial assessment, determine the timing of transport and the appropriate destination. Do an additional assessment, or on scene focused history and physical exam, then a detailed physical exam, only on stable patients in safe scene circumstances. All other patients deserve immediate transport with continuation of assessment on the way to the ED. Frequent reassessment is important in all injured patients. Transport severely injured pediatric patients to trauma centers rather than community hospitals when possi-

ble. Many state trauma programs have algorithms for directing patients, including children, to the appropriate level of care.

Stabilization and Splinting for Transport

Indications for spinal stabilization of children are the same as for adults and are indicated for any child with a concerning mechanism of injury, signs of significant head injury, or multisystem trauma. Stabilize the neck using a properly sized pediatric extrication collar and a head immobilizer, when available. Otherwise, use properly secured towel rolls and tape. For a step-by-step description of this procedure, see Spinal Stabilization, Procedure 21.

Preschool-aged children may not be able to localize or communicate the presence of neck or back pain. Anatomical differences, specifically the large size of an infant's or toddler's head, require modification of stabilization procedures. For example, placing a thin (1 inch) layer of padding beneath a child's body from shoulders to hips before securing the child to the spine board (**Figure 6-14**) will help to properly align the airway and the spinal column.

The spine does not stop at C-7, and spinal stabilization is not complete unless the entire body is secured. *Secure the patient against all axes of motion on the spine board.* Near-vertical positioning may be necessary during extrication. Secure the patient against <u>lateral</u> movement by padding along the sides of the body to eliminate all space

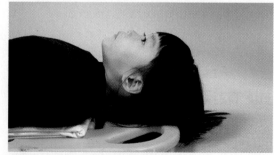

Figure 6-14 Keep the airway and spine in a neutral position by placing a layer of padding beneath the child's body from shoulders to hips before securing the child to the spine board.

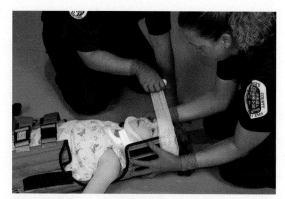

Figure 6-15 Vest-style extrication device.

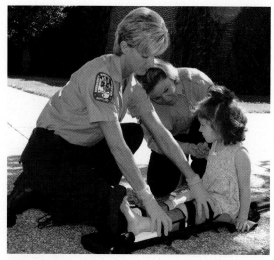

Figure 6-16 Splinting.

between the patient and the straps. Vest-style extrication devices can be effectively used to stabilize by rolling in the sides to provide side-to-side stabilization and using straps or tape across the pelvis, under armpits and across the lower extremities if needed. Do not place straps or tape over the lower chest or abdomen to avoid restriction of breathing. The device's head flaps can be brought up to the sides of the child's temples and secured with tape across the forehead (**Figure 6-15**).

Avoid chin straps and other spinal stabilization aides that might impair ventilation. Leave room for chest expansion during breathing when tightening chest straps or flaps. Make sure cervical collars fit properly, or use manual spinal stabilization until the child can be secured to the board if a properly sized collar is not available. Ensure that spinal stabilization equipment does not interfere with assessment and access to the patient. A child who does not have severe injuries may be frightened and fight the process vigorously. Reassure the child and offer relaxation or distraction techniques to minimize discomfort.

Splinting deformed or painful extremities is also an important prehospital intervention. Splinting has several important functions: pain control, hemorrhage reduction, and preservation of neurovascular function. Unless the extremity shows signs of neurovascular compromise or there is severe pain, splint bones that may be fractured or dislocated in an "as is" position (**Figure 6-16**). Leave exposed bone out, in order to avoid introducing further contami-

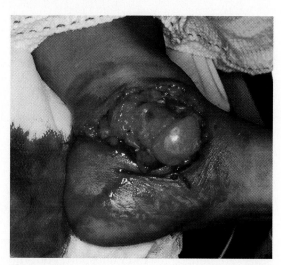

Figure 6-17 Leave exposed bone out. Do not attempt to reduce open fractures, unless circulation is compromised.

nation by forcing fractured bone fragments back under the broken skin (**Figure 6-17**).

Restraint of Children During Transport

Make sure all persons riding in an ambulance are appropriately restrained. Secure children with possible spinal injury in a supine position on a backboard, and secure the board to the stretcher (**Figure 6-18**). If the child has mild to moderate trauma without suggestion of spinal injury, use EMS system guidelines for age-appropriate restraint. Most states have well defined regulations on proper child restraint in a passenger vehicle. However, these regulations may not extend to ambulance transport.

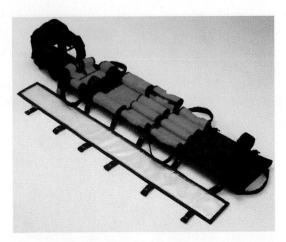

Figure 6-18 A pediatric spine board is an excellent stabilization device.

The use of specially designed pediatric spinal stabilization devices is more efficient than on scene modification of adult devices.

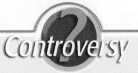

The use of car seats to transport injured children in ambulances remains controversial. Each EMS Agency should have consistent policy on this issue that conforms to local or state guidelines.

While spinal injures are not common in children, the high frequency of head injury means that spinal stabilization should be part of the care of most pediatric patients with a significant mechanism of blunt trauma.

The appropriate use of a child restraint seat in an ambulance is controversial. When "car seats" are utilized for EMS transport, both the device and the method of securing the seat to the gurney must conform to industry standards and meet local requirements. If EMS local policy allows, have the child's caregiver remain within view or speaking distance of the child, if the caregiver's presence does not compromise the child's treatment or crew safety. This is comforting for the conscious and <u>hemodynamically stable</u> child.

Pediatric Burn Patients

The assessment and management priorities for the burn patient are the same as for any other trauma patient. Make sure the scene is safe before approaching the child. Always anticipate exposure to hazardous materials and carbon monoxide, and use protective measures. Get technical help, if needed, from authorities on hazardous materials.

Assessment

Assess the scene for risk factors for airway and breathing. Important considerations in patients with fire and smoke exposures include the following:

- Enclosed space
- Heavy smoke
- Fumes
- Steam
- Hot vapors
- Chemical hazards
- Explosions with blunt or penetrating injury

Assess the patient for signs of smoke or particle inhalation and thermal burns of the airway. Give 100% oxygen for suspected carbon monoxide poisoning in children with abnormal appearance or ALOC, or in children exposed to fire or smoke in an enclosed space. Anticipate hidden injuries (especially abdominal) from a fall or a blast injury.

Make a quick estimation of burned body surface area. A modified anatomic diagram of children of different ages gives an approximation of burned body surface area, as

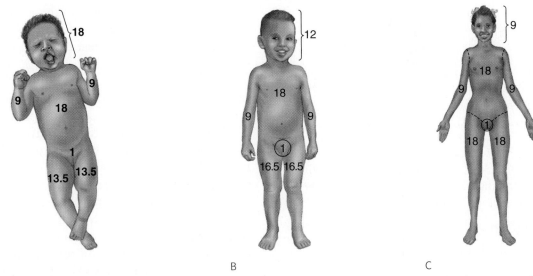

Figure 6-19 Modified anatomic diagrams of children of different ages give an approximation of involved body surface area for calculation of extent of burn in (A) infant, (B) child, and (C) adolescent.

shown in **Figure 6-19 A–C.** If such a diagram is not available, use the "rule of palms," which states that the patient's palm equals 1% of body surface area (**Figure 6-20**). The percent of burned body surface area is therefore roughly equal to the number of patient palm-sized areas burned.

Although most burns are unintentional, assess all burn patients for risk factors for intentional injury. <u>Scald</u> and <u>contact burns</u> are common in children and are frequent findings in child maltreatment victims, as explained in Chapter 12. A "pattern" burn (where there is a clear demarcation of an object in the burned skin), "glove" or "stocking" distribution of a scald burn (**Figure 6-21**), or a history that is inconsistent with the injury are suspicious circumstances for intentional injury.

Management

Remove any burning clothes. Give 100% oxygen to all patients with flame or blast burns. High-flow oxygen therapy is the only field treatment for suspected carbon monoxide poisoning. Because of the risk of hypothermia, do not flush or wet burned areas unless necessary to decontaminate or stop the burning process. Cover burned areas with clean dry sheets or nonstick

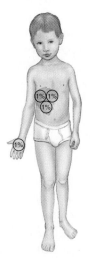

Figure 6-20 The palm is approximately 1% of the body surface area.

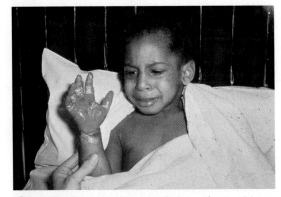

Figure 6-21 Consider intentional injury with a suspicious pattern of the burn, especially a "stocking" or "glove" distribution.

Do not apply ointments or creams to burn areas.

dressings. Covering helps to reduce pain by minimizing exposure to air currents. *Do not apply ointments or creams to burn areas.*

Advanced Airway Management of the Pediatric Burn Patient

Consider early (before edema starts) endotracheal intubation in any patient exposed to a fire in an enclosed space with a suspected inhalation injury to the airway. Such patients may have abnormal airway sounds, abnormal positioning, and respiratory distress or failure. Singed or burned nasal hairs and carbonaceous sputum may also indicate airway injury. Smoke inhalation may cause bronchospasm. If wheezing is present, give a bronchodilator, either SQ epinephrine or inhaled albuterol.

Pharmacologic Management of the Pediatric Burn Patient

Try to establish at least one IV line in patients with partial or full thickness burns greater than 5% body surface area. Insert IV catheters through a burn site if necessary. Initiate fluid resuscitation with 20 mL/kg boluses of crystalloid fluid. Both fluid and heat are rapidly lost through disrupted skin, with the rate of loss proportionate to the percent body surface area burned. Provide early analgesia and sedation and titrate to effect. For longer transports, contact the medical control to determine IV infusion rates.

Pain Management and Sedation

Fear and pain in children are frequently ignored or misinterpreted. Pain management is an important out-of-hospital priority, especially in trauma and burn patients with long transport times. Infants and young children experience the same degree of pain as older children and adults; they just can't express it in words.

Pain and anxiety are different things and require different treatments. Treat pain with a narcotic analgesic drug, such morphine or fentanyl. Treat anxiety with a sedative drug, such as a benzodiazepine (e.g., <u>diazepam</u> or <u>midazolam</u>). For example, a child with continued pain after stabilization of an isolated extremity fracture needs morphine to control the principal problem, which is pain. Narcotics such as morphine are pain killers, but also provide some sedation. On the other hand, a child who is anxious and has extreme psychomotor agitation, such as a child bucking an endotracheal tube, needs a sedative such as diazepam because anxiety is the problem, not pain.

IV analgesics such as morphine are appropriate in hemodynamically stable trauma patients with burns or with isolated long-bone fractures or dislocations. If serious blood loss or bleeding is suspected, or if assessment suggests hypoperfusion, avoid narcotics because they may contribute to hypotension. This is a special concern in a child with possible abdominal injury. Consider sedative drugs when transporting an awake, intubated child or a child who has received neuromuscular blocking agents (paralytics) during RSI to help with endotracheal intubation. Benzodiazepine drugs can also contribute to hypotension, so give them only to patients who are hemodynamically stable.

Table 6-10 lists common medications to treat pain or anxiety in a hemodynamically stable child after consultation with medical control as per local EMS protocol.

All IV sedatives and narcotics will cause respiratory depression. Give by slow IV push over 3 to 5 minutes. Give supplemental oxygen to all children receiving these medications. Place the child on a cardiac monitor and use pulse oximetry when available. Be ready to begin positive pressure ventilation with a bag-mask device if the child develops respiratory depression.

Naloxone (0.1 mg/kg/dose to a maximum single dose 2.0 mg IV/IO/SQ/ET) may temporarily reverse respiratory depression due to narcotic administration. Treat circulatory compromise with IV fluid boluses.

Tip

Pain and anxiety are different things and require different treatments.

Blip

Avoid narcotics in the multiple trauma patient because they may contribute to hypotension.

Table 6-10	ALS: Pharmacologic Management of Pain and Anxiety
Pain	
Morphine sulfate	*Neonates:* 0.05 mg/kg IM, IV, IO, or SQ *Infants and children:* 0.1–0.2 mg/kg IM, IV, IO, or SQ *Adolescents:* 3–4 mg IV or IO, repeat in 5 minutes as needed
Fentanyl	Dose: 1–5 μg/kg every 30–60 minutes
Anxiety	
Diazepam	Dose: 0.1 mg/kg IV (max 5 mg/dose) every 5–10 minutes
Midazolam	0.05–0.1 mg/kg IV, IM, or IO

Summary of Burns

Burns are common pediatric injuries, but usually are small and require only first aid. Burns involving the airway or more than 5% of body surface area require important field interventions, including possible airway protection, and vigorous fluid administration. Closed space burns raise the possibility of carbon monoxide poisoning. Pain is a universal feature of burns, and analgesia is usually a primary intervention.

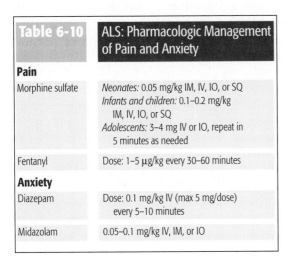

Case Study 3

You are dispatched to a child who has been run over by a vehicle. Upon your arrival you notice a full-size SUV parked in the middle of the road, and a 6-year-old girl, conscious and alert with a small laceration on her chin being held in her father's arms. She has no abnormal airway sounds or increased work of breathing, and her skin is pale. You notice the odor of alcohol on the man's breath. According to bystanders the child was riding on the fender and fell off. The patient is cool and clammy to the touch. Respiratory rate is 40 breaths/min, heart rate is 146 beats/min, and you are unable to obtain a blood pressure. Lung sounds are decreased in lower fields. While exposing the child you notice a tire track impression across the abdomen and sternum area. Pulse oximetry is 90% on room air.

1. What critical injuries do you suspect?
2. What are your treatment and transport priorities?

Case Study Answers

Case Study ❶ page 129

This patient will require immediate treatment and transport. The patient has sustained multisystem trauma to the head, chest and lower extremities, and the initial assessment confirms respiratory failure and shock. Snoring respirations are likely due to airway obstruction by soft tissues, blood, or broken teeth. Positioning the airway and suctioning may alleviate the problem. Perform rapid spinal stabilization.

The patient is hypoxic with abnormal breath sounds from either pulmonary contusion or tension pneumothorax.

Advanced Life Support

If the child does not respond to oxygen at 100% via positive pressure ventilation, consider needle decompression on the right side. Consider endotracheal intubation if the oxygenation does not improve with less invasive airway management.

Stabilize the femur with a traction splint. Start IVs en route to the hospital and initiate fluid resuscitation. Transport rapidly to a trauma center with pediatric expertise.

Case Study ❷ page 139

This child appears to have an isolated head injury and TBI. The child's rapid deterioration suggests an expanding intracranial hematoma, which may be life-threatening. As with any serious head injury, consider the risk of associated spinal injury. Stabilize the child's spine and be prepared for vomiting. Apply 100% oxygen. Rapidly transport.

Advanced Life Support

Establish an IV en route for the administration of medications and leave at TKO.

Transport to a facility with pediatric neurosurgical capability, or consider rendezvous with an air ambulance service if such care is not available in your community. This is a surgical emergency and immediate access to operative care may make the difference between the life and death of this child.

Case Study ❸ page 153

The injuries to this child are life-threatening and she appears to be in shock. Transport immediately after spinal stabilization and 100% oxygen.

Advanced Life Support

Do not prolong scene time with IV attempts. Give fluid resuscitation during transport.

This child is at risk for massive internal injury, including abdominal solid organ hemorrhage (liver, spleen, and kidneys), viscus rupture of the stomach, small bowel and large bowel, hemothorax, pneumothorax, and pulmonary contusion as well as pelvic fracture. The source of bleeding is not relevant to field care, but the recognition and treatment of compensated shock is critical.

Transport to the highest level of trauma care available in your community, based on local trauma triage protocol. This child requires rapid radiological assessment of the extent of injury and early operative intervention.

Suggested Readings

Textbooks

American Academy of Orthopaedic Surgeons: *Emergency Care and Transportation of the Sick and Injured,* 9th Edition. Sudbury, MA, Jones and Bartlett Publishers, 2005.

American Academy of Pediatrics and the American College of Emergency Physicians: *APLS: The Pediatric Emergency Medicine Resource,* 4th Edition. Sudbury, MA, Jones and Bartlett Publishers, 2004.

Barss P, Smith G, Baker S, Mohan D: *Injury Prevention: An international perspective,* 1st Edition. Oxford University Press, 1998.

Bledsoe B, Porter R, Cherry R: *Essentials of Paramedic Care.* New Jersey, Prentice Hall, 2003.

Campbell J: *BTLS for Paramedics and Other Advanced Providers,* 5th Edition. New Jersey, Pearson-Prentice Hall, 2004.

Articles

Adelson PD. Guidelines for the acute medical management of severe traumatic brain injury in infants, children, and adolescents. Chapter 4. Resuscitation of blood pressure and oxygenation and prehospital brain-specific therapies for the severe pediatric traumatic brain injury patient. *Pediatr Crit Care Med.* 1 Jul 2003; 4(3 Suppl):S12–18.

Morrison W. Pediatric trauma systems. *Crit Care Med.* Nov 2002; 30 (11 Suppl):S448–456.

Sadow KB. Prehospital intraveous fluid therapy in the pediatric trauma patient. *CPEM.* Mar 2001; 2(1):23–27.

Stafford PW. Practical points in evaluation and resuscitation of the injured child. *Surg Clin North Am.* April 2002; 82(2):273–301.

Stallion A. Initial assessment and management of pediatric trauma patient. *Respir Care Clin N Am.* Mar 2001; 7(1):1–11.

Toxic Emergencies

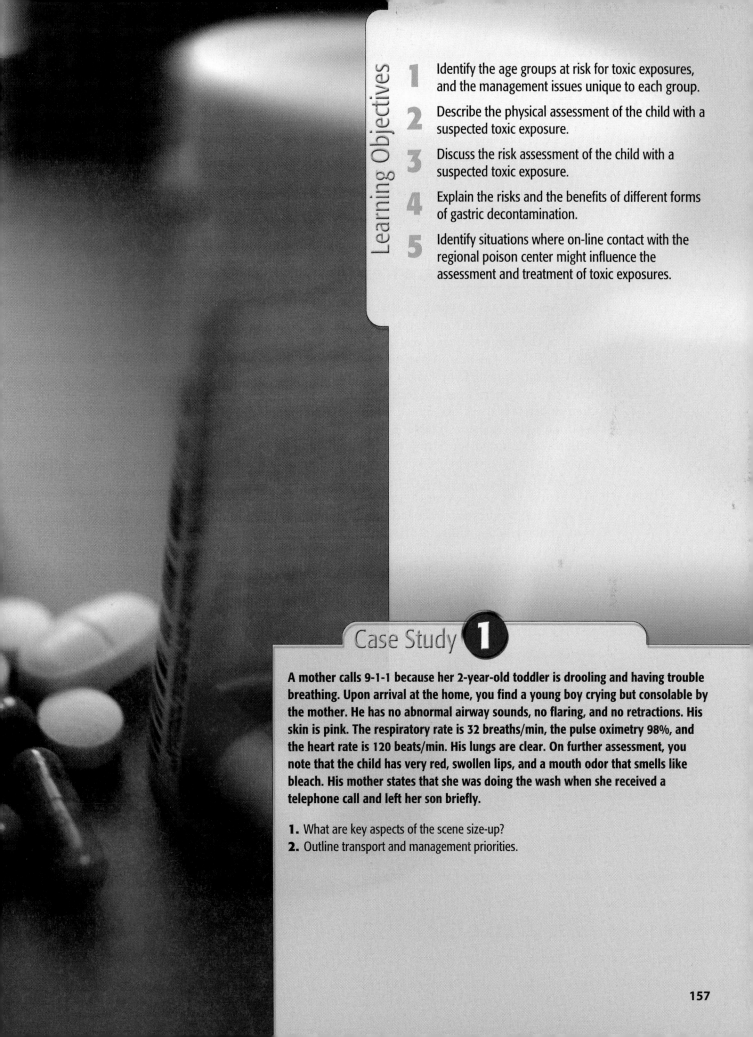

1 Identify the age groups at risk for toxic exposures, and the management issues unique to each group.

2 Describe the physical assessment of the child with a suspected toxic exposure.

3 Discuss the risk assessment of the child with a suspected toxic exposure.

4 Explain the risks and the benefits of different forms of gastric decontamination.

5 Identify situations where on-line contact with the regional poison center might influence the assessment and treatment of toxic exposures.

Case Study 1

A mother calls 9-1-1 because her 2-year-old toddler is drooling and having trouble breathing. Upon arrival at the home, you find a young boy crying but consolable by the mother. He has no abnormal airway sounds, no flaring, and no retractions. His skin is pink. The respiratory rate is 32 breaths/min, the pulse oximetry 98%, and the heart rate is 120 beats/min. His lungs are clear. On further assessment, you note that the child has very red, swollen lips, and a mouth odor that smells like bleach. His mother states that she was doing the wash when she received a telephone call and left her son briefly.

1. What are key aspects of the scene size-up?
2. Outline transport and management priorities.

Introduction

A TOXIC EXPOSURE is an ingestion, inhalation, injection, or application of any substance that causes illness or injury. There are a myriad of reasons that children experience such exposures, including unintentional ingestions of poisons, environmental misadventures, and deliberate intoxications. An example of an unintentional exposure is a toddler who ingests a caregiver's medication; an environmental misadventure might be a child who inhales carbon monoxide during a house fire, or a child with a systemic reaction to a skin contact with an insecticide. Deliberate intoxications include recreational exposures and attempted suicides.

Age-Related Differences

Toxic exposures are a common pediatric out-of-hospital complaint, but rarely result in death in children less than 6 years of age. In 2001 data from American Association of Poison Control Centers Toxic Exposure Surveillance System, there were 26 deaths in children under 6 years of age out of 1,169,478 reported total exposures (**Table 7-1**). Young children accounted for 51.6% of the total exposures for all age groups, but represented only 2% of all deaths. For the entire pediatric age group (<1 to 19 years), there were 1,496,712 exposures (66.0% of total), again highlighting young children as the age group at highest risk for exposure. While the number of reported exposures for the adolescent population (13–19 years) is relatively low, the mortality rate is much higher, comprising 10.7% of total deaths.

The majority of exposures in infants and preschool children less than 6 years of age are asymptomatic. The toddler is a fearless, curious individual who explores the world by placing objects in her mouth (**Figure 7-1**). Because toddler ingestions are unintentional, and the majority of non-food items ingested are not very palatable, poisonings in this age group generally involve small volumes of a single substance. The most common ingestions in young children include cosmetics and personal care products, cleaning substances, and analgesics. In this age group, analgesics cause the most fatalities.

Children 6–12 years of age are less likely to ingest non-food articles or non-prescribed medications, but in 2001 this age group still accounted for 156,612 exposures and 12 deaths. The majority of these deaths were due to carbon monoxide exposure.

Among adolescents (13–19 years), toxic exposures are usually intentional, either as recreational abuse or as a suicide gesture or attempt. *Intentional exposures lead to more ED visits and hospital admissions than unintentional exposures.* In suicide attempts,

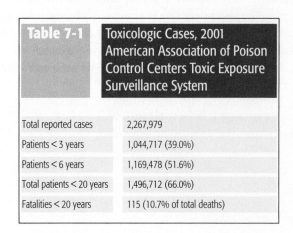

Table 7-1	Toxicologic Cases, 2001 American Association of Poison Control Centers Toxic Exposure Surveillance System
Total reported cases	2,267,979
Patients < 3 years	1,044,717 (39.0%)
Patients < 6 years	1,169,478 (51.6%)
Total patients < 20 years	1,496,712 (66.0%)
Fatalities < 20 years	115 (10.7% of total deaths)

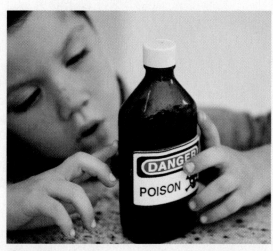

Figure 7-1 Toddlers are "oral explorers"—they will try to taste or swallow almost any substance.

adolescents usually ingest two or more substances, often in large quantities (**polypharmacy**). Recreational abuse often involves alcohol in addition to another recreational drug(s). The number of fatalities in this age group is increasing. Statistics represent an underestimation of the true incidence, since statistics only include those cases reported to the database.

An unusual form of abuse involves deliberate intoxication of infants or young children, a condition called Munchausen Syndrome by Proxy. This condition is a complex form of deliberate poisoning of a child by a caregiver. In these cases, the caregiver frequently possesses more than average medical information and is trying to induce a state of illness in the child in a disordered attempt to bring attention to herself. Children with such exposures may be especially difficult to identify, as the intoxication is secretive and often chronic.

Role of the Poison Center

Almost every state in the U.S. has at least one regional poison center. The telephone number within the state is usually toll-free. For ease of access, there is also a national toll-free number (1-800-222-1222) that forwards calls to the state poison center, when available. At the other end of the telephone is a specialist who can provide information about the potential toxicity of an item, adverse effects, and can recommend home or hospital management. Caregivers often call the poison center for advice prior to or while awaiting the arrival of the prehospital professional.

The regional poison center can also be a valuable resource to the prehospital professional when managing children with a toxic exposure. Local EMS system protocol should define the circumstances when contact with the poison center must be made via on-line medical control, and when the call can be made directly.

Table 7-2	Common Substances Responsible for Toxic Exposures
Children (< 6 yrs)	**Adults (> 19 yrs)**
Cosmetics and personal care products	Analgesics[a]
Cleaning substances	Sedative-hypnotics/antipsychotics
Analgesics[a]	Antidepressants
Foreign bodies	Bites/envenomations
Topical medications	Alcohols
Plants	Food products, food poisoning
Cough and cold preparations	Cosmetics and personal care products
Pesticides	Pesticides
Vitamins	Chemicals
Gastrointestinal preparations	Cardiovascular drugs

[a]Analgesics include aspirin, acetaminophen, ibuprofen, and narcotic analgesics such as methadone and morphine.

The poison center has a key role in community prevention and treatment of toxic exposures. Have the toll-free number (1-800-222-1222) posted near or on your telephone.

Common Substances Responsible for Serious Poisonings in Children

Most poisonings occur in the home. **Table 7-2** lists common substances responsible for serious poisonings.

Summary of Age-Related Differences

Most toxic exposures in children are minor and involve household products. The most common patient is the toddler who unintentionally ingests a single agent in small quantity and is asymptomatic. The second most common patient is the adolescent who uses recreational drugs or who is making a suicide attempt or gesture. Adolescent exposures often consist of more than one drug, and often involve large quantities. Common serious exposures in young children involve analgesics, while those in adolescents involve analgesics, alcohol, and recreational drugs. An unusual form of intoxication in young children involves a condition called Munchausen Syndrome by Proxy, a complex form of deliberate poisoning or abuse of a child by a caregiver.

Most patients with toxic exposures are toddlers or preschool-aged children. There is usually only one poison involved, the exposure is usually small and unintentional, and the child is asymptomatic.

Prearrival Preparation and Scene Size-up

Sometimes, at the time of dispatch, the toxin has already been identified by the caregiver, the poison center, or another health professional. In such cases, immediately contact medical control or the poison center, depending on local EMS protocol. They will help clarify the toxicity of the agent and priorities in assessment and treatment. In other cases, where the dispatch involves a toddler or adolescent with a sudden change in behavior, consider a toxic exposure.

On arrival, first perform the scene size-up. Note if there are potentially hazardous toxins in the area or on the patient's clothes or skin. If so, assess the scene and whether immediate patient decontamination is safe

Bring bottles, containers, plastic bags, suspicious substances, plants, or syringes to the ED.

to perform. The poison center or other public health agency may assist in defining risk and the need to mobilize other personnel (e.g., Hazardous Materials team).

If there is a possible toxin or hazardous material, secure the scene and minimize the risk of toxic exposures to the EMS crew through the skin, eyes, or lungs by use of personal protective equipment. Be aware of the possibility of a mass exposure to a toxic substance, either because of unintentional or deliberate action (e.g., bioterrorism). If a disaster or multicasualty event is suspected, implement disaster preparedness (Chapter 8).

Next, look over the surrounding area. Bring any bottles, containers, or plastic bags containing possible toxins as well samples of ingested plants or syringes to the ED along with the patient (**Figures 7-2 A and B**). If the caregiver refuses to let a poisoned child be

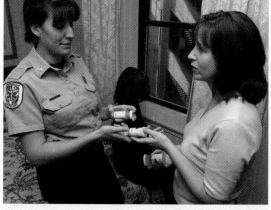

A

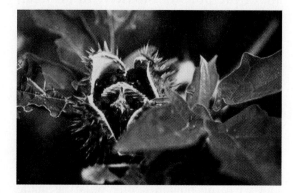

B

Figure 7-2 Bring any bottles or plant samples to the ED. (A) Bottles and containers. (B) The poisonous plant jimsonweed.

Tip

The adolescent who makes a suicide attempt or gesture must be transported to the ED for both medical and psychological assessment, even if the child refuses. This is true even if the injury or immediate medical risk is assessed as trivial.

Blip

Never forget about toxic hazards on scene. Watch out for absorbable toxins and protect skin and eyes by using gloves and other personal protective equipment.

transported to the hospital, ask medical control to talk to the caregiver over the telephone or radio. If this strategy does not work, then request assistance from law enforcement personnel.

Assessment of the Child with a Possible Toxic Exposure

General Assessment

After the rapid scene size-up and environmental evaluation for toxins, assess the child. Use age appropriate techniques to approach the patient, as outlined in Chapters 1 and 2, and conduct a general assessment (PAT), an initial assessment, and then an additional assessment when appropriate. If the child is unstable, treat the physiologic abnormalities detected in the general (PAT) and initial assessment, and then transport. En route, do a reassessment and also the additional assessment, if possible.

History is the best tool for overall assessment of risk and for determining urgency for treatment in pediatric poisoning. It is usually more accurate than a physical evaluation in

determining the specific type of toxic exposure. In the first few minutes, the important questions are: (1) the identity of the agent; (2) the route of exposure (ingestion, inhalation, injection); (3) the time since the exposure occurred; and (4) the amount of the agent involved in the exposure.

Special Considerations in the Initial Assessment

After the PAT, do the hands-on ABCDEs to complete the initial assessment, and then immediately treat any physiologic abnormalities. Special elements of the physical assessment that may help identify the type of poison include: breath odor, vital signs, pupillary size, skin temperature, and skin condition. An odor of bitter almonds may be due to cyanide, while garlic odor may be due to organophosphates. Also, look for stains and powders on the skin or clothes. Use assessment information to match the patient's signs and symptoms with possible "Toxidromes," identifiable clinical patterns of single agent intoxications. **Table 7-3** outlines the symptoms and signs of important toxidromes in pediatrics.

Airway

Clear, maintain, and control the airway in the child with a suspected toxic exposure who has altered level of consciousness (ALOC). This may happen in a child exposed to a <u>sedative/ hypnotic</u> drug, such as a benzodiazepine or a barbiturate. Beware of the child who has ingested a <u>caustic</u> agent, such as <u>lye</u>. This child may have severe burns of the esophagus and present with drooling, <u>dysphagia</u>, and signs of upper airway obstruction.

Breathing

Give 100% supplemental oxygen by a nonrebreathing mask if there is ALOC, respiratory distress, or a history of exposure to a toxic substance known to cause breathing problems. One example of this type of toxic exposure is <u>hydrocarbon</u> inhalation. Obtain pulse oximetry, but be aware that the reading will not be accurate for some toxic exposures, notably carbon monoxide poisoning. Sedative/hypnotic drugs, opiates, and

Table 7-3	Common Toxidromes	
Toxidrome	**Agent(s)**	**Signs and Symptoms**
Anticholinergics	antihistamines, cyclic antidepressants	"Hot as a hare, red as a beet (hot dry, skin, hyperthemia), blind as a bat (dilated pupils), mad as a hatter (delirium, hallucinations)"
Cholinergics	organophosphates	DUMBELS = Diarrhea, Diaphoresis, Urination, Miosis, Bradycardia, Bronchoconstriction, Emesis, Lacrimation, Salivation
Narcotics	morphine, methadone	bradycardia, hypoventilation, miosis, hypotension
Sympathomimetics	cocaine, amphetamines	tachycardia, hypertension, hyperthermia, mydriasis (dilated pupils), diaphoresis (sweating)
Specific Agents		
Gamma hydroxybutyrate	GHB, "date rape drug"	Initially drowsiness, dizziness, and disorientation; High doses result in bradycardia, hypoventilation, and even apnea.
Ecstasy	3,4 methylenedioxy-methamphetamine	Euphoria, increased energy, intense visual perceptions Complications: hyperthermia, hypertension, seizures, dehydration, myocardial infarction, intracerebral hemorrhage.

gamma hydroxybutyrate (GHB) may decrease the respiratory rate, while sympathomimetic agents (cocaine, amphetamines), phencyclidine (PCP), and aspirin may increase the respiratory rate.

Circulation

If the child has eaten or swallowed a possible cardiopulmonary toxin, place her on a cardiac monitor to watch for dysrhythmias. Drugs such as beta blockers, digoxin or calcium channel blockers may decrease the heart rate, while sympathomimetic agents, anticholinergic agents (scopolamine, antihistamines, amphetamines), jimson weed, and cocaine may increase heart rate. Skin can be warm and dry due to drugs such as antihistamines and anticholinergics, while the skin may be hot and sweaty from sympathomimetics, organophosphates, aspirin, and phencyclidine.

Disability

ALOC is a common effect of many different chemical exposures. Recreational drug use with sedative/hypnotics depresses the central nervous system (CNS). Sympathomimetic drugs may stimulate the CNS and cause excitement, agitation, paranoia, or hallucinations. Cyclic antidepressants may cause seizures or coma. In the comatose or unresponsive patient, always consider the other common causes of ALOC, such as a head injury, seizure, or hypoglycemia (which may accompany alcohol or beta blocker inges-

tion). *Check the bedside glucose level in any patient with ALOC, even if toxins are suspected.*

Exposure

Undress the child and look for evidence of toxic exposure to the eyes and skin. Many substances, such as hydrocarbons, irritate the eyes. Other toxic substances, such as hydrochloric acid, irritate the skin. Organophosphate insecticides enter through the skin and can cause a severe cholinergic crisis with diaphoresis (sweating), urination, miosis (small pupils), bradycardia, bronchoconstriction, emesis, tearing, and salivation. The mnemonic DUMBELS (**Table 7-3**) will help identify signs of cholinergic drug intoxication.

Initial Management of Toxic Exposures

After the initial assessment, determine the need for treatment and transport of the poisoned child by combining the physical assessment with a risk assessment. The physical assessment is a way to determine the child's physiological stability and the overall urgency for treatment and transport. The risk assessment evaluates the probability of serious toxicity—both early and delayed—from the exposure. *Perform the risk assessment with knowledge of the identity of the drug involved, time since ingestion/exposure, and amount of poison involved. The child's weight should also be considered (see*

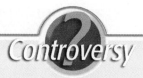

Controversy

If the child is stable and has a history of a single small ingestion of a low-risk agent, some EMS systems allow the transport to be canceled after agreement from medical control. While this approach may be medically sound, it eliminates an opportunity for assessment of psychosocial risk factors in the ED.

Tip

In suspected toxic exposures, perform risk assessment to determine the chances of serious toxicity.

Table 7-4	Risk Assessment

Assess the chances of serious toxicity from the following five pieces of information:

1. Identity of the agent involved and its lethality, usually through consultation with medical control or the poison center.
2. Amount of the poison ingested, in milligrams (mg).
3. Child's weight.
4. The per-kilogram amount of poison in the exposure, in mg/kg.
5. Time since the exposure.

Table 7-5	One Pill Can Kill: Potentially Lethal Toddler Ingestions
Medicine	**Lethal Dose**
Camphor	One teaspoon of oil
Chloroquine	One 500-mg tab
Clonidine	One 0.3-mg tab
Glyburide	Two 5-mg tabs
Imipramine	One 150-mg tab
Lindane	Two teaspoons of 1% lotion
Diphenoxylate/atropine	Two 2.5-mg tabs
Propranolol	One or two 160-mg tabs
Theophylline	One 500-mg tab
Verapamil	One or two 240-mg tabs

Table 7-4). Contact with the poison center can provide much of this information.

Common toxic agents such as aspirin, acetaminophen, or iron have predictable physiologic effects that are determined by how much of the drug was taken, time since exposure, and amount of drug per kg. By collecting information and evidence at the scene, the prehospital professional serves an important role in later ED testing and treatment.

Sometimes the prehospital professional's risk assessment determines that a child has had a potentially lethal exposure, although the child is physiologically stable. Indeed, in a small child, one ingested pill of some common

medications can kill. **Table 7-5** lists potentially dangerous agents where a tiny toxic exposure (e.g., one pill) may be fatal to a toddler.

The Transport Decision: Stay or Go?

After the initial assessment, initial treatment, and risk assessment, consider whether to transport immediately, doing additional

Case Study 2

You respond to a call for a 4-year-old who just ingested all of her mothers' prenatal iron tablets (approximately 30). Upon your arrival, the child is active, running around the room, but complaining that her "tummy hurts." She has no increased work of breathing, and her skin is pink. Her respiratory rate is 24 breaths/min, heart rate is 110 beats/min and blood pressure is 90/60 mm Hg. Her physical examination reveals no abnormalities.

1. Do you need to transport this child to the hospital?
2. Should you give activated charcoal?

assessment and treatment on the way to the ED, or to stay on the scene. If the results of the physical assessment and the risk assessment reveal an asymptomatic child the ingestion of a small amount of a single low-risk agent, consider canceling transport after appropriate consultation with medical oversight or the poison center. This is controversial; however, because some EMS systems consider hospital transport necessary in all toxic exposure cases. Other systems allow the poison center to manage minor ingestions exclusively over the telephone.

If the physical assessment indicates that the child has any physiologic abnormality, or if the risk assessment indicates that the toxic exposure is potentially harmful, transport and do additional assessment on the way to the ED, if possible. The onset of symptoms will vary with the substance involved. A child without symptoms on arrival of EMS may have ingested a lethal dose of a substance. For example, ingestions of iron and acetaminophen, two common household over-the-counter medicines, may be extremely dangerous but cause no early symptoms. History from the scene is critical to the management in the ED.

Most pediatric poisonings do not require any treatment in the field.

Additional Assessment

If the child has no physical abnormalities and is asymptomatic, and if the risk assessment indicates no serious toxicity, perform a complete assessment on scene. Additional assessment includes the focused history and physical exam and the detailed physical exam (trauma). Sometimes it is more appropriate to perform this additional assessment on the way to the ED. **Table 7-6** lists important history in a suspected toxic exposure, presented in the standard SAMPLE format. During the initial assessment and the risk

Table 7-6	The Pediatric SAMPLE for Toxic Exposures
Component	**Explanation**
Signs/Symptoms	Time of suspected exposure
	Behavior changes in child
	Emesis and content of vomitus
Allergies	Known drug reactions or other allergies
Medications	Identity of suspected toxin
	Amount of toxin exposure (count pills or measure volume)
	Pill or chemical containers on scene
	Exact names and doses of prescribed medications
Past medical problems	Previous illnesses or injuries
Last food or liquid	Timing of the child's last food or drink
	Type and time of home treatment (such as ipecac)
Events leading to the exposure	Key events leading to the exposure
	Type of exposure (inhaled, injected, ingested, or absorbed through the skin)
	Poison center contact

assessment, the prehospital professional will have already obtained some of the SAMPLE history.

Summary of Assessment of the Child with a Possible Toxic Exposure

Every child with a toxic exposure needs a careful physical assessment and risk assessment. The physical assessment includes all of the features of the standard assessment, with an emphasis on the history—which is usually the most important part of the toxicologic evaluation. Preparation begins on the way to the scene with dispatch information about the age of the patient, the type and potential toxicity of exposure, and the need for personal protective equipment. Preparation then continues with the scene size-up and environmental assessment. If multiple patients are involved, consider disaster plan activation.

After the physical assessment, the risk assessment will help determine if there might be serious toxicity based on the type of toxin involved, the amount of the toxin, the weight of the child, and the time since the exposure.

The risk assessment gives important information about expected physiologic effects, need for treatment, and timing of transport. The poison center often plays a key role in helping decide about treatment and transport.

Toxicologic Management

The prehospital professional has three possible options for toxicologic management of serious or potentially lethal exposures: (1) decontamination to reduce local and/or systemic exposure to the toxin; (2) enhancement of elimination, or increasing the speed of removal of the toxin; or (3) antidote administration to reverse the actions of the poison directly.

Decontamination

After the treatment and transport decision, consider decontamination. There are several ways to decontaminate, depending on the toxin and the type of exposure.

Skin

If there is a chance that the poison was <u>absorbed</u> through the skin, remove the child's clothing. The prehospital professional must protect her own skin and eyes by using gloves and protective gear. Flood the skin with large amounts of water, and then wash it well with mild soap and water.

Eyes

Immediately wash out the eyes if there has been direct eye contact (**Figure 7-3**). <u>Alkali</u> burns with caustic agents such as lye are the most dangerous. Flush the eyes for 20 minutes using normal saline or water. Attach IV tubing to the bag of normal saline and flush the eye with the end of the IV tubing. If this is not possible, hold the patient's head under the sink and pour water into the eye from a pitcher or cup. When the eyes are the main point of exposure, continue flushing during transport if possible.

Gastrointestinal Decontamination

Prior to any gastrointestinal decontamination, contact medical control or the poison center, depending upon EMS protocol. In some cases, it may be beneficial to dilute mild <u>acid</u> or alkali ingestions by asking the

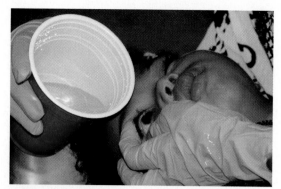

Figure 7-3 Immediately wash out the eyes if there has been direct eye contact.

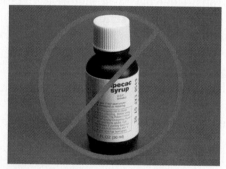

Figure 7-4 Ipecac has no role in prehospital professional treatment of pediatric poisoning.

alert patient to drink an 8-ounce glass of milk or water. *Dilution is contraindicated when there is absent gag reflex, airway compromise, diminished level of consciousness, or ingestion of a hydrocarbon corrosive, or caustics (strong alkalis and acids).*

<u>Ipecac</u>, an old time remedy for ingestions, may have been given in the home by the caregiver. Make note of this and the time it was given. The vomiting induced by ipecac does not remove significant amounts of ingested toxins from the stomach and it may cause prolonged emesis, delaying the administration of <u>activated charcoal</u> (**Figure 7-4**). *Ipecac is no longer advised for home use. Do not use in children.*

Blip

Do not give ipecac to a child with a suspected ingestion.

Table 7-7	Toxins Poorly Adsorbed by Activated Charcoal
"PHAILS"	
Pesticides	
Hydrocarbons	
Acid, Alkali, Alcohol	
Iron	
Lithium	
Solvents	

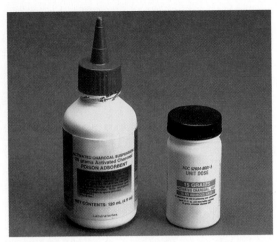

Figure 7-5 Activated charcoal is a treatment option for potentially serious ingestions of bindable toxins.

Activated Charcoal Most high-risk ingestions in toddlers and preschool children do not require any out-of-hospital treatment. In cases where <u>gastrointestinal (GI) decontamination</u> is necessary, consider using activated charcoal. Activated charcoal is made from burned wood products. Its surfaces are "activated" by steam or chemical treatment, so the material can irreversibly <u>adsorb</u> ingested toxins in the stomach and small bowel, and reduces bloodstream absorption of the toxins. Charcoal itself is not absorbed from the GI tract, nor is it metabolized. Activated charcoal has no odor or taste, but has a granular consistency that makes many children unwilling to drink it. Charcoal administration is messy, even with a cooperative child. In a child with altered or deteriorating mental status, aspiration of charcoal can lead to serious pulmonary consequences. There are limited data on the utility of activated charcoal in the prehospital setting, and the risks of prolonged scene time must be weighed against the potential benefits of rapid transport and early ED management. Some agents are not adsorbed by activated charcoal, as noted in **Table 7-7**.

Administration of Activated Charcoal The activated charcoal dose is 10 times the mass of the ingested substance. However, because the actual amount of ingested material is usually not known, use 1–2 g/kg of the child's body weight. Activated charcoal begins working immediately, and it is most effective when given within an hour of ingestion (**Figure 7-5**).

Never force a child to take activated charcoal because this may lead to aspiration and pulmonary complications. If local EMS policy allows, consider adding a flavoring agent (e.g., cola, juice, milk) to make the mixture more acceptable to drink, then transport the child. Some formulations of activated charcoal also contain <u>sorbitol</u>. However, there are dangers in giving charcoal with sorbitol to infants less than 1 year of age. **Table 7-8** summarizes activated charcoal and guidelines for use.

Advanced Life Support

The child must be stable and cooperative to receive activated charcoal. Because young children or adolescents may not want to drink the activated charcoal, some EMS systems use a nasogastric tube as an alternative method of delivery if the ingestion is potentially serious or lethal. Delivery of activated charcoal by nasogastric tube can be dangerous and must be reserved for highly unusual circumstances where transport time is long and risk assessment indicates severe toxicity.

Blip

Delivery of activated charcoal by nasogastric tube can be dangerous and must be reserved for highly unusual circumstances where transport time is long and risk assessment indicates severe toxicity.

Table 7-8	Activated Charcoal: Guidelines for Use
Product Information	A highly adsorbent, harmless, tasteless material made from wood pulp.
Indication	To limit amount of drug absorbed by the body in most toxic ingestions (i.e., intestinal decontamination). Repeated doses may enhance the elimination process.
Technique	Mix 1–2 g/kg patient weight with water to form a <u>slurry</u>. If the quantity of ingested substance is known, give 10 times the ingested dose of toxin by weight (max dose: 100 g). Administer orally (or by nasogastric tube in rare situations). Consider adding a flavoring agent to make the slurry more acceptable.
Contraindications	Loss of gag reflex. Altered level of consciousness. Unwillingness voluntarily to take the drug. <u>Corrosive</u> substance ingestion. Drugs not adsorbed by charcoal.
Adverse Effects	<u>Constipation</u> or intestinal <u>bezoar</u> (large foreign-body mass in gut). Pulmonary aspiration. Diarrhea and dehydration may occur in young children given a combined <u>cathartic</u> (e.g., sorbitol) and activated charcoal.

Table 7-9	Common Antidotes
Poison	**Antidote**
Carbon monoxide	Oxygen
Organophosphate	Atropine/2-PAM
Tricyclic antidepressants	Bicarbonate
Opiates	Naloxone
Beta blockers	Glucagon
Calcium channel blockers	Calcium
Benzodiazepine	Flumazenil

Tip

The biggest problem with field use of activated charcoal is the difficulty getting children to take it.

Blip

Sorbitol may cause nausea, vomiting, abdominal discomfort, and diarrhea in children, and therefore should not be used in pediatric patients.

Enhancement of Elimination

<u>Sorbitol</u> is a cathartic that is mixed with many commercial activated charcoal preparations. Cathartics have been promoted to clear the bound toxin from the gut and help speed up elimination. The effectiveness of cathartics has not been proven. Sorbitol is not an approved drug in most EMS systems. Prehospital professionals may think they are giving pure activated charcoal when the preparation actually is a mixture of activated charcoal and sorbitol. Sorbitol may cause nausea, vomiting, abdominal discomfort, diarrhea, and electrolyte disturbances in young children. *Therefore, never use a cathartic in children in the prehospital setting.*

Table 7-9 lists the few commonly available antidotes for several chemical exposures.

Antidotes

Antidotes are medications that reverse or treat the side effects of toxic ingestions. Prehospital providers carry several antidotes (**Table 7-9**) that may be life-saving for poisoned patients. Use these medications with knowledge of the type of ingestion/exposure, patient's clinical status, and possible adverse effects associated with the antidote.

<u>Naloxone</u> is an antidote used frequently in adult patients with suspected opioid overdose. It can have a therapeutic as well as diagnostic effect in selected pediatric patients. If the child has signs of an opioid ingestion/overdose (bradycardia, coma, small pupils, respiratory depression), administer 0.1 mg/kg. Maximum dose is 2 mg. Although IV is the preferred route, it can be given IM, IO, ET, or SQ. However, ET or SQ administration is less effective. The child may then awaken slightly or fully, with improvement in vital signs. The duration of action of naloxone is 20 to 60 minutes, so repeat doses may be necessary if a longer acting narcotic (e.g., methadone) is involved.

Although <u>flumazenil</u> is an effective benzodiazepine antagonist, do not use this antidote routinely for patients with ALOC of unknown cause. One of the most common causes of ALOC in children is the postictal state following a seizure. If flumazenil is given and the child has further seizures, benzodiazepines will not be effective. Also, flumazenil may precipitate seizures if administered to the patient who is on chronic therapeutic doses of a benzodiazepine.

<u>Sodium bicarbonate</u> will help reverse the adverse cardiac effects seen with cyclic antidepressant overdoses, including conduction abnormalities. It alkalinizes the blood to reverse the sodium channel blockade caused by the drugs. The dose is 1–2 mEq/kg IV slowly.

Beta blockers are drugs commonly used for treatment of hypertension and adult cardiac disease. Overdose in children can cause bradycardia and hypotension. <u>Glucagon</u>, a familiar drug to prehospital professionals because of its role in treatment of hypoglycemia, will help reverse toxicity from beta blocker overdose. Although there are no good pediatric studies, the suggested dosage of glucagon is 0.03–0.15 mg/kg followed by 0.07 mg/kg/hr (maximum 5 mg/hr). Beta blocker overdose can also cause hypoglycemia in young children, so check the bedside glucose level and treat hypoglycemia if present.

Calcium channel blockers are another frequently prescribed medication for hypertension in adults. Pediatric ingestions may result in severe toxicity that is similar to beta blocker overdose, including bradycardia and hypotension. There can be secondary respiratory and neurologic effects (respiratory depression, decreased level of consciousness). IV fluids are the first line of therapy, and calcium can be beneficial. Give either <u>calcium chloride</u> or <u>calcium gluconate</u>. Glucagon is another potential therapy for refractory hypotension in such patients.

Organophosphates

DUMBELS (**Table 7-3**) is the mnemonic that summarizes the clinical hallmarks of organophosphate poisoning toxidrome. Treatment involves several steps:

1. Ensure your personal protection (use gloves and other protective clothing to prevent exposure).
2. Perform the initial assessment and ensure adequate oxygenation and ventilation.
3. Decontaminate the patient (flush the skin with large amounts of water, wash the skin, hair, and under the nails well with soap and water).
4. Flush exposed eyes with large amounts of warm water or saline.
5. If the child has refractory bradycardia, consider treatment with the antidote <u>atropine</u>. The drug will help reverse the "muscarinic" organophosphate effects (salivation, bronchorrhea, bronchospasm, bradycardia, respiratory depression, seizures, coma). The initial pediatric atropine dose is 0.01–0.02 mg/kg IV. Repeat doses until the airway is dry and the child has adequate perfusion. The specific antidote is <u>pralidoxime (2-PAM)</u>.

With the advent of possible chemical terrorism incidents, there has been much attention to the side effects of organophosphates,

Tip

Poison centers have the capability to follow up with continuing reassessment by telephone.

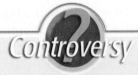

Controversy

The value of activated charcoal for out-of-hospital treatment of ingestions is unproven. While the drug has a possible advantage of early binding of toxins in the gut, there are potential complications such as aspiration and bowel obstruction.

which are the same as those for nerve agents such as sarin gas. Since some EMS agencies have distributed MARK 1 or MARK 2 kits to their providers for management of chemical terrorism, it is important to realize that the medication doses in these autoinjector kits are for adults. However, in severe, life-threatening pediatric cases, administer the contents of these kits for children by IM injection.

Summary of Toxicologic Management

Most children with toxic exposures do not require treatment of any kind in the field. Consider cancellation of EMS transport after consultation with medical control and/or the poison center only if the child is asymptomatic, has ingested a small amount of a single low-risk substance, and there are no "red flags" for child neglect or abuse. In other circumstances, when physical assessment and risk assessment together show physiologic instability or possible toxicity, treatment is indicated. After managing the ABCDEs, consider toxicologic management by decontamination or, in special situations, administering an antidote. Perform skin and eye decontamination when indicated. Attempt gastrointestinal decontamination for serious or potentially fatal ingestions based on local protocol. Activated charcoal is a useful binding agent for many types of toxic ingestions, but can be safely administered only to a cooperative child. Sorbitol is contraindicated in children. Several antidotes carried by prehospital professionals may be diagnostic, therapeu-

tic, and even life-saving. Remember to educate the family or caregiver on poisoning prevention if circumstances allow, as discussed in Chapter 1.

Medicolegal Issues

There are several scenarios where medicolegal issues play an important role in the management of toxiologic emergencies in children. If the caregiver refuses therapy and transport to the hospital, ask medical control to talk to them over the telephone. If this strategy does not work, then request assistance from law enforcement personnel.

The adolescent who makes any suicide attempt or gesture must be transported to the ED. An individual who has attempted suicide is legally incompetent to make treatment decisions, and cannot refuse transport. In some cases, law enforcement must become involved in scene management. Place the patient in temporary protective custody and transport to the hospital (see Chapter 13).

The adolescent can also present legal problems because of issues such as the ability of a dependent minor to <u>consent for care</u>, and illegal use of alcohol and/or recreational drugs. If an adolescent has taken a potentially toxic dose of medication, or has life-threatening complications of drug use or overdose, treat based on the emergency exception rule (the doctrine of implied consent) as explained in Chapter 13. Leave the legal issues of alcohol or drug use to law enforcement officials.

Case Study 3

You respond to a call about an unconscious female. Upon arrival, you find a group of high-school students surrounding one of their friends who has "passed out" at the party. The patient is a 17-year-old female who is lying on a couch, is unresponsive to voice and not moving. Work of breathing is normal but her skin is pale. Her respiratory rate is 8 breaths/min and shallow, heart rate is 50 beats/min, and blood pressure is 110/70 mm Hg. Her pupils are 3 mm and sluggishly reactive. There is no evidence of head trauma. The remainder of her examination is negative. There is an empty vodka bottle on the kitchen counter.

1. What are your initial management priorities?
2. Can you treat and transport this patient without parental consent?

Chapter Review

Case Study Answers

Case Study ❶ page 157

The sudden onset of mucous membrane changes in a previously healthy toddler is concerning for a caustic or acid ingestion. Laundry detergents and bleach are caustics, with alkaline pH values that can cause severe tissue damage and swelling of the lining of the mouth, pharynx, and esophagus when ingested, especially if the agent is industrial strength. Given the circumstances of this event, and the tell-tale odor on the child's breath, a bleach ingestion is most likely. Undertake skin and eye decontamination if indicated, and protect yourself with gloves and goggles.

Rapidly transport this child to the hospital, frequently reassessing his airway. Bring the bottle to the ED. Allow the child to sit upright in a position of comfort. Administer blow-by oxygen, as a face mask will not likely be tolerated. Contact with medical control or the regional poison center can provide information on potential complications to anticipate in transport, such as airway edema, stridor, or wheezing. Do not give anything by mouth, including charcoal or fluids to dilute the bleach, as this will increase the risk of vomiting with the potential to further damage the esophagus as the alkaline stomach contents are regurgitated.

Bleach is a strong alkali whose corrosiveness depends upon the pH (>12.5 is very corrosive). Most household detergents and bleaches (pH 11–12) are not as problematic as industrial strength cleaners. Because the exact nature of this product is unknown, it should be assumed to be highly corrosive. Given the oral mucous membrane findings, this child may undergo esophagoscopy and bronchoscopy (fiber optic inspection of the esophagus and airways while under anesthesia) in the operating room to assess the degree of damage and need for further treatment.

Case Study ❷ page 163

Although this child appears well, this is a potentially dangerous ingestion. Iron is one of the most common fatal ingestions in children. There are four phases to an iron ingestion. The initial phase begins with the ingestion and lasts 6 hours. Common signs and symptoms in mild ingestion include nausea and vomiting. Stage 2 (at 6–12 hours) is the quiet phase during which the child appears well. It is not until stage 3 (12–24 hours after ingestion) that the child begins to show signs of toxicity, including gastrointestinal hemorrhage, hypotension, altered mental status, and renal and hepatic failure. Stage 4 is the post-recovery phase, during which gastrointestinal strictures can still occur. Because the extent of toxicity cannot be predicted from early symptoms, a cautious approach is warranted. Transport any child who has ingested iron-containing pills to the hospital for further evaluation unless the regional poison center has been contacted and has determined that this is a nontoxic ingestion based on the nature and number of pills taken. This is commonly the case with ingestion of children's multivitamins, where the concentration of iron is low. The ingestion of prenatal vitamins, on the other hand, can be very serious. Bring any pill bottles to the ED to ensure proper identification and risk assessment. Because iron is not absorbed by activated charcoal, do not attempt gastrointestinal decontamination.

Case Study ③ page 169

The first priority is to establish an effective airway, and begin bag-mask ventilation with 100% oxygen, as respiratory failure is present based on rate and depth of respirations.

Some questions to ask her friend include a SAMPLE history:

- Signs and symptoms: Did anyone see her before she passed out? Was she acting normal?
- Allergies: Any known drugs reactions or other allergies?
- Medications: Does she take any medications? Was she drinking any alcohol? Does she use illicit drugs? Did anyone see other drugs being passed around?
- Past medical problems: Does she have any medical problems?
- Last food or liquid: When was the last time anyone saw her with something to eat or drink?
- Events: Did anyone see her fall? When she passed out, did she hit her head?

The triad of respiratory depression, decreased level of consciousness, and pinpoint pupils is typical of an opiate ingestion, but can also occur with sedative hypnotics and gamma hydroxybutyrate (GHB)— a popular party drug. This can also be a mixed overdose, as there is evidence of alcohol on the scene. Consider naloxone, and transport the patient to the emergency department, supporting airway, breathing, and circulation as needed based on frequent reassessments.

Even without the girl's assent or her parents' consent, you are legally bound to treat and transport this patient, because she has a life-threatening condition.

Suggested Readings

Textbooks

American Academy of Pediatrics and the American College of Emergency Physicians: *APLS: The Pediatric Emergency Medicine Resource,* 4th Edition. Sudbury, MA, Jones and Bartlett Publishers, 2004.

Dieckmann R: Toxic Exposures. In: Seidel J, Henderson D, *Prehospital Care of Pediatric Emergencies,* 2nd Edition. Boston, MA, Jones and Bartlett Publishers, 1997: 122–129.

Olson K: *Poisoning & Drug Overdose,* 4th Edition. McGraw-Hill Professional, 2003.

Article

Watson W. 2002 Annual report of the American Association of Poison Control Centers Toxic Exposure Surveillance System. *Am J Emerg Med.* Sep 2003; 21(5):353–421.

8

Children in Disasters

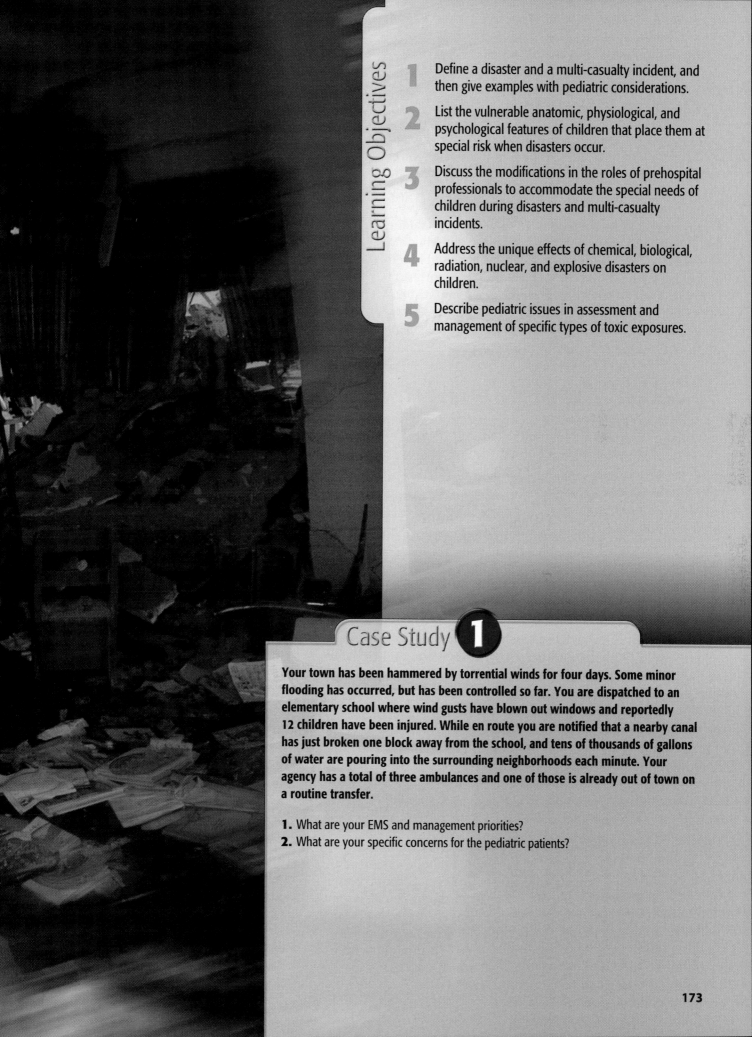

1 Define a disaster and a multi-casualty incident, and then give examples with pediatric considerations.

2 List the vulnerable anatomic, physiological, and psychological features of children that place them at special risk when disasters occur.

3 Discuss the modifications in the roles of prehospital professionals to accommodate the special needs of children during disasters and multi-casualty incidents.

4 Address the unique effects of chemical, biological, radiation, nuclear, and explosive disasters on children.

5 Describe pediatric issues in assessment and management of specific types of toxic exposures.

Case Study 1

Your town has been hammered by torrential winds for four days. Some minor flooding has occurred, but has been controlled so far. You are dispatched to an elementary school where wind gusts have blown out windows and reportedly 12 children have been injured. While en route you are notified that a nearby canal has just broken one block away from the school, and tens of thousands of gallons of water are pouring into the surrounding neighborhoods each minute. Your agency has a total of three ambulances and one of those is already out of town on a routine transfer.

1. What are your EMS and management priorities?
2. What are your specific concerns for the pediatric patients?

Children in Disasters

DISASTERS HAVE ALWAYS been a dramatic part of human history, and community responses to disasters have been a highly visible feature of modern emergency care systems. Indeed, catastrophic events have offered much affirmation of the essential role of the EMS system, as well as its limitations. Disasters present unique difficulties to prehospital professionals, and children present complex additional challenges because of their special medical, psychological, and transportation needs. There is limited data on the types and frequencies of children's injuries and illnesses during disasters, nor are there national guidelines on disaster treatment triage, and transport of children. However, in such uncommon circumstances, chaos and system overwhelm are common, so planning and preparation are imperative. Hence, all prehospital professionals must have a basic understanding of the unique pediatric issues in disasters, and EMS agencies must possess a thorough, well-rehearsed disaster response plan that addresses children. Some disasters, such as school mayhem, may primarily victimize children, and the horrific vision of prehospital professionals responding to their own children is also a distinct possibility. Post-event Critical Incident Stress Management (CISM) is becoming an intricate part of long-term disaster response.

What Is a Disaster?

Disasters are always a local issue but often also have county-wide, state-wide, or regional impact. The definition of a disaster varies by the size and location of the event. For example, a bus crash in a large city will not have much of an impact on that EMS system, but the same incident in a small rural town may exceed the community's response capabilities. Therefore, a <u>disaster</u> is an event or series of events that overwhelms the capabilities of the local emergency system and its mutual aid agreements.

Disasters are community emergencies that disrupt normal function and threaten the safety of the citizens. Because the United States emergency care system is designed primarily to care for adults, the infrastructure for caring for children in a disaster in most communities is likely to be inadequate—fewer hospital beds, fewer specialists, and less experience with pediatric critical illness.

A <u>multi-casualty incident (MCI)</u> is an occurrence with at least three or more patients to treat and transport. An MCI may require two or more ambulances or additional help from another EMS provider agency. In some circumstances, an MCI may have an enormous impact on the EMS system. An MCI and a disaster are components on a spectrum of major community unto-ward events, rather than distinctly different types of emergency situations.

A Level I MCI occurs when local medical resources are available and adequate and regional backup resources may be put on alert. A Level II MCI requires multi-jurisdiction medical mutual aid. Mutual aid agreements should be able to provide backup plans for jurisdictions stripped of their local resources. A Level III MCI involves activation of the state disaster plan. Requests for federal assistance may be necessary.

There are two basic types of disasters: natural and man-made. **Table 8-1** lists common examples. Natural disasters are events caused by non-human, usually environmental perturbations such as earthquakes, severe storms, flooding, and natural epidemic disease outbreaks. Man-made disasters result

Table 8-1	Common Natural and Man-made Disasters	
Natural	**Man-made**
Earthquake	Hazardous material spill
Hurricane	Structure fire
Tornado	Biological exposure
Flood	Chemical exposure
Wildland fire	Nuclear exposure
Disease epidemic	Structural failure
	Terrorism

from human errors, such as toxic spills, structural collapses, terrorism, or mass shootings. Regardless of origin, disasters typically cause significant increases in incidence of both pediatric injuries and illnesses.

Natural Disasters

Earthquakes

North America is situated atop multiple seismically active fault lines. Faults are seams in the earth's crust along which geological plates slide. An earthquake is a sudden, rapid shaking of the earth caused by the breaking and shifting of rock beneath the earth's surface along these fault lines. This shaking can cause buildings and bridges to collapse; disrupt gas, electric, and phone service; and sometimes trigger landslides, avalanches, flash floods, fires, and huge, destructive ocean waves (tsunamis). Ground movement during an earthquake is seldom the direct cause of death or injury. Most earthquake-related injuries result from collapsing walls, flying glass, and falling objects.

Damage from earthquakes can be extensive, and multiple types of injuries may occur. These injuries usually include blunt and multisystem trauma. Penetrating injuries are less frequent. *Seismic events also trigger illnesses, especially asthma.* Environmental disasters presumably release environmental antigens that are associated with bronchospasm and respiratory illness. The additional psychological stress during earthquakes can also contribute to increases in prevalence of childhood wheezing.

Floods

Many environmental events can cause flooding (**Figure 8-1**). Unlike earthquakes, flooding is usually somewhat predictable and typ-

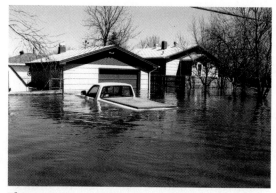

Figure 8-1 Flooding is a yearly concern in many areas of the country.

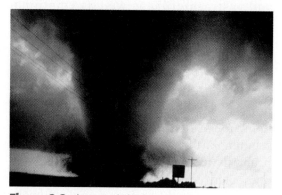

Figure 8-2 The central plains experience tornados.

ically has a more gradual development, so dislocation can be anticipated and flooding tends not to separate families unexpectedly. However, separation can occur during flash flooding. An additional public health consequence of flooding is contamination of drinking water and outbreaks of disease. Children may be at a greater risk of dehydration from vomiting and diarrhea associated with contamination.

Hurricanes, Tornados, and Severe Storms

Severe storms are different depending on the geographical region. Coastal areas have hurricanes, while the central plains experience tornados (**Figure 8-2**). Much of the continent is at risk from blizzards, heavy rains, and high winds, and these often wreak havoc on communities. Prehospital professionals must be aware of the potential for pediatric patients to experience cold temperature emergencies during severe storms because infants and young children have a higher body surface area and lose heat more

Tip

A natural disaster and environmental disturbance, such as an earthquake, often causes a major increase in pediatric respiratory ailments, especially asthma.

quickly than adults when their skin is wet or cold.

Hurricanes, tornados, and severe storms can lead to structural damage, loss of power, communication outages, and isolation. Floods may result. EMS providers must coordinate efforts with other local agencies, like search and rescue, to help the victims. These events will place children and the elderly at the greatest risks of injury from environmental conditions and structural damage. There are also added problems of asthma exacerbations, respiratory ailments, and gastroenteritis as well as emotional crises over separation of families.

Many types of disasters will damage the infrastructure and often separate family members. Depending on the time of day the event occurs, there may be heavy concentrations of children in schools and other locations. Younger children will have little understanding of the events. Instead, they may be primarily focused on separation from loved ones. Being separated from their parents and uncertain about the coming events will make the management of their emotional needs difficult. *EMS systems must anticipate these emotional crises and have a plan in place to establish communications and restore unity of families as quickly as possible.*

EMS systems must anticipate emotional crises in children who are separated from their families during a disaster and have a plan in place to establish communications and restore unity of families as quickly as possible.

Disease Epidemics

Every year there are significant communicable disease outbreaks. Typically, the pediatric population is at the heart of these outbreaks. Non-immunized children become victims then disease vectors, and increase the likelihood of epidemic outbreaks of infections such as influenza, chicken pox, measles, polio, and hepatitis. Sometimes new viruses, especially influenza, may attack a community and greatly elevate requirements for prehospital and hospital services. Occasionally, the prehospital professional may be at risk for disease transmission from contact with an infected patient.

Man-made Disasters

Disasters can also be man-made, such as hazardous material incidents, structure failures, and criminal activities such as mass shootings, or terrorism. These events have an extensive impact on children.

Hazardous Materials Exposures

In daily life, **hazardous materials** are everywhere (**Table 8-2**). Examples of these hazards are chemicals used in refrigeration, swimming pool maintenance, and fuels as well as petroleum-based agricultural products. All of these materials are present in schools and other public facilities, as well as in homes. A new hazard in recent years is home-based, illegal methamphetamine labs. Materials used in creation of recreational methamphetamines are highly explosive and may cause burns and serious injuries to bystanders—which may include unsuspecting children.

Children have a higher body surface area and thin skin, which makes them more susceptible to injury from burns, chemicals, and absorbable toxins.

Table 8-2	Examples of Common Hazardous Materials	
Diesel fuels		Insecticides
Gasoline		Fertilizers
Motor oil		Propane
Herbicides		Natural gas

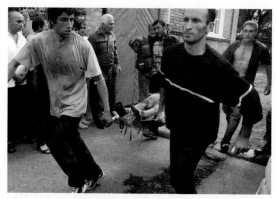

Figure 8-3 Evacuating an injured child during the school terrorism attack in Russia.

A new and troubling trend is the targeting of children, sometimes by their peers, for school shootings and terrorism.

Table 8-3	Vulnerable Pediatric Characteristics
Pediatric Characteristic	**Special Risk During Disaster**
Respiratory	Higher minute volume increases risk from exposure to inhaled agents. Nuclear fallout and heavier gases settle lower to the ground and may affect children more severely.
Gastrointestinal	May be more at risk for dehydration from vomiting and diarrhea after exposure to contamination.
Skin	Higher body surface area increases risk of skin exposure. Skin is thinner and more susceptible to injury from burns, chemicals, and absorbable toxins. Evaporative loss is higher when skin is wet or cold, so hypothermia is more likely.
Endocrine	Increased risk of thyroid cancer from radiation exposure.
Thermoregulation	Less able to cope with temperature problems with higher risk of hypothermia.
Developmental	Less ability to escape environmental dangers or anticipate hazards.
Psychological	Prolonged stress from critical incidents. Susceptible to separation anxiety.

Structural Failures

Buildings, bridges, and platforms sometimes fail. These collapses typically cause multiple injuries. Victims may be hysterical and confused, and individuals may be buried under other victims. Sometimes, children are the primary victims, especially when structural failures involve schools or recreational facilities.

Criminal Activity and Terrorism

A new troubling trend is the targeting of children by their peers for criminal acts. These disasters may have horrific mass casualties. School shootings are the most obvious of these types of disasters. School shootings pose many unique difficulties because of safety issues for prehospital professionals, communication requirements, emotional responses of victims and providers, and gross overextension of emergency resources.

Terrorism is an emerging threat for all regions of the world. Children are frequent targets, sometimes because of the desired psychological impact of death and injury of vulnerable victims by the perpetrators (**Figure 8-3**).

Vulnerable Pediatric Physiological and Psychological Characteristics in Disasters

Because of their younger anatomy and physiology, children are especially vulnerable to the effects of disasters. In addition, their immature behavioral and psychological characteristics place them at higher risk for immediate injury and longer term effects. **Table 8-3** summarizes vulnerable physiologic and psychological characteristics of children that place them at high risk during disasters.

Emotional Responses of Children

Response to a disaster or MCI must include an assessment of the emotional states of a child and the child's family. The mental health needs of children also must be recognized in the incident command system and planning for disasters. *Appropriate mental health personnel with pediatric expertise should participate in the aftermath of disasters,* to help ensure adequate sheltering and secure places to begin the stress debriefing and counseling services. Reuniting children with their families is key to family-centered care. Children and families' emotional responses range from fear and anxiety to depression, grief, and symptoms of posttraumatic stress. Children may be especially vulnerable to posttraumatic stress reactions. Pediatric aspects of shelter management need to be considered if children are separated from their parents. Each child responds differently to disasters, depending on his age and maturity. However, children of all ages experience anxiety from disasters. Younger children may interpret the disaster as a personal danger to themselves and those whom they care about.

Roles of the Prehospital Professional in a Disaster

Phases of Disaster Response

There are three phases of disaster response. The first phase is the <u>activation phase</u>. This occurs with notification and initial response and includes organization of command structure (Incident Command System) and scene assessment. This is followed by the <u>implementation phase</u>, during which there is search and rescue, victim triage, initial stabilization and transport, and definitive management of scene hazards and victims. Finally, the <u>recovery phase</u> occurs with scene withdrawal, return to normal operations, and debriefing.

Overall Response Strategy

Disasters often overwhelm prehospital professionals and the EMS system. First, prehospital professionals must recognize that the incident will probably exceed their individual capabilities, and they should immediately activate special response plans. These response plans must be part of a unified command/management structure. Prehospital professionals must immediately establish the <u>Incident Command System (ICS)</u> and an <u>Incident Commander (IC)</u> to set the stage for efficient management of the event. The goal in a disaster response is to do the most good for the most victims, and these actions allow optimal organization of the response.

Second, prehospital professionals must refrain from rushing into the scene and becoming victims themselves. This task is even more daunting when the victims are children and the impulse to help is powerful. *Remember that you cannot help if you become injured.* Use appropriate safety equipment and personal protective equipment (PPE) on every call when there is potential that the rescuer may come in contact with contaminated patients. Chemical, biological, and radiological incidents require specific and specialized equipment. Therefore, before entering any scene, be sure it has been cleared by the appropriate authorities (law enforcement, fire). Most experts agree that Level C protection (facemask with canister filtration system) is adequate for most conventional disasters, while

Case Study 2

You are the first to arrive on the scene of a reported shooting at a local middle school. The dispatch information said at least four people have been shot and the perpetrators have been apprehended. When you arrive on scene, law enforcement has secured the area. Three students in the cafeteria and one adult on the second floor in the principal's office are seriously injured.

1. As you and your partner park and begin to pull your gear from the ambulance, what are your first considerations?
2. What pediatric issues are important?

Prehospital professionals must refrain from rushing into the scene and becoming victims themselves. Injured and dead rescuers will not be able to save anyone.

Because prehospital professionals often have trouble locating pulses on some children, the pulse step can be skipped in triage if the provider believes that there is evidence of perfusion. Move right on to giving the five breaths and reassess.

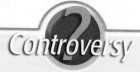

The JumpSTART system has not been field tested in any large scale incidents.

some experts contend that Level B may be necessary (hose-supplied air).

Third, prehospital professionals must exercise the highest vigilance in securing communications between victims and families. This is especially important for children during disaster triage, treatment, and transport.

Specific Response Strategies

After initial recognition and general responses to a disaster, the subsequent organization consists of four specific components: staging, triage, treatment, and transport.

Staging

Staging occurs when ambulances arrive on the scene of a recognized disaster. The prehospital professionals meet in an assigned location and await the instructions from the staging officer. This will ensure quick deployment. Providers assigned to staging must remain close to their ambulances. In order for the ICS to function properly, all prehospital professionals need to coordinate their efforts to ensure proper and timely patient care.

Triage

Triage is the process of prioritizing patients based on the severity of their injuries and available resources. The goal of triage in the disaster setting is to make a seemingly impossible task manageable. The pediatric population is a challenge, as many patients are nonverbal, frightened, separated from family members, and may have injuries with

which rescuers are unfamiliar (e.g., crush injuries, hypothermia, bomb blasts). Proper triaging of pediatric patients requires triage algorithms. The START (Simple Triage And Rapid Treatment) triage system developed by the Newport Beach (CA) Fire and Marine Department and Hoag Hospital is one identified method for triage of disaster patients. The START triage system categorizes patients by color to allow the prehospital professional to categorize a patient rapidly for treatment. It is difficult to apply the START concepts to young children because the system requires that victims have the ability to verbally communicate and ambulate.

The JumpSTART triage system, designed for children under 8 years of age or under 100 pounds, is another possible pediatric triage tool for disasters. This triage system uses important assessment characteristics of infants and children to distinguish them from older patients. JumpSTART uses breathing as the cornerstone for triage decisions (**Figure 8-4**).

There are four triage categories in the JumpSTART system, designated by colors corresponding to different levels of urgency for treatment. Decision points include: able to walk (except infants), presence of spontaneous breathing, respirations less than 15 or

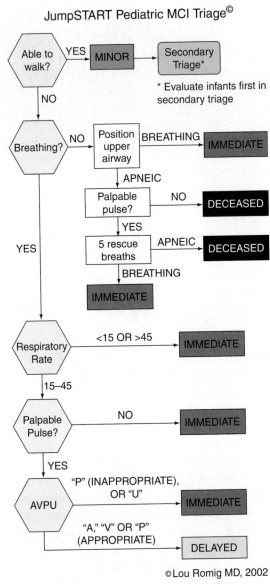

JumpSTART Pediatric MCI Triage©

© Lou Romig MD, 2002

Figure 8-4 The JumpSTART triage system.

ignated as Red for Immediate intervention. Children who are both apneic and without pulse, or apneic and unresponsive to rescue breathing are designated as Black and considered deceased or expectant deceased.

Treatment

<u>Decontamination</u> is the physical process of removing or neutralizing potentially harmful substances from personnel, equipment, and supplies. A person or piece of equipment may become contaminated by contacting vapors, mists, solids, or liquids from a source of contaminant or from others already contaminated. *Perform decontamination whenever an individual is actually or potentially contaminated with a hazardous substance.* One objective of patient decontamination is to minimize the amount of a hazardous chemical on a victim's skin that is available for absorption. Another objective is to prevent contamination of the rescuers. Families are likely to be kept together during this process. However, lack of adequate protocols or preplanning may require that other adults or older children be recruited to assist in decontaminating younger children.

Whenever the number of patients exceeds the number of ambulances available for transportation, assign treatment areas and attempt to keep families together. Once these patients have arrived at the treatment area, conduct a secondary triage to determine if the child's initial triage status has changed. Essential medical equipment is vital in maintaining a functional treatment area. Each of the different JumpSTART triage divisions—red, yellow, green, and black—needs to have its own treatment area. Have the most experienced providers treat the red and yellow designated patients.

Treatment of pediatric patients in disaster situations varies greatly depending upon the specifics of the disaster, the exposure of the patient, and the availability of resources of the responding agencies. Treatment should always include removing the patient

greater than 45 breaths/min, palpable peripheral pulse, and appropriate response to painful stimuli on the AVPU.

Patients who are able to walk are designated as Green for Minor and not in immediate need of treatment. Those breathing spontaneously, with a peripheral pulse and appropriately responsive to painful stimuli, are designated as Yellow for Delayed treatment. Children that have apnea responsive to positioning or rescue breathing; respiratory failure; breathing but without pulse; or with inappropriate painful response, are des-

Table 8-4	Common Chemicals Detrimental to Human Health	
Bleach (laundry)	Oven cleaner
Pesticides	Rubbing alcohol
Paint thinner	Paint
Ammonia	Laundry soap
Nail polish	Asbestos
Furniture polish	

Table 8-5	Biological Agents That Pose a Threat to Humans	
Anthrax	E. coli
Smallpox	Salmonella
Ricin	Botulism
HIV	Cholera
Plague	Influenza

from the source of the threat or agent as immediately as possible with due consideration to hot, warm, and cold zones, secondary threats, and the prehospital professional's safety.

Special care is indicated for children because they are at an increased risk for hypothermia when exposed to the environment during decontamination. Make sure there are pediatric-sized clothes to dress the children after decontamination is completed. This procedure also reduces the risk of secondary contamination to responding health care providers and public safety personnel. Time is a critical consideration in effective decontamination of skin exposed to liquid chemical agents. Even if large amounts of time have elapsed since the initial exposure, perform decontamination on the patient to eliminate the exposure to others.

Transport

The transport officer's duty is to get patients into ambulances and routed to hospitals. The transport officer must be flexible in order to ensure that the proper patients are transported to the proper facilities. Prehospital professionals must be cognizant of destination policies, so that children go to hospitals prepared for pediatric emergencies. Do not give pediatric patients priority for transport just because they are children. Assign transport priority based on the patient's condition.

Effects of Chemical, Biological, Radiation, Nuclear, and Explosive Disasters on Children

Chemicals

Millions of different chemicals in the world are detrimental to human health (**Table 8-4**). Chemicals are transported throughout the country every day by trucks, trains, and planes. Chemical weapons may cause death and disease. These chemicals range from mustard gas to VX.

When chemical spills are identified, government officials working in hazardous materials (HazMat) are a key resource for identification of toxicity and relative risk, decontamination procedures, and specific treatment.

Biological Agents

There are many different biological agents that pose a threat to humans (**Table 8-5**). They can be as common as influenza or as deadly as HIV. Biological weapons used by terrorists can cause widespread disease and death. Typical weapons include anthrax, smallpox, botulism, and plague. Terrorists use these agents because they are fairly easy to purchase or make. An added incentive is that most of the agents are extremely contagious and are often spread to a large number of people, which can include children in schools and childcare facilities.

Radiation

Radiation disasters, while rare, can occur wherever radioactive materials are used, stored, or transported. In addition to nuclear power plants, hospitals, universities, research laboratories, industries, major highways, railroads, or shipping yards are possible sites. Radioactive materials are dangerous because of the harmful effect certain types of radiation have on the cells of the body. The longer a person is exposed to radiation, the greater the risk. Children may be more susceptible to radiation injury. Radiation weapons include nuclear and "dirty" bombs. Radiation cannot be detected by sight, smell, or any other sense.

Nuclear

A <u>dirty bomb</u>, also known as a radiological weapon, consists of a conventional explosive such as dynamite packaged with radioactive material that scatters when the bomb explodes. A dirty bomb kills or injures through the initial blast of the conventional explosive and by airborne radiation and contamination—hence the term "dirty."

A <u>nuclear bomb</u> uses the power of nuclear fission or fusion to produce an intense pulse or wave of heat, light, air pressure, and radiation. In a nuclear blast, injury or death may occur as a result of the blast itself or as a result of debris thrown from the blast. Children may experience moderate to severe skin burns, depending on their distance from the blast site. Those who look directly at the blast may experience eye damage ranging from temporary blindness to severe burns on the retina. Individuals near the blast site may be exposed to high levels of radiation and develop symptoms of radiation sickness.

There are two types of exposure from radioactive materials from a nuclear blast: external exposure and internal exposure. External exposure occurs when people are exposed to radiation outside of their bodies from the blast or its fallout. Internal exposure occurs when people eat food or breathe air that is contaminated with radioactive fallout. Both internal and external exposure from fallout can occur miles away from the blast site.

Perform decontamination whenever an individual is possibly contaminated with a hazardous substance

Be sure children do not get hypothermic after decontamination. Dry them and give them warm clothes right away.

Explosives

Explosive devices are frequently employed for terrorism. Children are at risk for blast injury due to their size and susceptibility to head and abdominal injuries. The blast wave, flying debris, and injuries from being thrown may have more deadly results.

Pediatric Issues in Assessment and Treatment of Specific Toxic Exposures

Nerve Agents

Characteristics of <u>nerve agents</u> are that they are extremely toxic and they have very rapid effects. Common agents may include: tabun, sarin, soman, VX, or organophosphates. The nerve agent, either as a gas, aerosol, or liquid, enters the body through inhalation or through the skin. These two characteristics pertain to children because of their faster respiratory rates and larger skin surface area-to-mass ratio. Poisoning may also occur through consumption of liquids or foods contaminated with nerve agents. All nerve agents cause toxic effects by preventing the proper operation of the chemical that acts as the body's "off switch" for glands and muscles.

Case Study 3

It is 7:00 AM. You are dispatched to a large downtown hotel. Upon arrival you are presented with two adult and three pediatric patients, all tourists from a neighboring state. They all have some level of respiratory distress, tightness in their chests, and coughing. Some complain of weakness and joint pain, and two of the children and one adult are cyanotic especially around their lips. They state the only thing they can relate this to, is being sprayed in the subway at 10:00 PM last night by a group of protesters. The patients state they thought it was just air in the aerosol cans. There was no odor or color. They also state that there are 36 of them traveling together but the others haven't shown up for the breakfast as planned.

1. Would you suspect a biological or chemical agent in this case?
2. How would you treat and transport these patients?

Without an "off switch," the glands and muscles are constantly being stimulated, causing the victim to tire and no longer be able to sustain breathing. Due to the extremely rapid onset of symptoms, it is likely that children exposed to these agents will develop symptoms before exposed adults.

The initial signs and symptoms of a nerve agent exposure include: frontal headache, eye pain, miosis (pupil constriction), runny nose, anorexia (loss of appetite), nausea, excessive sweating, tightness in the chest, and heartburn. If the patient is exposed to large amounts of nerve agents, abdominal cramps, vomiting, profuse sweating, dyspnea, diarrhea, drooling and tearing, urinary frequency, involuntary urination or defecation, and/or excessive bronchial secretions may occur. Children are more prone to dehydration due to gastrointestinal fluid losses, further complicating their management.

Treatment for nerve agents includes use of atropine, pralidoxime (2-PAM), and benzodiazepines. These can all be given IM with effective absorption. Use antidotes only for severe exposures with signs and symptoms listed above. Treat skin contact by decontamination with copious amounts of water. Pralidoxime dosing is 25–50 mg/kg over 5–30 minutes with a maximum dose of 1 g IV. Most packaging of 2-PAM is available to prehospital professionals in auto-injectors. In order to manipulate the dosing for children, discharge the auto-injector into a sterile vial and then draw

Blip

Inhalation of nerve gas may occur without the knowledge of the victim.

Tip

Children may be more susceptible to nerve gas because of their faster respiratory rates and larger skin surface area-to-mass ratio.

up for administration. Children are challenging to care for by personnel wearing PPE, because it is difficult for rescuers to perform procedures while at the same time having to battle their own environmental conditions. In addition, prehospital personnel wearing PPE may frighten children and render the assessment more confusing.

Cyanide

Cyanide is a rapidly acting, potentially deadly chemical that can exist in various forms. Cyanide can be a colorless gas or in a crystal form. Cyanide sometimes is described as having a "bitter almond" smell, but it does not always give off an odor, and not everyone can detect this odor. Cyanide is released from natural substances in some foods and in certain plants. It is in cigarette smoke and the combustion products of synthetic materials such as plastics. Patients may be exposed to cyanide by breathing air, drinking water, eating food, or touching soil that contains cyanide. The extent of poisoning caused by cyanide depends on the amount of cyanide a patient is exposed to, the route of exposure, and the length of time that a patient is exposed.

Breathing cyanide gas causes the most harm, but ingesting cyanide can be toxic as well. Cyanide prevents the cells of the body from using oxygen. When this happens, the cells die. Cyanide is more harmful to the heart and brain than to other organs because the heart and brain use a lot of oxygen. Children exposed to a small amount of cyanide by breathing it, absorbing it through their skin, or eating foods that contain it may have some or all of the following symptoms within minutes: tachypnea, restlessness, dizziness, weakness, headache, nausea and vomiting, and tachycardia. Exposure to a large amount of cyanide by any route may cause convulsions, hypotension, bradycardia, loss of consciousness, lung injury, and respiratory failure leading to death.

Cyanide is highly volatile and removing the patient from the environment is often all that is needed to decontaminate them. If the child is soaked from a spill, remove the clothing and wash the child with soap and warm water. Even though cyanide inhibits cellular oxygen usage, administration of 100% oxygen probably is still useful. Most cases of cyanide poisoning will respond to these simple steps.

In the case of a significant exposure, locate cyanide antidote kits. Cyanide antidote kits are available at most hospitals; however, it is unlikely that in the event of a large MCI involving cyanide exposure that there will be enough kits available. Kits contain three components; amyl nitrate ampoules, sodium nitrate, and sodium thiosulfate. Administer amyl nitrate by inhalation of 30 seconds every 2 minutes until signs of recovery occur. The amyl nitrate is supplied in 0.3-cc thin glass capsules (similar to ammonia inhalants) that can be crushed and placed by the patient's mouth and nose or into an oxygen mask. Sodium nitrate is usually given when a methemoglobin concentration of 12 g/dL, is documented. The dose is 0.33 mL/kg of the standard 3% solution given slowly, IV, over 5 to 10 minutes. The initial thiosulfate dose for pediatric patients is 1.65 mL/kg of the standard 25% solution, IV. Second treatments with each of the two antidotes may be given at up to half the original dose if needed.

Although the combination of sodium nitrate and sodium thiosulfate may save victims exposed to lethal doses of cyanide and are effective even after breathing has stopped, many patients will recover even without specific antidotal treatment if they receive vigorous general supportive care. Administration of antidotes, especially if not given slowly enough or if given in extremely large doses, is also associated with morbidity and even mortality. Do not withhold antidotes in a patient in whom cyanide poisoning is suspected, but be sure infusion rates are slow and the drugs titrated to effect. Avoid overdosage.

Pulmonary Intoxicants

Pulmonary intoxicants produce pulmonary edema. The most widely known agents are phosgene and chlorine. The effects of these agents are not immediate. In most cases, patients will have shortness of breath caused by pulmonary edema hours after exposure. Patients will typically exhibit eye and airway irritation, dyspnea, and chest

Patients exposed to a small amount of cyanide by breathing it, absorbing it through their skin, or eating foods that contain it may have symptoms within minutes.

tightness. Without treatment, patients can go into respiratory failure.

Vesicants

<u>Vesicants</u> are chemicals that cause blistering of the skin, irritation and inflammation of the airways, vomiting and diarrhea, convulsions, and lethargy. Exposure to vesicants can be through inhalation, absorption, or ingestion. The most common vesicants are sulfur mustard (mustard gas) and Lewisite. Mustard has no immediate effects. Blistering will usually occur hours after contact. Lewisite causes immediate irritation to eyes, skin, and upper airways. Within seconds, Lewisite liquid causes pain and burning on any surface it comes in contact with.

Treatment for these chemicals includes decontamination with large volumes of warm water at low pressure, airway control, and oxygen administration. Bandage wounds with dry dressings. Providers may consider administration of British Anti-Lewisite (BAL) as an antidote for Lewisite at a dose of 3 mg/kg. However, there is little experience with this in children.

Biological Pathogens

<u>Biological pathogens</u>, released intentionally, accidentally, or naturally occurring, can result in disease or death. Human exposure to these agents may occur through inhalation, cutaneous exposure, or ingestion of contaminated food or water. Following exposure, physical symptoms may be delayed and sometimes confused with naturally occurring illnesses. Biological agents may persist in the environment and cause problems some time after their release.

Smallpox

<u>Smallpox</u> is caused by variola virus. The incubation period is about 12 days (range 7–17 days) following exposure. Initial symptoms include high fever, fatigue, and head and back aches. A characteristic rash, most prominent on the face, arms, and legs, follows in 2 to 3 days (**Figure 8-5**). The rash starts with flat red lesions that evolve at the

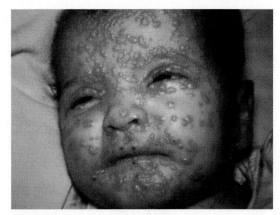

Figure 8-5 Smallpox.

same rate. Lesions become pus-filled and begin to crust early in the second week. Scabs develop and then separate and fall off after about 3 to 4 weeks. The majority of patients with smallpox recover, but death occurs in up to 30% of cases. Smallpox is spread from one person to another by infected saliva droplets that expose a susceptible person having face-to-face contact with the ill person. Persons with smallpox are most infectious during the first week of illness, because that is when the largest amount of virus is present in saliva.

Anthrax

<u>Anthrax</u> is an acute infectious disease caused by the spore-forming bacterium *Bacillus anthracis*. Anthrax most commonly occurs in hoofed mammals and can also infect humans. Symptoms of disease vary depending on how the disease was contracted, but usually occur within 7 days after exposure. *The serious forms of human anthrax are inhalation anthrax, cutaneous anthrax, and intestinal anthrax.* Initial symptoms of inhalation anthrax infection may resemble a common cold. After several days, the symptoms may progress to severe breathing problems and shock. Inhalation anthrax is often fatal. The intestinal disease form of anthrax may follow the consumption of contaminated food and is characterized by an acute inflammation of the intestinal tract. Initial signs of nausea, loss of appetite, vomiting, and fever are followed by abdominal pain, vomiting of blood, and

The serious forms of human anthrax are inhalation anthrax, cutaneous anthrax, and intestinal anthrax.

Plague is an infectious disease carried by rodents and their fleas in many areas around the world.

severe diarrhea. Direct person-to-person spread of anthrax is extremely unlikely.

Plague

Plague is an infectious disease of animals and humans caused by the bacterium *Yersinia pestis. Y. pestis* is found in rodents and their fleas in many areas around the world. Pneumonic plague occurs when *Y. pestis* infects the lungs. The first signs of illness in pneumonic plague are fever, headache, weakness, and cough productive of bloody or watery sputum. The pneumonia progresses over 2 to 4 days and may cause septic shock and, without early treatment, death. Person-to-person transmission of pneumonic plague occurs through respiratory droplets, which can only infect those who have face-to-face contact with the ill patient.

Ricin

Ricin is a potent protein toxin derived from the beans of the castor plant (*Ricinus communis*). The beans are available worldwide and the toxin is fairly easily produced. When inhaled as a small particle aerosol, this toxin may produce pathological changes within eight hours and have severe respiratory symptoms followed by respiratory failure in 36 to 72 hours. *When ingested, ricin causes severe gastrointestinal symptoms like vomiting and bloody diarrhea.* Ingested ricin exposure will eventually cause hallucinations, seizures, low blood pressure, followed by vascular collapse and death. Ricin cannot be transmitted from person to person.

Specific Treatment of Biological Disease

Table 8-6 summarizes the specific treatment of diseases caused by biological agents, including pediatric doses.

Critical Incident Stress Debriefing

A **critical incident stress management (CISM) team** can provide support and counseling for prehospital professionals who have been exposed to stressful incidents in the course of providing emergency medical services. The need for this may be especially acute after dealing with pediatric patients in disasters. A mental health professional may be part of the CISM team. The debriefing process is intended to be educational, and CISM is not psychotherapy. The effectiveness of CISM after disasters, for prehospital professionals and for children, is not known.

Summary

Disasters are fortunately a rare occurrence, but when they happen they will often involve children. Preparation is the key to providing good care. Using the National Incident Management System and ICS will ensure the incoming resources will be able to communicate and interact with the incident commander on scene. Triaging of patients can be done using a number of methods. The JumpSTART system may provide distinctive features for young children.

Because of their physiological, anatomical, and psychological aspects, children present a challenge to the prehospital professional. Both natural and man-made disasters will require EMS to pre-plan their response and rehearse their roles in an ever changing world.

Table 8-6	Medical Management of Bioterrorism Infections			
Vaccine and Dosage	**Treatment (adolescents)**	**Treatment (children)**	**Prevention (adolescents)**	**Prevention (children)**
Anthrax				
Bioport vaccine, 0.5 mL SC at weeks 0, 2, and 4, and months 6, 12, and 18, then annual boosters	Ciprofloxacin, 400 mg IV twice daily *or* Ciprofloxacin, 500 mg orally twice daily *or* Doxycycline, 200 mg IV, then 100 mg IV twice daily for 60 days *or* Penicillin, 4 million units IV every four hours for 14 days	Ciprofloxacin, 10 to 15 mg per kg IV twice daily (maximum: 1 g per day)	Ciprofloxacin, 500 mg orally twice daily for 60 days; *or* Doxycycline, 100 mg orally twice daily for 60 days, plus vaccination	10–15 mg/kg (max 500 mg) POg 12 hours for 60 days *or* Doxycycline (> 8 years), 2.5 mg per kg IV or orally twice daily for 60 days (max dose 100 mg)
Smallpox				
Wyeth calf lymph vaccinia, one dose by scarification	No current treatment other than supportive; cidofovir is effective in vitro; animal studies are ongoing	Same as adult treatment	Vaccinia immune globulin, 0.6 mL/kg IM within 3 days (most effective within 24 hours) of exposure. Usually given to immunocompromised persons	If available, give vaccine
Plague				
Vaccine is no longer available	Streptomycin, 30 mg per kg per day IM in two divided doses for 10 to 14 days *or* Gentamicin, 5 mg per kg IM or IV once daily for 10 to 14 days *or* Ciprofloxacin, 400 mg IV twice daily until clinically improved, then 750 mg orally twice daily for a total of 10 to 14 days *or* Doxycycline, 200 mg IV, then 100 mg IV twice daily until clinically improved, then 100 mg orally twice daily for a total of 10 to 14 days	Streptomycin, 15 mg per kg IM twice daily for 10 days (maximum: 2 g per day) *or* Gentamicin, 2.5 mg per kg IM or IV three times daily for 10 days *or* Doxycycline (< 45 kg), 2.2 mg per kg orally or IV twice daily for 10 days Doxycycline (> 45 kg), adult dosage	Doxycycline, 100 mg orally twice daily for 7 days or duration of exposure *or* Ciprofloxacin, 500 mg orally twice daily for 7 days *or* Tetracycline, 500 mg orally four times daily for 7 days	Doxycycline, 2.2 mg/kg (max 100 mg) orally twice daily for 7 days Ciprofloxacin, 20 mg/kg (max 500 mg) orally twice daily for 7 days Chloramphenicol, 25 mg/kg (max 1 g) orally every 6 hours for 7 days

Abbreviations are: SC = subcutaneously; IV = intravenously; PO = orally; IM = intramuscularly; FDA = U.S. Food and Drug Administration; CDC = Centers for Disease Control and Prevention.

Chapter Review

Case Study Answers

Case Study ❶ page 173

Confirm that your position is safe and identify all other potential initial responders.

Ask for determination whether the school is in a flood zone and consider the necessity of an evacuation order. Establish the Incident Command System and identify your casualty collection point at the nearest safe location. Begin rescue and evacuation operations. Establish your disaster operations plan and activate your mutual aid agreements as necessary. Have dispatch notify your local medical facilities of the MCI/disaster and assure the necessary notifications are made to emergency relief agencies.

During your assessment of the children, determine the severity of injuries and triage them using an appropriate system, such as the JumpSTART triage system. Maintain the psychological support of the children by remaining calm and attempt to reunite families when possible. Pediatric patients will require additional care to maintain thermal balance during a weather related emergency. Providing blankets and protection from the wind and rain are important aspects of caring for these patients.

Case Study ❷ page 178

Scene safety must be the primary consideration. Law enforcement should provide notification of a safe scene and provide clear access to the patients. Establish Incident Command if it has not already been established by the initial officers on scene, and determine staging and triage areas. Request an adequate (ALS/BLS) response and transportation or additional resources such as helicopters.

Use an appropriate triaging system, such as JumpSTART, to assist with rapid triage and transport. Concentrate resources on salvageable patients (red and yellow categories) and transport children to appropriate hospitals. Consider transporting the children to a trauma center with pediatric capabilities.

Case Study ❸ page 183

These patients may have been exposed to a toxic agent, dispersed in the aerosol spray. More likely it would be a biological agent because most chemical agents work within minutes of contact. Biological agents, in contrast, must have time to incubate.

Begin by donning personal protective equipment such as gowns, gloves, and masks. Treatment must begin by securing the scene in order to contain the spread of the potential disease. Have someone make contact with the other guests from the group and determine if additional concerns exist. Contact medical command to determine the best location for transport of the patients. Make sure to notify law enforcement authorities, because events of terrorism are first and foremost a crime scene. Determine if additional notifications must be made to the health department or other governmental agency.

Suggested Educational Resources

Textbooks

Hogan D, Burstein J: *Disaster Medicine.* Philadelphia, PA, Lippincott Williams & Wilkins, 2002.

Bledsoe B, Porter R, Cherry R: *Essentials of Paramedic Care.* Upper Saddle River, NJ, Prentice Hall, 2003.

Articles

Ball J, Allen K. Consensus recommendations for responding to children's emergencies in disasters. *Natl Acad Pract Forum.* 2000; 2:253–257.

Lovejoy J. Disaster medicine: Initial approach to patient management after large-scale disasters. *Clin Ped Emerg Med.* 2002; 3(4):217–223.

Waeckerle JF, Seamans S, Whiteside M, et al. Executive summary: Developing objectives, content, and competencies for the training of emergency medical technicians, emergency physicians, and emergency nurses to care for casualties resulting from nuclear, biological, or chemical (NBC) incidents. *Ann Emerg Med.* 2001; 37:587–601.

Holbrook PR. Pediatric disaster medicine. *Crit Care Clin.* 1991; 7:463–470.

Emergency Delivery and Newborn Stabilization

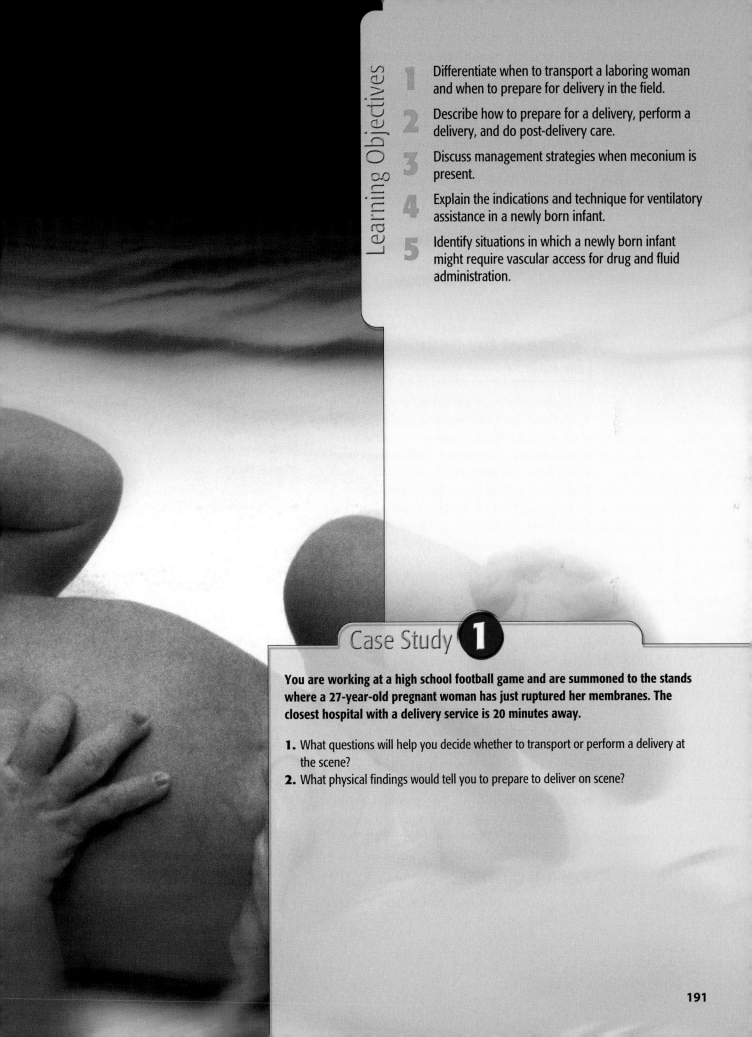

Case Study **1**

You are working at a high school football game and are summoned to the stands where a 27-year-old pregnant woman has just ruptured her membranes. The closest hospital with a delivery service is 20 minutes away.

1. What questions will help you decide whether to transport or perform a delivery at the scene?

2. What physical findings would tell you to prepare to deliver on scene?

Introduction

ALTHOUGH MOST DELIVERIES in the field or home occur without complications, there are increased risks for perinatal morbidity and mortality in the out-of-hospital setting. The probability of death or lifelong brain injury is higher when the child is born after a precipitous, out-of-hospital delivery compared to a controlled, in-hospital delivery. Furthermore, when a perinatal complication does occur, the treatment during an infant's first few minutes after birth may make a great difference in the child's functional outcome and quality of life. Emergency deliveries are more common for preterm babies, and prematurity significantly increases the risk of early complications for the child. Emergency delivery and care of the infant in the first 24 hours (the child is termed the "newly born" during this vulnerable period) can be challenging to the prehospital professional. The presence of two patients—the mother and the newly born infant—adds another dimension to this challenge.

Triage of the Patient in Labor

The safest place for the laboring mother and the baby is in a delivery room of a hospital staffed by physicians, nurses, or midwives with extensive experience with both normal and complicated deliveries. Sometimes, however, labor is fully in progress when 9-1-1 is activated. Emergency delivery in a moving vehicle is dangerous. When treating a woman in labor, the prehospital professional must first decide whether to transport the mother to an ED or to prepare for an out-of-hospital delivery.

A special problem is an emergency delivery with multiple births—twins, triplets, or more. Multiple births are likely to involve preterm infants who often require more extensive resuscitation. Sometimes the mother does not know that there is more than one baby. In these situations, use the rules for triage of mothers with single births and consider calling for a second ambulance.

In order to properly triage the laboring patient, ask two simple questions and then perform a brief physical assessment of the mother's perineum. This information will tell whether delivery is imminent (**Table 9-1**).

Two Key Questions

First, get a good history from the woman and/or her partner about the number and type of prior deliveries. Typically, the time in active labor is longer for first-time mothers

Table 9-1	Determining if Delivery Is Imminent
Questions	
Is this your first delivery?	
If you have delivered before, how long was the labor?	
Do you feel the "urge to push"?	
Physical findings	
Is the child's head crowning?	
Is the head or scalp visible at the perineum during contractions?	

(primiparas) than for women who have had prior deliveries (multiparas). If this is not a first time delivery, ask the woman the length of her previous labor(s). A history of short labor with prior pregnancies may repeat itself.

Second, ask the mother if she has an "urge to push." Most women experience this feeling at the end of labor. *In general, if the mother has the urge to push, the delivery will take place within an hour in first pregnancies, but within 30 minutes in second, third, or later pregnancies.*

Assessment of the Perineum

Next, perform a brief physical assessment of the perineum. Look for crowning—the visible appearance of the fetal head at the vaginal introitus (**Figure 9-1**). Crowning is a sign that delivery is near.

If the child's head is not immediately visible, inspect the mother's perineum during a contraction and note if the head

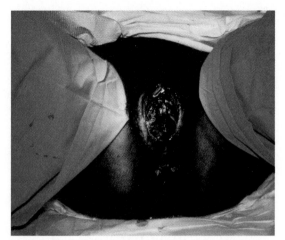

Figure 9-1 Use the presence or absence of crowning to help decide whether to transport or prepare for delivery.

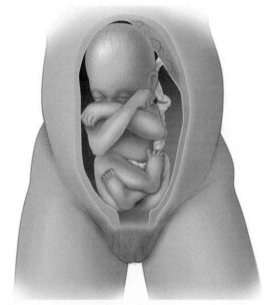

Figure 9-2 Breech birth.

becomes visible. If the infant is crowning or if the baby's head is visible at the perineum with contractions, prepare for delivery unless the transport time is extremely brief (less than 5 minutes).

Breech Deliveries

Four percent of term deliveries are <u>breech</u> deliveries (**Figure 9-2**). Inspection of the perineum will not show a head crowning, but another anatomic part, such as the feet or buttocks, might be visible. In this situation, transport immediately to the nearest ED. Breech deliveries carry a much higher risk

to both the infant and mother than <u>vertex</u> deliveries. *Given the risk of complications and the potential need for an emergency cesarean section to safely deliver the baby, initiate transport to the hospital as soon as a breech presentation is identified, even if delivery appears imminent.*

Tip

The "urge to push" experienced by most women at the end of labor is a sign that delivery is near, usually within 30 to 60 minutes.

Blip

Never try to deliver a baby with a breech presentation in the field. Initiate transport to the hospital as soon as a breech presentation is identified, even if delivery appears imminent.

Summary of Triage of Patient in Labor

The responses to the two questions (first delivery? feeling urge to push?) and the visual assessment of the perineum will provide the essential information to triage a laboring woman in the field. Look for crowning and estimate time to the hospital to decide whether to transport or prepare for delivery. Breech births are especially difficult and require immediate transport. If delivery is near in multiple-birth situations, plan to deliver on scene and call for another ambulance.

Preparation for Delivery

Resuscitation-Oriented History

Many factors in the mother's medical history will affect the outcome of the baby and help predict the need for newly born resuscitation. However, once the decision has been

Table 9-2	Resuscitation-Oriented History: Three Essential Questions
1. Do you have twins or multiple fetuses?	
2. When are you due to deliver?	
3. What color is the amniotic fluid?	

Tip

A large number of out-of-hospital deliveries will be preterm, and the need for resuscitative efforts rises with the number of days of prematurity.

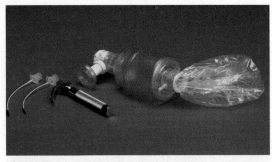

Figure 9-3 Special equipment for premature infant resuscitation: Mask, size 0 laryngoscope blade, and endotracheal tubes sizes 2.5 and 3.0.

made to deliver on scene, only three questions are pertinent for the immediate safety of the baby (**Table 9-2**).

1. *Do you have twins or multiple <u>fetuses</u>?*

   If twins or multiple newborns are expected, prepare for more than one delivery. This may mean finding extra equipment, preparing an additional warm environment, and planning the management of the first baby while delivering the second. This usually requires calling for a second ambulance.

2. *When are you due to deliver?*

   A significant number of out-of-hospital deliveries will be preterm (less than 36 weeks <u>gestation</u>), and the earlier the expected delivery date, the greater the chances of delivering a depressed newly born. Knowing the due date is important for preparing the right resuscitation equipment for airway management and breathing support. Make sure there are masks sized for preterm infants less than 30 weeks gestation. Have a size 0 <u>laryngoscope</u> blade and endotracheal tubes in sizes 2.5 and 3.0 ready as well (**Figure 9-3**).

3. *What color is the amniotic fluid?*

   Greenish color in the <u>amniotic fluid</u> is a sign of passage of <u>meconium</u>,

which is fetal stool. Meconium release by the fetus may indicate intrauterine stress, especially hypoxia. If meconium is observed, be prepared to deal with a depressed baby and/or airway obstruction. Thorough suctioning of the baby's mouth and oropharynx before delivery to clear the airway of thick meconium will usually prevent meconium aspiration and respiratory distress. Overly aggressive suctioning, however, may cause vagal stimulation and lead to bradycardia.

Tip

The presence of meconium may herald complications in the newly born: cardiorespiratory depression and/or airway obstruction.

Assembling Equipment

If the triage decision is to deliver on scene, get the appropriate equipment ready. **Table 9-3** lists the essential ambulance equipment, best organized in a portable <u>obstetric</u> pack (**Figure 9-4**).

Warming the Environment

Avoiding hypothermia is an important part of newly born management. Before delivery, make the room or ambulance as warm as possible. Turn up the heat until it is uncom-

Table 9-3	Contents of a Portable Obstetric Pack for Vaginal Delivery
Number	**Item**
1	Sterile disposable scalpel or scissors
3	Disposable towels
1	Receiving blanket
1	Sterile disposable bulb syringe
2	Sterile umbilical clamps or ties
1	Large plastic bag with twist tie (to store the **placenta**)
2	Plastic lined underpads
1	Disposable plastic apron, mask, and protective eyewear

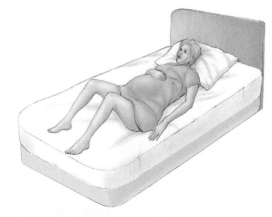

Figure 9-5 A safe position for delivery is with the mother lying supine on one side of a bed, allowing her to deliver the baby onto the bed with minimal handling.

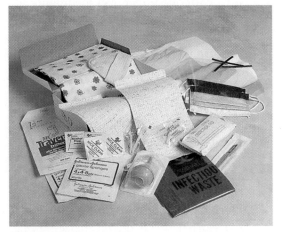

Figure 9-4 Obstetric pack.

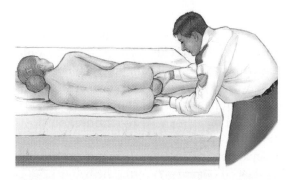

Figure 9-6 The Sims position has the mother on her side with her back toward the attendant and her knees drawn toward her chest. This position allows for easy suctioning.

fortable for an adult! Turn off the air conditioning. Air blowing across the newly born can lead to heat loss, so turn off all fans. If the setting allows, consider having a family member warm towels in the dryer in anticipation of the delivery.

Positioning the Mother

Although it is a medical emergency for the patient and the family, the delivery of a baby is also a highly personal and emotional event. Establish a plan for positioning for delivery with the mother, but let her stay in a comfortable position and covered prior to crowning.

A safe maternal position for the delivery is lying supine (on her back) on one side of a bed. *Allow her to deliver the baby onto the bed*

with minimal handling (**Figure 9-5**). However, suctioning the baby's mouth and nose before delivery of the body is difficult with the mother in this position because most infants are born face down. Another technique involves raising the mother's buttocks with a stack of folded towels in order to allow oropharyngeal suctioning of the baby.

Another safe position is the <u>Sims position</u>, in which the mother lies on her side with her back toward the attendant and her knees drawn toward her chest (**Figure 9-6**). In this position, the infant's head is easy to reach for suctioning before delivery. This is a big help in deliveries complicated by meconium-stained amniotic fluid where complete suctioning of the infant's mouth, nares, and oropharynx before delivery of the body is

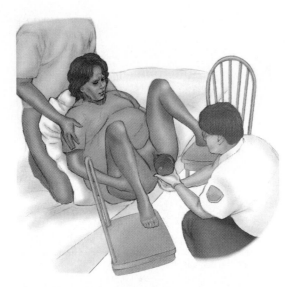

Figure 9-7 Alternate delivery position. The woman is perpendicular to the bed with each foot on a separate chair and her perineum at the end of the bed.

necessary. In this position, the mother's perineum is still over the bed, so delivery onto the bed with minimal handling is still possible.

A third position to consider, in situations where oropharyngeal suctioning is necessary, is with the woman lying supine and positioned sideways on the bed, with each foot on a separate chair and her perineum at the edge of the bed (**Figure 9-7**). After the baby's head is delivered, this position provides enough space to suction the mouth and nose before delivering the body. The disadvantage of this position is the lack of a supportive surface under the perineum, so that the prehospital professional must actually "catch" the baby.

Do not interfere unnecessarily with the delivery process.

Selecting a Clean Delivery Surface

Select a surface that is as clean as possible to conduct the immediate care of the child. *Make sure everyone involved in the child's care has washed her hands and has several pairs of gloves.*

Vaginal Delivery

Performing the Delivery

Most babies deliver themselves without assistance, especially if the laboring mother is lying supine or in the Sims position in bed. While the prehospital professional may attempt to control the delivery as described below, only minimal interference with this natural process is necessary in most cases.

Use the following sequence for all deliveries:

1. Allow the mother to push the head out of the vaginal opening.
2. Next, with one finger, feel the infant's neck for the <u>umbilical cord</u> (**Figure 9-8**). If it is there, gently lift it over the baby's head. Do not pull hard on the cord because it may lead to <u>avulsion</u> of the cord with severe hemorrhage.
3. If the woman is delivering in bed, let the delivery proceed without intervention. Place one hand around the infant's neck <u>posteriorly</u> and one hand underneath the infant to help control the delivery (**Figure 9-9**). On occasion, the infant's anterior shoulder needs to be pulled posteriorly to clear the mother's <u>symphysis pubis</u>. Place a hand on

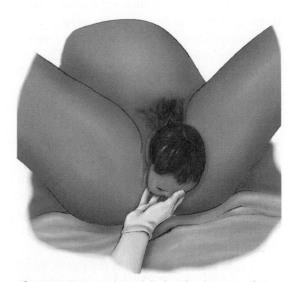

Figure 9-8 Ensure the umbilical cord is not wrapped around the baby's neck.

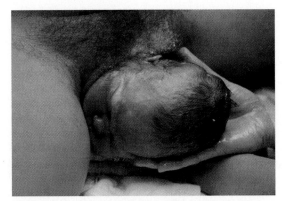

Figure 9-9 Placing a hand around the neck posteriorly and one underneath the infant may help control the delivery.

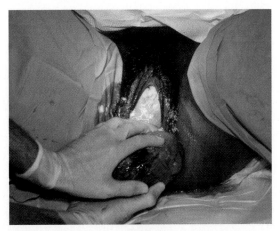

Figure 9-10 On occasion, the infant's anterior shoulder may need to be pulled posteriorly to clear the mother's symphysis pubis. This can be accomplished by placing a hand on either side of the infant's head and gently pulling downward.

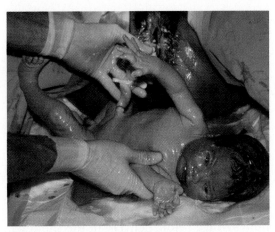

Figure 9-11 Tie/clamp the cord in two places (approximately 3 and 4 inches from its insertion into the baby). Cut the cord between the two ties/clamps.

either side of the infant's head and gently pull downward (**Figure 9-10**).

4. Keep the infant lying on the bed at the level of the <u>vaginal introitus</u> until the umbilical cord is clamped or tied. Do not hold the baby higher than the <u>uterus</u> or <u>womb</u> prior to clamping the cord because this may lead to transfusion of blood from the baby to the placenta (<u>fetal placental transfusion</u>), hypovolemia, and anemia. Alternatively, holding the baby with an unclamped cord below the level of the uterus can lead to transfusion of blood from the placenta to the baby, leading to a dangerously high <u>hematocrit</u>.

5. Suction the baby's mouth and nose using a rubber bulb syringe. Suctioning will help clear the airway of mucus and amniotic fluid and make the transition to breathing easier.

6. Tie or clamp the cord in two places, approximately 3 inches and 4 inches from its connection to the baby. Cut the cord between the two ties (**Figure 9-11**).

7. Dry and warm the baby with clean, warm towels. This will remove amniotic fluid, prevent heat loss and stimulate the newborn to breathe. Remove damp towels or blankets from around the baby and replace them with clean, dry ones.

8. The last step in the delivery process is the delivery of the placenta. This generally occurs spontaneously 10 to 15 minutes after birth. Delivery of the placenta is not an emergency procedure and must not delay the transport of the mother and infant. Do not pull on the umbilical cord to hurry the process.

Separation of the placenta from the uterus is often signaled by a "gush of blood" from the vagina. After the placenta has separated from the uterine wall, gentle pulling on the cord will remove it from the vagina. Too much pulling before it has separated naturally may lead to avulsion of the cord and bleeding. Place the placenta in a plastic bag and transport it with the patient for pathological evaluation.

Tip

Delivery of the placenta is a natural act that requires no assistance in the field.

Blip

Do not hold the baby higher than the womb prior to clamping the cord, because this may lead to hypovolemia and anemia from transfusion of the baby's blood back to the placenta.

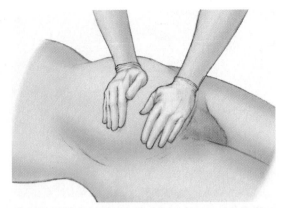

Figure 9-12 To massage the uterus, place one hand with fingers fully extended just above the mother's pubic bone, and use your other hand to press down into the lower abdomen and gently massage the uterus until it becomes firm.

Complications During Vaginal Delivery

Meconium

<u>Meconium</u> is fetal stool passed in the uterus. It can be thin and watery or thick and sticky. If the mother passes thick meconium-stained amniotic fluid, take the additional step of thoroughly suctioning the baby's mouth, nose, and pharynx with a bulb syringe before delivery of the shoulder. If the newly born is vigorous (normal respiratory effort, muscle tone, and a heart rate greater than 100 beats/min) simply use a bulb syringe or large-bore catheter (12F or 14F) to clear the secretions and any meconium from the mouth and nose. *On the other hand, if the newly born is depressed and has meconium, airway management requires an extremely careful approach.* Although tracheal suctioning is recommended for in-hospital management of the depressed newly born with meconium, it has unproven value in the out-of-hospital setting, where there is a large variability in comfort and skill levels of prehospital professionals. The practice options for clearing the airway of thick meconium and providing effective ventilation in the depressed newly born should be addressed by local EMS systems based upon local training and provider capabilities.

Postpartum Hemorrhage

The most common <u>postpartum</u> maternal complication is excessive bleeding. Usually, pregnant women will lose 500 mL of blood with a vaginal delivery. Symptoms such as tachycardia and orthostatic hypotension start to appear in the mother with 1200 to 1500 mL of blood loss. Estimating blood loss is difficult, so monitor the postpartum mother's vital signs carefully.

If a postpartum mother has excessive vaginal blood loss, perform uterine massage (**Figure 9-12**). To massage the uterus, place one hand with fingers fully extended just above the mother's pubic bone and use the other hand to press down into the lower abdomen and gently massage the uterus until it becomes firm. This should take from 3 to 5 minutes. As the uterus firms up, it should feel about the size of a softball or large grapefruit. If the infant is stable, encourage breastfeeding to increase uterine tone and to slow the uterine bleeding.

Advanced Life Support

Treatment of Postpartum Hemorrhage

Begin volume resuscitation with crystalloid fluid in the mother who continues to bleed after the placenta is delivered and has dizziness, pallor, tachycardia, or low blood pres-

Case Study **2**

You are called to a residence by a woman in labor who has no transportation to the hospital. Upon arrival, the baby is crowning and the mother has an urge to push.

1. What three questions are most appropriate to ask at this time to best prepare for delivery?
2. Discuss appropriate positioning of the woman for delivery.

sure. Give 1 to 2 liters over 30 to 45 minutes during transport. A blood transfusion may be necessary in the hospital.

Summary of Vaginal Delivery

Delivery is a natural process that usually does not require much intervention. The birth attendant must simply control the environment to avoid things happening too fast. However, delivery of an infant is not a common procedure in the out-of-hospital setting, so the level of anxiety for both the laboring patient and the prehospital professional is often high. A history of prematurity, multiple fetuses or meconium-stained amniotic fluid suggests higher probability of a depressed newly born. Review the steps for performing a vaginal delivery while on the way to the scene. Have the proper equipment ready, control the temperature of the environment, and position the mother to facilitate childbirth and early newborn care. If the child has meconium-stained amniotic fluid, carefully suction the mouth and nose before delivering the shoulder. Control postpartum bleeding with uterine massage and encouragement of breastfeeding.

Table 9-4	Organized Approach to Assessment and Care of the Newly Born
Dry and warm the baby.	
Clear the airway.	
Assess breathing.	
Assess heart rate.	
Assess color.	

Immediate Care of the Newly Born

Although most term babies are healthy and need little treatment, follow a well-organized plan for assessment and immediate care of all babies. **Table 9-4** lists the five essential steps to care for every newly born in every setting. Most term newly borns will not require any ALS interventions.

Dry and Warm the Baby

At birth the baby is covered in amniotic fluid and can lose a lot of heat through <u>evaporation</u> unless immediately dried. Heat loss drastically increases the metabolic demand and

Encourage the mother to breastfeed the active, vigorous infant.

Perform the initial steps of drying, suctioning, and positioning on all infants, whether active or depressed.

oxygen consumption. Thoroughly dry every infant, healthy, or depressed. Remove wet towels or blankets from around the baby after drying and replace them with clean, dry ones. This will take no more than 5 to 10 seconds.

Clear the Airway

The newly born's head is larger than an older child's or adult's compared to its overall body size, which leads to flexion of the neck in a supine position. This may cause airway occlusion. Extend the head slightly to place the airway in a neutral position. Repeat nasopharyngeal suctioning to make sure there is a patent airway.

Assess Breathing

Next, assess breathing. Most babies will be crying, indicating adequate respiratory effort! Breathing effort may be slightly irregular in normal newly borns. Gasping or grunting are signs of increased work of breathing and respiratory distress.

An apneic baby, with no visible respiratory effort, requires immediate treatment. Most apneic newly borns will start breathing simply with tactile stimulation. If the baby is apneic or has gasping respiration after drying and suctioning, further stimulation is not likely to improve respiratory effort. Begin bag-mask ventilation with 100% oxygen (see "Depressed Newly Born Resuscitation").

Advanced Life Support

A special situation occurs when the prehospital professional encounters a newly born with respiratory depression after delivery by a narcotic-addicted mother. Do not give naloxone to the baby if the mother is addicted to narcotics because the drug may

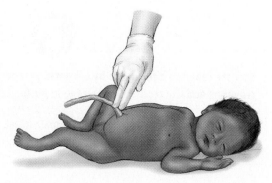

Figure 9-13 Feel for a pulse at the base of the umbilical cord.

precipitate acute narcotic withdrawal and seizures. Assist ventilation with bag-mask and follow the guidelines for care of a depressed newly born.

Assess Heart Rate

In the newly born, a low heart rate is usually due to hypoxia, not primary cardiac disease. The crying, active baby usually has an adequate heart rate. Assess heart rate carefully in a baby who is not active or who requires assisted ventilation. This is most easily accomplished by palpating a pulse at the base of the umbilical cord (**Figure 9-13**). Count the number of beats over 6 seconds and multiply this number by 10. Sometimes the umbilical vessels are constricted so that the pulse is not palpable. Therefore, if a pulse cannot be felt, listen for the heartbeat over the left side of the chest using a stethoscope.

Treat heart rates of less than 100 beats/min with a bag-mask device, even if the respiratory effort appears normal. Bradycardia usually responds rapidly to bag-mask venti-

Do not give naloxone to the newly born if the mother is addicted to narcotics.

Assist ventilation in an infant with a heart rate less than 100 beats/min with a bag-mask device. Bradycardia usually reflects inadequate respiratory effort.

lation, in which case no further treatment is necessary (see "Depressed Newly Born Resuscitation").

Assess Color

Skin color assessment in newly borns has several unique features. In utero, the fetus depends on placental delivery of oxygen, and blood oxygen concentrations are very low compared to conditions after birth. Therefore, prior to the initiation of respiration after delivery, the infant will appear cyanotic.

If the cyanotic newly born is apneic, immediately begin bag-mask ventilation. If the baby is breathing, but appears blue, determine if the cyanosis is central (on the trunk and face) or peripheral (limited to the hands and feet). This difference will help with decision making and therapy. If central cyanosis is present, true hypoxia is present. Administer supplemental oxygen at 15 L/min via a mask held loosely over the baby's face.

Peripheral cyanosis is also termed acrocyanosis. This is a common finding in newly borns through the first 24 to 48 hours of life and requires no therapy.

Apgar Score

All hospitals and some EMS systems use the Apgar score for newly born assessment. This score measures the baby's overall cardiopulmonary and neurologic function at 1 and 5 minutes of life, then every 5 minutes thereafter in the unstable baby. The APGAR may be helpful in assessing the effectiveness of resuscitation.

Depressed Newly Born Resuscitation

Depressed newly born resuscitation refers to the series of interventions used to stimulate spontaneous respiratory effort. When the baby remains depressed after drying, warming, and clearing the airway, begin resuscitation. Use the following sequence:

1. Dry the infant and place in the supine position in a warm environment.
2. Suction her mouth and nose.
3. Position the head in slight extension.
4. Assess breathing. If respiratory effort is absent or irregular, start bag-mask ventilation with 100% oxygen at 40 to 60 breaths/min.
5. Assess heart rate. If less than 100 beats/min, start bag-mask ventilation (**Figure 9-14**).
6. Assess heart rate after 30 seconds of ventilation. If less than 60 beats/min, proceed with chest compressions. Deliver 90 compressions and 30 ventilations (120 events per minute). Continue bag-mask ventilation.
7. Continue positive-pressure ventilation until heart rate is above 100 beats/min and spontaneous breathing is present.

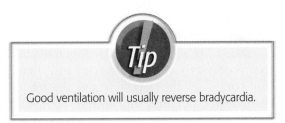

Good ventilation will usually reverse bradycardia.

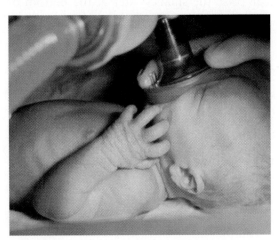

Figure 9-14 Using a bag-mask device on a newly born.

Endotracheal Intubation and Epinephrine Administration

Check the heart rate after 30 seconds. If less than 60 beats/min, prepare for endotracheal intubation and administration of <u>epinephrine</u> (0.01–0.03 mg/kg = 0.1–0.3 mL/kg of 1:10,000 solution). The endotracheal route may be associated with lower blood levels of the drug. Therefore, consider using the higher end of the dosage range when administering it via the endotracheal route. However, there is no evidence that use of a higher concentration of epinephrine results in a better outcome, and there is some concern that higher concentrations/dosages in the newly born may result in brain and heart damage.

Continue chest compressions and give repeated doses of epinephrine every 3 to 5 minutes until heart rate is above 60 beats/min.

The Inverted Pyramid

The inverted pyramid (**Figure 9-15**) illustrates the relative need for interventions in depressed newly borns.

Basic life support (BLS) is usually all that is required during deliveries and therefore comprises the largest area at the top of the inverted pyramid. In contrast, advanced life support (ALS) interventions such as chest compressions, intubation, and medication administration are rarely required, and comprise the smallest area at the bottom of the inverted pyramid.

Meconium Aspiration

A child born with thin meconium staining who appears active and without respiratory

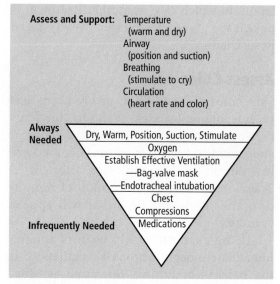

Figure 9-15 Guidelines for neonatal resuscitation as recommended by the American Academy of Pediatrics and the American Heart Association. Reproduced with permission from the American Heart Association. ©2003 *Pediatric Advanced Life Support.*

distress needs only routine oral and nasal suctioning and standard newly born care. On the other hand, a child born with thick meconium staining who has respiratory distress despite suctioning on the perineum needs further aggressive suctioning of the mouth and nose. *However, suctioning of meconium should not distract from the need for emergent oxygenation and ventilation of the newly born.* In the patient with meconium aspiration and respiratory failure or apnea, quickly suction meconium and then begin bag-mask ventilations.

A meconium aspirator device may facilitate endotracheal suctioning in an intubated newly born with absent or ineffective respiratory effort. However, the use of this device has not been studied in the prehospital setting and its impact on clinical outcome is unknown.

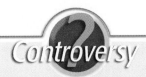

Shock

Shock at birth is most commonly due to <u>asphyxia</u> (severe hypoxia in the womb or during delivery) and <u>acidosis</u>. Blood loss during delivery due to umbilical cord avulsion or fetal-placental transfusion is an uncommon cause of shock in the newly born. Signs and symptoms of shock, whatever the cause, include abnormal appearance (lethargy, hypotonia), abnormal color (pallor, mottling), tachycardia, and prolonged capillary refill time. Hypothermia may also mimic these findings.

Advanced Life Support

Treatment of Shock

Because intrauterine or perinatal asphyxia is the most common cause of depression in the newly born, initial resuscitative efforts should ensure adequate oxygenation and ventilation. Volume resuscitation is rarely needed. In exceptional circumstances where hypovolemic shock is suspected, consider placing an IO line. Fluid resuscitation should be limited to avoid precipitating congestive heart failure. The only medication likely to be used in newly born resuscitation is epinephrine, which may be administered via the endotracheal tube or through an IO line.

Summary of Depressed Newly Born Resuscitation

The typical newly born response to hypoxia is apnea and bradycardia. *The primary treatment of the depressed newly born therefore involves reversal of hypoxia with immediate bag-mask ventilation.* If the child does not improve, begin chest compressions and perform endotracheal intubation on the scene before transport. Shock is rare, and is most commonly the result of asphyxia. Hypovolemia is an uncommon cause of shock in the newly born. If hypovolemic shock is suspected, transport immediately and initiate volume resuscitation via IV or IO line on the way to the hospital.

Advanced Life Support

Vascular Access

Vascular access is rarely needed in newly borns in the field because resuscitation is largely focused on airway management and breathing.

In reality, establishing vascular access is challenging in the newly born and its benefits must be carefully weighed against prolonged on scene time and potential complications. IV access may be attempted in the <u>antecubital fossae</u> or the <u>saphenous vein</u> at the ankle. Intraosseous infusion is an alternative.

When there is no IV or IO access, give resuscitation medications such as epinephrine through the endotracheal tube. Do not

Tip

Treat a hypovolemic newly born like an acute trauma patient with life-threatening blood loss.

give other solutions such as sodium bicarbonate or dextrose through the endotracheal tube, as these are damaging to the lungs.

Umbilical catheterization in the field is a controversial procedure. While this route of vascular access is widely used in the neonatal intensive care unit, there will be very few opportunities for the prehospital professional to practice and maintain this skill, and serious complications can occur. *Intraosseous infusion may be preferable if vascular access is clearly necessary for resuscitation, and a peripheral IV cannot be placed.*

Stabilization for Transport

The active term infant requires no intervention or electronic monitoring during transport. Be sure the child is restrained as per local EMS system policy. In some systems it is acceptable to restrain the mother appropriately and allow her to hold the baby during transport. Encourage her to breastfeed the active infant if possible. This may prevent hypoglycemia and promote maternal-infant bonding, uterine contractions, and decreased uterine bleeding. Provide a warm environment in the ambulance.

Transport of the Compromised Newly Born

Oxygen Therapy

Give supplemental oxygen if the newly born is hypoxic (pulse oximetry < 95% on room air).

Monitoring

After resuscitation, reassess the status of the infant throughout transport. Place cardiac leads in the same position as in an adult. A heart rate between 120 and 160 beats/min is normal in a newly born. If heart rate decreases, follow the procedures for depressed newly born management.

Attach an infant pulse oximetry probe on a finger or toe. If unable to get an accurate reading, the probe may have to be placed around the hand or the foot. Saturations between 90% and 100% are normal. Although there are negative effects of hyperoxia (high oxygen saturation) in the newly born, if the baby is distressed, the goal in the field should be to ensure adequate oxygenation through administration of supplemental oxygen and assisted ventilation when needed.

Hypothermia

Hypothermia develops quickly in newly borns. Oxygen demand triples when skin temperature drops by 1 degree. Signs of hypothermia are similar to those of shock. Keep the baby warm during transport. Have a small knit cap available to cover the infant's head. Turn the heat on in the ambulance even at the risk of discomfort to the mother and crew. Place the baby on the mother's bare chest (skin-to-skin contact) and cover both of them to maintain the infant's temperature.

Blip

If commercial warm packs are used to prevent or treat hypothermia in the newly born, place a towel between the infant's skin and the device. The combination of thin skin, little subcutaneous fat, and an inability to communicate discomfort puts them at high risk for burns.

Transport of the Compromised Newly Born: Hypoglycemia

The depressed newly born or prematurely delivered baby is at risk for hypoglycemia, but this complication is unlikely to develop in the first 30 minutes of life. If transport times are longer, measure a bedside glucose level at approximately 30 minutes after birth, or immediately in any baby who has a drastic change in responsiveness or perfusion. If a serum glucose of less than 40 mg/dL is documented in a depressed newly born, and an IV or IO line can be established in transport, give 10% dextrose in a 2 mL/kg push. Re-check serum glucose every 30 minutes during long transports. If the infant has documented hypoglycemia but is active, in no respiratory distress, and has a <u>suck reflex</u>, allow her to breastfeed or offer her 20 to 30 mL of 5% dextrose by bottle.

Case Study 3

Upon arriving at the home of a family who had called 9-1-1 for labor, you find a woman has just delivered an apparently term female infant that is still attached to the umbilical cord and is not crying or moving.

1. Discuss the scene management of the baby.
2. What is the role of vascular access?

Chapter Review

Case Study Answers

Case Study page 191

First decide whether to transport the mother to the nearest hospital or to prepare for delivery of the newly born. Ask if this is a first pregnancy and if the mother feels the urge to push. If the mother feels the urge to push, then examine for the presence of crowning.

If you decide to deliver at the scene, obtain a resuscitation-oriented history. Are twins present? What is the due date? What color was the amniotic fluid when the membranes ruptured? These questions will assist you in preparation.

If the child is crowning at the perineum, prepare the obstetric delivery pack, familiarize yourself with the contents, and make sure all necessary equipment is present. Warm the environment and get clean towels to dry the baby. Get or make a cap to place over the child's scalp to reduce heat loss from the head. Find a clean delivery surface for the baby.

Case Study 2 page 199

If time allows, review the procedure for a vaginal delivery while on the way to the scene. On arrival, first plan for appropriate positioning of the mother. Discuss the position with the patient ahead of time so that she understands the plan for delivery.

Clear amniotic fluid implies there is no meconium. Meconium is released by the fetus in conditions of stress. While the presence of clear fluid does not rule out the possibility of a depressed newly born, it is a reassuring sign and increases the chances of an active child who will need only the five steps of standard newly born care.

The woman should be lying supine with an object (stack of towels or a phone book) under her hips to allow for suctioning the mouth and nose. Alternatively, she can lie on her side facing away from you with her knees drawn towards the chest (Sims position).

Case Study 3 page 205

The baby is in acute distress and needs immediate intervention. Thoroughly dry the baby, position her on her back, and suction the mouth and nose. Tie or clamp the umbilical cord at 3 inches and 4 inches from the baby and cut it. At this point, if the infant is still not breathing, begin bag-mask ventilation with 100% oxygen at 40 to 60 breaths/min and observe for chest rise. Suction the mouth and nose again, and adjust the mask seal if there is inadequate chest rise. After 30 seconds of assisted ventilation, reassess the heart rate. If the heart rate is less than 60 beats/min, begin chest compressions at 90 compressions and 30 breaths/min. Administer three compressions followed by a bag-mask ventilation.

If the infant does not respond to these efforts with improvement in tone, color, and heart rate within 30 seconds, have one member of the team prepare for intubation and administration of epinephrine. Optimal cardiopulmonary resuscitation requires three individuals, one to assist ventilation, one to administer chest compressions, and one to prepare for intubation and possible administration of medications. If only two prehospital professionals are present, as is frequently the case, get help from another adult to perform chest compressions.

While vascular access is not usually needed for newly born resuscitation, this baby is at high risk for hypoglycemia and hypotension during transport and may benefit from intravenous access. Attempt an IV or IO line in transport. Check the serum glucose at 30 minutes of life and treat for a level of < 40 mg/dL. Since further resuscitation may be necessary, secure the infant on a gurney and transport with continuous ECG and oxygen saturation monitoring. Consider transport to a facility with a neonatal intensive care unit, as this baby may need ongoing critical care.

Suggested Readings

Textbooks

American Academy of Orthopaedic Surgeons: *Emergency Care and Transportation of the Sick and Injured,* 9th Edition. Sudbury, MA, Jones and Bartlett Publishers, 2005.

Bledsoe B, Porter R, Cherry R: *Essentials of Paramedic Care.* New Jersey, Prentice Hall, 2003.

Kattwinkel J, Denson S, Zaichkin, et al: *Textbook of Neonatal Resuscitation.* American Academy of Pediatrics and American Heart Association, 4th Edition. Elk Grove Village, IL, American Academy of Pediatrics, 2000.

Articles

Burchfield D. Advances in pediatric resuscitation: Newborn resuscitation. *Clinical Pediatric Emergency Medicine.* June 2001; 2(2):119–123.

Lane B, Finer N, Rich W. Duration of intubation attempts during neonatal resuscitation. *Journal of Pediatrics.* July 2004; 145(1).

10

Children with Special Health Care Needs

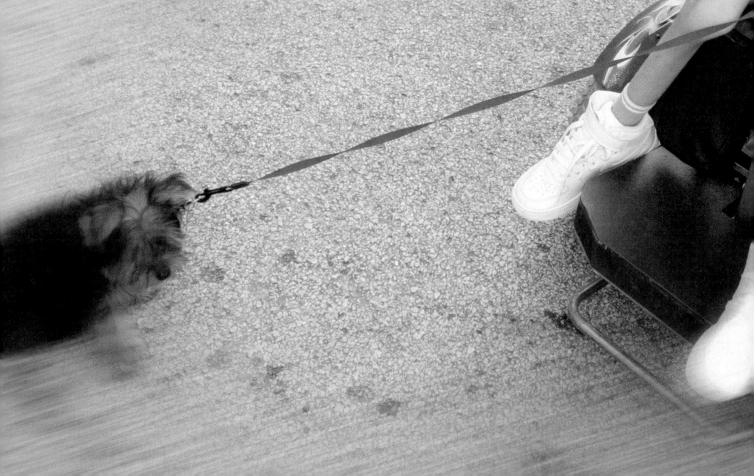

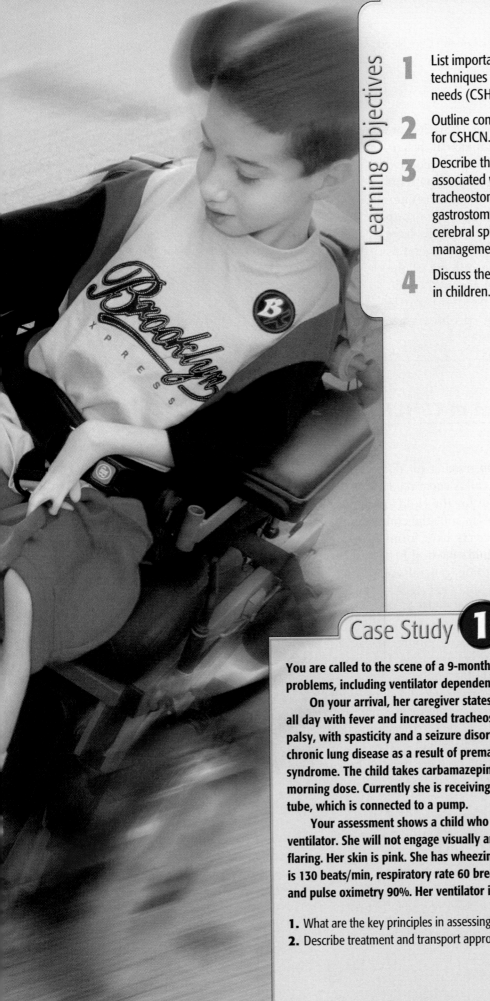

1 List important modifications of field assessment techniques for children with special health care needs (CSHCN).

2 Outline common transport considerations for CSHCN.

3 Describe the most common complications associated with assistive devices—including tracheostomy tubes, central venous lines, gastrostomy tubes or gastric feeding tubes, and cerebral spinal fluid shunts—and the emergency management of those complications.

4 Discuss the management of behavioral emergencies in children.

Case Study ❶

You are called to the scene of a 9-month-old girl with multiple underlying medical problems, including ventilator dependence at night through a tracheostomy tube.

On your arrival, her caregiver states that the girl has had difficulty breathing all day with fever and increased tracheostomy secretions. The child has cerebral palsy, with spasticity and a seizure disorder. She is ventilator dependent because of chronic lung disease as a result of prematurity at birth and respiratory distress syndrome. The child takes carbamazepine for her seizures and received her morning dose. Currently she is receiving her feedings through her gastrostomy tube, which is connected to a pump.

Your assessment shows a child who is in bed and connected to a home ventilator. She will not engage visually and has subcostal retractions and nasal flaring. Her skin is pink. She has wheezing and crackles on lung exam. Her heart rate is 130 beats/min, respiratory rate 60 breaths/min, blood pressure 85 mm Hg/palp, and pulse oximetry 90%. Her ventilator is set at 20 breaths per minute.

1. What are the key principles in assessing this child?
2. Describe treatment and transport approaches.

Introduction

CHILDREN WITH SPECIAL health care needs (CSHCN) are children with chronic physical, developmental, behavioral, or emotional conditions that are either acquired or congenital. They are a diverse group of patients who frequently need out-of-hospital emergency assessment and treatment. This high user group includes children who were born prematurely, have suffered closed head injury and have central nervous system injuries, or have chronic problems of the lungs, brain, or kidneys. Examples of acquired conditions include cerebral palsy or <u>posttraumatic epilepsy</u>. Examples of <u>congenital</u> problems are <u>cyanotic heart disease</u> or <u>spina bifida</u>.

Technology-assisted children (TAC) or technology-dependent children are a subgroup of CSHCN who depend on medical devices for their survival. Common devices include tracheostomy tubes, home ventilators, indwelling central venous lines, feeding tubes, pacemakers, and cerebral spinal fluid (CSF) shunts.

Today CSHCN are surviving longer and often live at home. They need emergency medical care more frequently than children without special health care needs. Because of their abnormal baseline status, CSHCN pose unique problems in field assessment and treatment. Therefore, prehospital professionals must recognize common types of CSHCN, know modifications in assessment, and understand management of frequent problems.

Assessment of CSHCN

Modifications

The most important resource for the prehospital provider is the child's caregiver. He usually knows how to care for the child's particular condition and understands the child's equipment. Often caregivers have forms or cards that outline the child's medical history, medications and <u>baseline</u> general appearance, oxygen saturation, and vital signs.

Begin evaluation of CSHCN with emergency pediatric assessment techniques adjusted to the child's developmental level, rather than his chronological age. Caregivers can usually provide the child's developmental age, weight, and baseline vital signs. *With TAC, do not become distracted by their specialized equipment.* Care for the child, not the machinery. Caregivers are often extremely helpful in figuring out the base-

line status of CSHCN or in operating or troubleshooting the equipment. *Ask for assistance from the caregiver!*

The assessment of CSHCN has the following important modifications:

1. Baseline status: Ask the caregivers what "normal" is for their child. Most likely, they will know the child's baseline better than any medical record.
2. Rely on the caregivers' opinions: What do they think is wrong? In what ways is the child "acting differently?"
3. If the child is physiologically stable, take a focused history on scene. Caregivers usually know the child's medical history, health problems, medications, medical devices, and current complaints. They are also aware of what approaches work best.
4. The child may be slow to answer questions or may be unable to talk. Use a patient approach to the stable child and begin by talking directly to the child, rather than to his caregiver.
5. Seemingly minor illnesses can be life-threatening in some CSHCN. An example is a cold in a child with chronic lung disease who is ventilator-dependent. The child may have little reserve and may become hypoxic easily.

Do not become distracted by the specialized equipment used by TAC. Care for the child, not the machinery.

6. Communicate with the child using developmentally appropriate language, gestures, and techniques, as discussed in Chapter 2.

7. If a caregiver is not present, find out if the child has a form or card with information about his medical problem, normal vital signs, medications, and other important medical data. Several states recommend that CSHCN carry information cards, such as Wisconsin's Child Alert 10-33, New Mexico's ChUMS (Children's Updated Medical Summary), New Hampshire's SKIPS (Special Kids Information Program) and the Washington DC EMS Outreach program. An Emergency Information form has also been developed by the American Academy of Pediatrics (AAP) and the American College of Physicians (ACEP).

8. Look for a Medical Alert bracelet.

9. The normal baseline vital signs for a CSHCN may be "out of the normal range" compared to a child of the same age who does not have special health care needs. Standard vital signs may have limited value in assessment of CSHCN. Pay more attention to the PAT and observations from the caregiver.

10. Do not assume that a child with a physical disability is cognitively impaired. Many children with cerebral palsy, for example, have <u>spasticity</u> but do not have cognitive abnormalities. Discreetly ask the caregiver about the child's normal level of functioning, understanding, and interactions.

11. Be polite and professional. Listen to the caregiver and take his concerns seriously. Families of CSHCN often have had a lot of experience with the medical system. If most of their experience has been positive, they will view the prehospital professional as an ally. However, if they have had bad experiences with the medical system, they may be suspicious or aggressive.

12. Keep in mind the amount of stress caregivers of a CSHCN may be experiencing.

13. Ask the caregivers what therapies or interventions have been already undertaken in response to their child's emergency.

14. If possible, try to transport CSHCN to their "medical home" facility. Always follow local EMS protocols.

Pediatric Assessment Triangle

The PAT is a good way to look and listen for signs that will help figure out the type of physiologic problem and the urgency for treatment of a CSHCN. However, because CSHCN often have altered baseline physiology, there are several limitations and modifications to the PAT.

Approach the developmentally delayed child using techniques appropriate to his developmental level, not his age in years.

Appearance

Although the child's overall appearance reflects the adequacy of oxygenation, ventilation, perfusion, and CNS status, this is the part of the PAT that may differ the most in CSHCN. The underlying medical problem may cause abnormal muscle tone, such as the increased tone and spasticity in a child with cerebral palsy or the decreased tone seen in children with <u>Down syndrome (DS)</u>. There may be decreased interactiveness, a common behavioral state in a child with brain damage or developmental delay. Look or gaze is helpful because most CSHCN can recognize their caregiver by looking or by hearing their voice. A CSHCN may be unable to speak, but the

Assess appearance by asking the caregiver about the child's baseline.

Do not assume that a child with a physical disability is mentally impaired. Many children with cerebral palsy, for example, have spasticity but not cognitive abnormalities.

strength and quality of his cry or facial expressions may be a useful sign of health or distress. For example, a high-pitched cry in a child with a CSF shunt may mean obstruction.

Work of Breathing

Many CSHCN have respiratory problems. Children with chronic pulmonary disease, such as **bronchopulmonary dysplasia (BPD)**, have rapid respiratory rates and increased work of breathing. When such children have a fever or experience an added respiratory illness or injury such as pneumonia or chest trauma, they have less reserve. Therefore, work of breathing in these patients increases rapidly with any acute illness or injury.

Assess abnormal breath sounds (stridor, wheezing, or grunting) from across the room. Some "abnormal" airway sounds may be normal for a CSHCN. For example, a child with a tracheostomy tube usually has noisy breathing, and an infant with BPD may have slight expiratory wheezing. Children with BPD or congenital heart disease are much more likely to develop respiratory infections, especially from **respiratory syncytial virus (RSV)**, in the winter. They can decompensate quickly. CSHCN who have developmental delay and neurologic problems are at high risk for aspiration, pneumonia, and respiratory failure.

Abnormal positioning, such as tripoding and head bobbing, are important visual signs of increased work of breathing and hypoxia, and usually indicate serious breathing problems. For the child who usually has mild retractions, the degree or location of retractions will provide clues to increased work of breathing. For example, the baseline retrac-

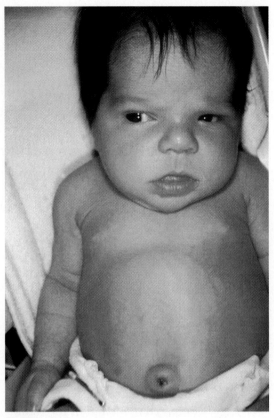

Figure 10-1 Ask a caregiver to describe the child's baseline color.

tions may be mild and only **subcostal**, but are now severe and also **suprasternal**. *Nasal flaring is not usually a baseline condition because this sign suggests significant hypoxia that is rarely permitted in children at home.*

Circulation to Skin

The skin color may appear abnormal in CSHCN, such as in infants with cyanotic congenital heart disease, chronic lung disease, cancer, or liver failure. A child with cyanotic congenital heart disease or chronic lung disease may have bluish lips and mucous membranes, nail beds, and extremities at baseline. A child with cancer may appear pale, whereas the skin of a child with liver disease may appear yellow. Ask a caregiver to describe the child's baseline color (**Figure 10-1**).

Adaptations in the Hands-on ABCDEs

After performing the PAT, complete the initial assessment by adjusting the evaluation of the ABCDEs to the child's baseline.

Airway

Open and maintain the airway. Keeping an open airway may be more difficult with the CSHCN. The child may have poor muscle tone and head control, or copious <u>secretions</u>. Getting, and then keeping, the right head position may require several maneuvers: a shoulder roll to correctly position the head in a neutral axis with the airway, and a chin lift or jaw thrust to open the airway. Always have suction available.

Advanced Life Support

Special Management in CSHCN: Tracheostomy Care   A child with a tracheostomy has an artificial airway that is easily blocked by secretions or by dislodgment of the device. The tracheostomy section of this chapter addresses specific management techniques for these children.

Breathing

Count the respiratory rate. Listen to the lungs for <u>bilateral</u> air movement and abnormal chest sounds. Listening may not give accurate results in the CSHCN who cannot sit still or who has noisy breathing. Also, obtain pulse oximetry and compare to baseline. Keep the child in a position of comfort. Give supplemental oxygen to any CSHCN with increased work of breathing or increased respiratory rate by blow-by, face mask, or bag-mask device. If the caregiver knows the usual baseline oxygen saturation, only give oxygen to achieve baseline levels. Children with chronic lung disease or some forms of congenital heart disease can get worse if too much oxygen is given. For CSHCN, the caregiver may know the best way to give oxygen to the child. For infants or children already on home oxygen, increase the flow rate. For a patient with a tracheostomy tube, place the oxygen directly over the tube or stoma.

Advanced Life Support

Special Management in CSHCN: Bronchodilator Administration   If a CSHCN has a history of breathing problems or uses bronchodilators at home, give a nebulized bronchodilator when wheezing is present.

Circulation

Assess heart rate, pulse quality, skin temperature, and capillary refill time. These are not usually different in CSHCN and require no modifications in clinical interpretation. If the child's age is 3 years or less, consider obtaining a blood pressure. However the value may be hard to obtain and interpret in this age group. Attempt to measure blood pressure at least once in all children *over* 3 years of age. Tachycardia is a common baseline finding in some CSHCN, and by itself does not indicate shock. This is diagnosis-dependent so asking the child's caregiver about the child's usual heart rate can be helpful. To evaluate heart rate and blood pressure, assess with the other key characteristics of circulation, as outlined in Chapter 3.

Management of shock in CSHCN is no different than for normal children. Standard management includes oxygen, positioning, and bag-mask support as needed.

CSHCN in shock usually need volume replacement, unless the child has a congenital heart defect and possible heart failure. The CSHCN has the same fluid requirements as a normal child. If the patient is injured, transport immediately and attempt vascular access. Give 20-mL boluses of crystalloid fluid on the way to the ED. If the child is ill, and if he has compensated shock, transport, and attempt access and fluid administration on the way. If the ill child has decompensated shock, make one attempt at vascular access on scene, if possible. In extreme cases, intraosseous access may be necessary. When a child has a vertical chest scar or a history of congenital heart disease, consider cardiogenic shock as an explanation for poor perfusion. Because a CSHCN may be more difficult to assess accurately, and because vascular access is often troublesome, always transport a child with suspected shock as soon as possible.

Advanced Life Support

Special Management in CSHCN   Bradycardia is not normal for CSHCN. *It is a sign of hypoxia or inadequate brain perfusion.* Suspect hypoxia in a child with BPD or other chronic cardiopulmonary condition who has a HR below normal for chronologic age. Suspect increased intracranial pressure in a child with a CSF shunt.

The normal baseline vitals for a CSHCN may be different or "out of the normal range" for the child's chronological age.

Bradycardia is not usually a normal finding in CSHCN.

Disability

The CSHCN often has an abnormal baseline neurologic status. Assess neurologic status by looking at appearance as part of the PAT, and establishing level of consciousness with the Alert, Verbal, Painful, Unresponsive (AVPU) mnemonic. Compare the findings to the child's baseline. In the assessment of motor activity, assess purposeful movement, symmetrical movement of extremities, seizures, posturing, or flaccidity. Treat altered level of consciousness if it is a change from baseline. The Glasgow Coma Scale may not be applicable for assessment of CSHCN because many CSHCN have baseline cognitive and physical problems that would affect the score. It is better to describe the child as being different from baseline.

Exposure

Be sure to inspect the child's entire body, but respect his modesty. Do not allow the child to become cold. Many CSHCN have minimal body fat and can become hypothermic quickly.

Summary of Assessment of CSHCN

Listen carefully to the caregiver when assessing CSHCN. Ask about the child's baseline status: What is "normal" for this child? Such children may present a confusing picture, with unexpected behaviors, communication difficulties, extensive medical histories, and complicated equipment. The child's neurologic status is often abnormal. If the caregiver is not present, look for sources of baseline information, such as a medical information form or Medical Alert bracelet. Use standard assessment techniques and developmentally appropriate approaches modified by baseline comparisons to evaluate and manage acute problems. Transport early.

The Glasgow Coma Scale may not be applicable for assessment of CSHCN because many CSHCN have baseline cognitive and physical problems that affect the score.

Transport

Table 10-1 lists key principles of transport of CSHCN. *Always restrain children in the ambulance.* The best type of restraint device and the best method for securing the device in the ambulance are controversial issues.

In general, if the child is critically ill or injured, restrain the child on his back secured on a gurney. Try to use a backboard for spinal stabilization if the child has suffered an injury to the head or if he has a spinal injury. Check with the caregiver about positioning and availability of any special car seat. In some children, the supine position may compromise the airway due to an abundance of secretions, poor tone, or anatomic abnormalities. The child's specially designed child restraint system or car seat may be the best option if it can be safely secured to the ambulance.

Table 10-1	**Principles of Transport of a CSHCN**

1. Transport a CSHCN who is on home oxygen with the oxygen (except for liquid oxygen). If the child has no respiratory distress, continue the same rate of oxygen flow.

2. Transport a child on a home ventilator with the ventilator if there are no equipment problems. If there is a concern about the ventilator, provide assisted ventilation via bag-mask. Regardless of the method of ventilation, always secure the child's home ventilator in the ambulance and transport with the child, so that it can be assessed by hospital personnel for potential problems and appropriate settings.

3. If the child has poor muscle control, or increased muscle tone, immobilize the child as needed in a position that is comfortable for him. If he has a special seat, wheelchair, or other equipment (e.g., feeding pump, suctioning device), transport these items to the ED if these items can be safely secured in the ambulance while still allowing enough room to safely care for the child during transport.

Many CSHCN have supplemental oxygen and oxygen delivery equipment. It is unsafe to transport liquid oxygen in an ambulance. Consider transporting non-liquid (or gaseous) oxygen and the child's personal devices or equipment to the ED.

Summary of Transport

CSHCN often have special transport considerations. Make sure the child is safely restrained in the ambulance. This may require using a special seat. Address the issue of transport with the caregiver and consider bringing supportive equipment to the ED if it can be safely secured in the ambulance.

Technology-Assisted Children

Technology-assisted children (TAC) have devices that may malfunction at home. The most common devices are <u>tracheostomy tubes</u>, <u>cerebral spinal fluid (CSF) shunts</u>, <u>indwelling central venous catheters</u>, and <u>feeding tubes</u>. Equipment malfunction can cause a range of problems. Some malfunctioning may have minor or no immediate effects, such as loss of a feeding tube or clotting of an indwelling central venous catheter. Other malfunctioning may cause serious physiologic effects, such as respiratory distress from loss of a tracheostomy tube or intracranial pressure elevation from obstruction of a CSF shunt.

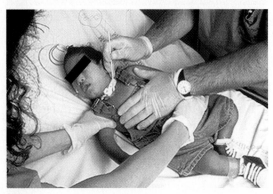

Figure 10-2 A tracheostomy.

Tracheostomy Tubes

A tracheostomy is a surgical opening (stoma) in the front of the neck into the trachea. A tracheostomy tube (sometimes called a "trach tube") is an artificial airway passed through this opening that allows the child to breathe (**Figure 10-2**). Infants and children may have a tracheostomy for several reasons, as noted in **Table 10-2**.

There are several types of tracheostomy tubes, and they come in many sizes. The size is written on the wings or flanges of the tube. The size and name (indicating type of tube) are also on the box. The inner and outer diameters are often on the wings as

Table 10-2	**Indications for a Tracheostomy**

1. To bypass an obstruction in the upper airway due to trauma, surgery, or a birth defect

2. To allow clearance of secretions

3. To provide long-term mechanical ventilation of children with chronic respiratory problems, injuries to the lungs, major central nervous system deficits, or severe muscle weakness

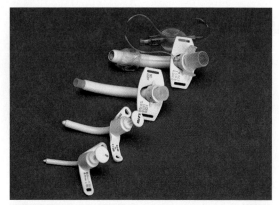

Figure 10-3 Sizes and inner and outer diameters are often written on the wings of tracheostomy tubes.

well (**Figure 10-3**). The most common pediatric tube sizes are 2.5 mm to 10.0 mm (sizes 000-10). All tracheostomy tubes have a standard outer opening or hub outside the neck so a bag-mask device can be attached. For some tubes, an adapter may be needed to make this connection.

Types of Tracheostomy Tubes

The main types of tracheostomy tubes are fenestrated, double lumen, and single lumen (**Figure 10-4**). Tubes can also come with or without a cuff. These cuffs can be filled with air or foam. All tubes have an <u>obturator</u>, which is a solid plastic guide placed inside the tube to make insertion easier. Use the obturator to clear the tube of secretions in an emergency if a suction catheter is not available.

A single-lumen tracheostomy tube has one hollow tube or cannula for both airflow and suctioning of secretions. Uncuffed, single lumen tubes are usually for neonates,

If the inner cannula of a double-lumen tracheostomy tube has been removed, a bag-mask device will not secure to the outer lumen of the tube. In order to ventilate a tracheostomy tube with the inner cannula removed, secure an infant face mask onto the bag, and then cover the tracheostomy tube's opening and seal the face mask on the neck.

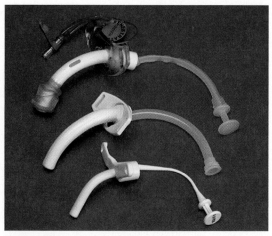

Figure 10-4 Fenestrated, double-lumen, and single-lumen tracheostomy tubes (top to bottom).

infants, and young children. A double lumen tube has both a hollow outer cannula and a removable (also hollow) inner cannula. Remove the inner cannula for cleaning, and keep it in place to provide mechanical ventilation. Never remove the outer cannula unless the entire tube must be replaced.

A fenestrated tube has holes (fenestrations) for air to flow upward through the vocal cords and mouth. This lets the child talk and breathe naturally. Fenestrated tubes have a decannulation plug attached to the outer cannula that blocks airflow through the stoma. If the child cannot breathe through his nose or mouth, remove this plug, so breathing is possible through the stoma. In addition, many fenestrated tubes also have a hollow inner cannula that must be in place for mechanical ventilation.

Oxygen Delivery and Assisted Ventilation through a Tracheostomy Tube

A child with a functioning tracheostomy tube can receive oxygen by the blow-by method, a face mask or tracheostomy mask placed directly over the tube opening, or by manual ventilation with a bag-mask device.

1. Provide blow-by oxygen. Place a stoma mask or pediatric face mask a short distance above the tracheostomy tube or stoma and give oxygen at 10 to 15 L/min.

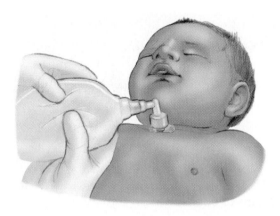

Figure 10-5 Bag-mask device attached directly to the external end of the tracheostomy tube.

2. Secure a face or tracheostomy mask directly over the tracheostomy tube opening and secure the straps around the neck.

3. Attach a bag-mask device to tracheostomy tube adapter. Attach a bag-mask device directly to the outer end of the tracheostomy tube (**Figure 10-5**).

For a child who has a stoma (surgical opening in the neck) but no tracheostomy tube, or when a tube cannot be reinserted, apply a seal with a mask over the stoma and ventilate through the stoma; or block the stoma with a <u>sterile</u> gauze and finger, and ventilate with a mask to the mouth or mask to the mouth and nose technique. Begin bag-mask ventilation as needed.

Tracheostomy Complications: Obstruction

Obstruction of the tracheostomy tube is a life-threatening emergency for CSHCN. Obstruction can be due to secretions, incorrect insertion (tube malposition), improper positioning of the child's head, or mechanical problems with the tube. Obstruction causes respiratory distress and failure.

The most common complication of a child with a tracheostomy tube is respiratory distress due to obstruction of the tube.

Assessment When a child has an obstructed tracheostomy tube, the chest is not rising and the child cannot breathe on his own. The PAT shows poor appearance, increased work of breathing, and cyanosis in cases of respiratory failure. The ABCDEs will further indicate poor air movement and bradycardia.

Treatment: Clearing an Obstructed Tube To clear an obstructed tracheostomy tube, follow these steps:

1. Position the child's head with a towel roll under the shoulders. Ensure that the outer opening of the tube is clear.

2. Check that the tube is in the proper location. The wings or flange should be against the neck, and the obturator should not be in place.

3. If the child has a fenestrated tube, remove the decannulation plug.

4. If the child has a double lumen tracheostomy tube, remove the inner lumen to clear secretions.

5. If none of these maneuvers work, suction the tube with a suction catheter.

Treatment: Suctioning a Tracheostomy Tube If efforts to clear the obstruction are unsuccessful, suction the tracheostomy tube using the following procedure (**Figures 10-6 and 10-7**):

1. Ask the caregiver if they have suction catheters, equipment, and supplies. If

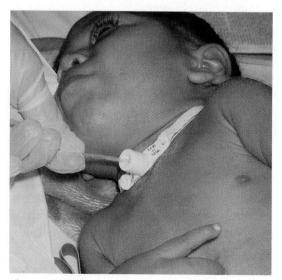

Figure 10-6 Suctioning a tracheostomy tube.

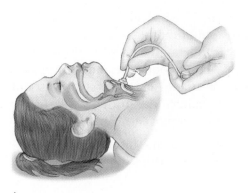

A

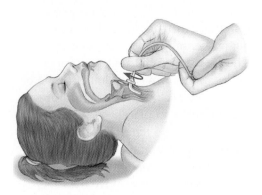

B

Figure 10-7 (A) Insertion of suction catheter to proper depth; suction port remains open. (B) Suctioning airway in circular motion as catheter is removed; suction port is closed.

so, use these. Otherwise, choose a suction catheter small enough to pass through the tube. (A size 1.0 [or 3.0-mm] tube will take a size 6 to 8 French catheter.) The caregiver may know the right size catheter. If equipment is not immediately available, insert the obturator to try to clear the obstruction.

2. If using a portable suction machine, set it to 100 mm Hg or less.

3. Give oxygen (over the tracheostomy tube) with a mask, and then loosen secretions by placing up to 1.0 to 2.0 mL of normal saline into the tube.

4. Insert the suction catheter approximately 2 inches (5 cm) into the tube. If the child begins to cough, the catheter is through the tube and into the trachea, and the depth of insertion is too deep. Do not use suction while inserting the catheter, and never force the catheter.

5. Cover the suction port (hole) and suction for 3 to 5 seconds, while slowly

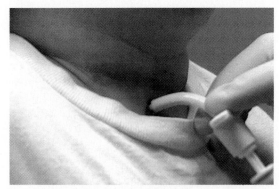

Figure 10-8 Replacing a tracheostomy tube.

removing the catheter. Never suction for longer than 10 seconds. Always monitor the child's heart rate and color during this procedure. Stop suctioning immediately if the heart rate begins to drop or the child becomes blue.

6. If the obstruction is removed, and the child can breathe on his own, do not suction further. If additional suctioning is needed, apply oxygen (by blow-by or direct ventilation) and repeat steps 3 to 5.

7. Always provide supplemental oxygen after suctioning by using the blow-by method or with manual ventilations.

Replacing a Tracheostomy Tube
Treatment of a tracheostomy problem usually requires simple techniques to establish a patent airway, such as suctioning or removal of the old tracheostomy tube and replacement with a new tube (**Figure 10-8**). Occasionally it is impossible to ventilate a child through an existing tracheostomy tube because of decannulation or complete obstruction. Under these conditions, the prehospital professional must place a new tracheostomy tube to save the child's life. For a step-by-step explanation of this procedure, see Removing and Replacing a Tracheostomy Tube, Procedure 23.

Central Venous Catheters

Many children receive nutritional support or medications at home through a <u>central venous catheter</u>. This includes children with poor weight gain due to gastrointestinal or liver problems, children with cancer who require chemotherapy, and children with infections who are receiving antibiotics at home.

Most central venous catheters require a surgical incision, but some can be placed percutaneously or through intact skin. They can enter through the skin of the chest, neck, or groin, but the internal end usually lies in or near the <u>superior vena cava</u> or right <u>atrium</u>. Some are single-lumen lines. Others are double lumen, with two separate external openings, but only one internal opening or port.

Types of Catheters

Central venous catheters may be inserted into the femoral, internal jugular, and subclavian veins (**Figure 10-9**). The skin entry site for the catheter is usually on the chest or arm. These are <u>partially implanted devices</u>.

<u>Totally implanted devices</u> are catheters attached to totally implanted injection ports or reservoirs. The catheter is in a central vein, such as the superior vena cava. Instead of coming out of the skin, as in partially implanted catheters, the end is attached to a reservoir (dome or port) that is in a subcutaneous pocket, usually on the chest. Therefore, there are no external parts visible, just a bulge or bump where the device rests.

If the bleeding is from the catheter and the catheter is in place, inspect the catheter and its end. If a cap is missing, replace the cap, if possible.

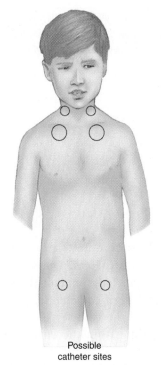

Possible
catheter sites

Figure 10-9 Possible insertion sites for a central venous catheter.

Tip

The most common complication in a TAC with a partially implanted central venous catheter is a broken or dislodged catheter.

Case Study ❷

You are called to the home of a 6-year-old boy whose central venous catheter has bleeding around the insertion site. His mother panicked because it is a new catheter and she is not used to taking care of it. She tells you that he has a history of short-gut syndrome due to an infarcted bowel sustained 6 months ago. He also has a gastrostomy tube through which he receives some medications, but he is totally reliant on his central venous catheter for his nutrition.

Upon arrival, you note a thin 6-year-old boy sitting quietly on the family's couch. His skin is yellowish. He has no increased work of breathing. His respiratory rate is 22 breaths/min, his heart rate is 95 beats/min, and his blood pressure is 90/50 mm Hg. Pulse oximetry is 98%. There is a tiny ooze of blood from the insertion site of the catheter in the right neck.

1. What are the key historical points?
2. Outline the assessment and management priorities.

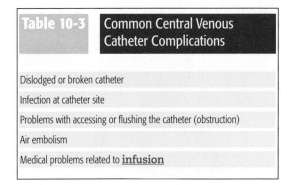

Table 10-3	Common Central Venous Catheter Complications
Dislodged or broken catheter	
Infection at catheter site	
Problems with accessing or flushing the catheter (obstruction)	
Air embolism	
Medical problems related to **infusion**	

Complications of Central Venous Catheters

Table 10-3 lists common complications of central venous catheters. *The most common problem with partially implanted devices is a broken or dislodged catheter.* Check the site for bleeding. If the catheter is in place, but there is bleeding from the entry site, apply direct pressure with sterile gauze. Likewise, if the catheter has been completely pulled out, and there is bleeding, apply direct pressure with sterile gauze.

Advanced Life Support

Clamping a Leaking Central Venous Catheter If the child is bleeding through a hole or cut in the catheter, clamp the exposed end. The caregiver usually has a clamp available, but if this has been misplaced, wrap the tips of a hemostat with gauze and apply to the catheter. If no **hemostat** is available, open the emergency delivery kit and use an umbilical clamp. If there has been bleeding, estimate the amount of blood loss.

Provide appropriate fluid therapy if there are signs of poor perfusion or shock. Do not use the central venous catheter.

Infection at Catheter Site Infection can occur at the site where a partially implanted catheter enters the skin or in the pocket where a totally implanted device is placed. Signs of infection are redness, tenderness, swelling, warmth, or yellow discharge (pus) from the site.

The child can also have a blood infection with fever, chills, and shock. In this case, treat for **septic shock**, as described in

Blip

If the indwelling central venous catheter site appears infected, do not use it for vascular access.

Chapter 4. If the line is possibly infected, do not use it for vascular access.

Obstruction A problem with accessing or flushing the catheter usually means obstruction. This complication can occur with all types of catheters. All that is required is patient assessment and transport. The major concern is a child who depends on hyperalimentation (IV nutrition) for calories and glucose. If the line is malfunctioning, and the child has not received any nutrition, his blood glucose may be low.

Treatment of Hypoglycemia Perform a quick fingerstick check of the blood sugar if there are signs or symptoms of hypoglycemia. For low blood sugar, BLS providers can give oral glucose per local protocols or ALS providers can and treat with IV dextrose or IM glucagon as described in Chapter 5.

Air Embolism This complication can occur if air accidentally gets into a central venous catheter when the line is being flushed or if the catheter breaks. Symptoms of air embolism include shortness of breath, chest pain, and coughing. Sometimes there is cardiovascular collapse and cardiopulmonary arrest.

Advanced Life Support

Treatment of Suspected Air Embolism Clamp the catheter or ask the caregiver to clamp the catheter, provide the child with oxygen, place the child on his left side in the head down position, and transport to the ED.

Medical Problems Related to Infusion Because of the various fluids and medications delivered through central venous catheters, several medical problems can develop. These include allergic reactions, abnormal heart rate or rhythms, or respiratory problems. Treat the appropriate problem, and bring the fluids that were being infused to the ED for analysis.

Feeding Tubes

A feeding tube (also called a gastrostomy tube or G-tube) supplies nutrition and medications to CSHCN who are unable to eat by mouth. A feeding tube allows the child to take in enough calories for adequate growth and nutrition.

Types of Feeding Tubes

Feeding tubes go through the nose (nasogastric [NG]) or, occasionally, through the mouth (orogastric [OG]) and into the stomach or small intestine (nasojejunal [NJ], orojejunal [OJ]) (**Figure 10-10**). These tubes are usually long catheters that are taped in place on the child's face. Another type of feeding tube goes directly into the stomach from an external site on the abdomen. There are several names for this type: <u>Gastrostomy tube</u>, <u>G-tube</u>, or <u>button</u>.

Tip

In a child who depends on <u>hyperalimentation</u> for calories and glucose, if the line is malfunctioning and the child has not received any nutrition, his blood glucose may be low.

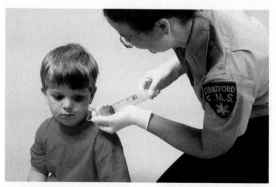

Figure 10-10 Nasojejunal catheter taped in place on the child's face.

Tip

The main complication of feeding tubes is dislodgment.

Complications of Feeding Tubes

The main complication of a feeding tube is dislodgment. The child may have aspirated fluid if a feeding tube has come out. Perform an assessment, paying special attention to the work of breathing, chest auscultation, and pulse oximetry.

Treatment

If an implanted tube (G-tube) comes out, check the site for bleeding and apply direct pressure with a sterile dressing. If the insertion site around the implanted tube appears irritated or infected (the skin appears red, warm, or swollen), apply a sterile dressing to the site.

Whenever a tube dislodges or there is evidence of infection, transport the child to the ED.

Ask the caregiver to bring the tube that fell out with the child to the hospital for sizing purposes. If the child was on an infusion of fluid or medication, ask the caregiver to disconnect the pump (infusion device) and transport it with the child. If the child has received fluid through a feeding catheter within 30 minutes of EMS arrival, consider transporting the child in a sitting position to prevent reflux and possible aspiration.

Advanced Life Support

Removing a Feeding Tube

If the NG or OG tube appears to be in place but the child is having respiratory difficulty, ask the caregiver to check its position. If position cannot be confirmed, remove the tube.

CSF Shunts

A CSF shunt is a device that drains excess cerebrospinal fluid from the brain. It usually runs from a ventricle (in the brain) under the skin, then down the neck into the <u>peritoneum</u> of the abdomen (ventriculoperitoneal shunt) or into the heart

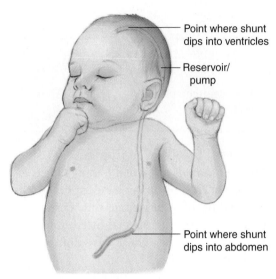

Point where shunt dips into ventricles

Reservoir/ pump

Point where shunt dips into abdomen

Figure 10-11 A CSF shunt directs cerebrospinal fluid from a ventricle in the brain to the skin and then down the neck to either the abdomen or the heart.

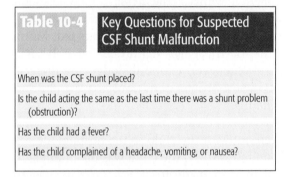

Table 10-4	Key Questions for Suspected CSF Shunt Malfunction

When was the CSF shunt placed?

Is the child acting the same as the last time there was a shunt problem (obstruction)?

Has the child had a fever?

Has the child complained of a headache, vomiting, or nausea?

(ventriculoatrial shunt) (**Figure 10-11**). Its path (or track) can usually be felt on one side of the head and down the neck until the track reaches a scar on the chest wall or abdomen. A CSF shunt helps a child with <u>hydrocephalus</u> maintain normal brain pressure. The hydrocephalus may be due to a congenital problem or to an acquired condition such as bleeding, trauma, or infection.

Complications of CSF Shunts

The major complications with a CSF shunt are obstruction and infection. *The most common complication is a shunt obstruction and malfunction.* **Table 10-4** lists key questions to ask during assessment to evaluate the severity of the complaint and the urgency for treatment.

Assessment of a Child with a Possible CSF Shunt Obstruction or Infection

Symptoms of a CSF shunt obstruction are the same as those of increased intracranial pressure and include headache, lethargy, sleepiness, irritability, nausea or vomiting, or trouble walking. Fever is usually a sign of a shunt infection or an <u>intercurrent</u> illness, but can occur with a shunt malfunction alone. Signs of a shunt obstruction are abnormal appearance, high-pitched cry, seizures, or altered level of consciousness.

A child with a shunt infection may have a fever, headache, feeding difficulty, or altered behavior. Signs of a shunt infection include abnormal appearance, altered level of consciousness, and septic shock.

Treatment

Make sure the child has a clear airway and effective breathing. Supply supplemental oxygen and transport the patient. Keep head in midline position and elevate 30° to 45° whenever possible. If the child has bradycardia, irregular respirations, and elevated blood pressure, there is increased intracranial pressure and herniation is imminent. Begin bag-mask ventilation and rapidly transport.

Advanced Life Support

Hyperventilation for Suspected Increased Intracranial Pressure Hyperventilation is a treatment for children with impending or frank herniation. However, the role of hyperventilation in treating out-of-hospital intracranial pressure elevation from hydrocephalus is not well understood. Hyperventilation, through rapid carbon dioxide reduction and vasoconstriction, will reduce brain perfusion. On the other hand, overly aggressive ventilation may dangerously decrease perfusion and cause brain ischemia. If a child with a CSF shunt has signs of impending or frank herniation, treat with mild hyperventilation at a rate of 5 breaths/min more than normal rate for age (35 breaths/min in an infant, 25 breaths/ min in a child). This is the same treatment as outlined for traumatic brain injury in Chapter 6.

Summary of Technology-Assisted Children

TAC may encounter many challenging problems with their equipment. The prehospital

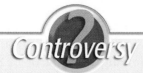
professional must be familiar with the basic purpose, design, and common complications of tracheostomy tubes, central venous catheters, feeding tubes, and CSF shunts. Always ask the caregiver about the equipment, and transport all devices and infusions with the child to the ED.

Behavioral Emergencies in Children

There has been an increase in the number of children suffering from behavioral and psychiatric conditions and a concomitant rise in the number of children presenting to EDs with these complaints. These children are a subset of CSHCN. There are many barriers to effective treatment including few resources for inpatient and outpatient treatment of mental health problems, a lack of tools for screening in the emergency department setting, and a lack of education of health care providers. Many hospitals do not have psychiatrists or other mental health workers on staff to perform emergency evaluations. Psychiatric conditions are sometimes present in cognitively impaired children as well as in children with normal intelligence. Sometimes these children's behavior is "out of control" or violent. The child may be at school or at home at the time of the crisis.

Assessment and Transport of the Child with a Behavioral Emergency

First, consider provider safety. Attempt to establish a rapport with the child while assessing the likelihood for violence (**Fig-**

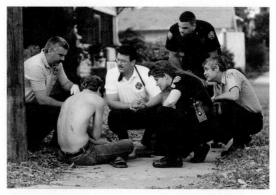

Figure 10-12 Establish a rapport with the child while assessing for the likelihood of violence.

ure 10-12). If the child appears cooperative and gives permission to be touched for examination purposes, do a focused history and physical exam. Next assess mental status. Is this child a risk to himself or others? Lastly, determine the need to transport the child. Consider restraints if the patient is a danger to himself or others. Always bring or ask the caregiver to follow the ambulance to the hospital.

Using Restraints for Assessment and Transport

Explain to the child's caregivers what you are doing as well as why you are restraining their child. Enlist their assistance. Talk to the child. Explain what you are doing and why, but do not negotiate. Do not attempt restraint placement alone. Prior to restraining a child, consider calling law enforcement officials. Do not allow the child to become positioned near an escape route. Should this happen, the child can escape or worse, attempt to injure the provider who has lost the ability to quickly escape. Apply restraint humanely, allowing the child as much dignity as possible. Document carefully the reasons for and the types of restraints in the medical record. Do periodic assessments. Keep restraints as loose as possible to avoid injury.

There may be conflict between parental wishes and the needs of the child. If the child is in immediate danger of self-harm or is an immediate danger to others, notify law enforcement officials to help restrain if necessary and transport to the closest appropriate facility.

Additional EMS Considerations for CSHCN

1. Many children with special health care needs, especially those with spina bifida, have a sensitivity or allergy to latex. Always use latex precautions with these patients. Reactions to latex can range from a localized skin reaction to anaphylaxis.

2. Speak quietly and calmly to the child, and explain what he can expect by using words appropriate for that child's developmental level. This approach will both decrease the child's anxiety and increase cooperation. Recognize that most CSHCN respond best with slower movements and firm, secure contact.

3. Children with musculoskeletal conditions such as cerebral palsy or muscular dystrophy need special care during preparation for transport. Children with cerebral palsy are often contracted and stiff. Do not force movements. Secure these children in their natural position. Children with paralysis or muscular dystrophy may not have normal sensation, and so special care should be taken to ensure that their limbs are secured on the stretcher and do not hang off the edges.

4. Assess pain in CSHCN. If the child cannot communicate, then ask the caregiver if the child is in pain. Position the child for comfort. Use blankets under vulnerable areas of the body. If local protocols allow, administer medications for pain control after ensuring the caregivers did not give the child any pain medication prior to EMS arrival.

5. When leaving the home of a CSHCN:
   - Ask the parents for the child's "Go Bag." This bag contains all of the supplies necessary (and which aren't routinely stocked on ambulances) to manage the child's tracheostomy tube, feeding catheter, or central venous line.
   - Ask the parents for the child's daily medical information form, which contains pertinent medical information regarding the child's medical condition, baseline vital signs, allergies, doctor's names and numbers, medications, therapies, and necessary home support equipment.
   - Ensure any compressed air or oxygen in the home is turned off prior to departure.

6. Request that the child's direct caregiver accompany the child to the hospital to continue assisting with the child's care. The caregiver will not only become a valuable resource for repeated assessments and interventions, but will also provide familiarity and reassurance to their child in the midst of an unfamiliar and potentially chaotic environment.

7. Recognize when the caregiver is overwhelmed with emotion or exhaustion. In these circumstances, it may be best to offer the caregiver a more passive role in their child's care while allowing them to continue to be with their child.

Case Study 3

A distraught mother calls 9-1-1 because her infant son is having difficulty feeding and appears more blue than usual. She tells you that the child is a 2-month-old boy with Down syndrome and a heart defect. He has been home for a few weeks and is being allowed to grow prior to surgery to repair his heart. His mother confirms that he normally has a pulse oximetry reading in the 80s. She hands you a card with the child's medical history, medications and hospital information, and states that he has been vomiting since the day before and has not kept down any of his medications.

You approach the child and note that he is cyanotic and poorly interactive. There are retractions and nasal flaring. The chest has crackles and the pulse oximetry is 75%. His heart rate is 130 beats/min, respiratory rate 70 breaths/min and blood pressure 86 mm Hg/palp.

1. What is the likely physiologic problem?
2. What are your primary interventions?

Case Study Answers

Case Study page 209

Assessment of the airway, breathing, and circulation suggests respiratory distress. Ask the child's caregiver about her baseline vital signs and activity level. Ask if there have been any changes and, if so, what is different.

Take the child off the ventilator and manually ventilate with a bag-mask device. Determine the ease of air entry through the tracheostomy tube and determine if aided respirations help the child's respiratory distress. Ask the caregiver when was the last tracheostomy tube change and the frequency of suctioning. Suction the tracheostomy to determine if this helps the child's breathing. Consider a tracheostomy tube change if there are copious secretions and/or there is difficulty with air entry during manual ventilations.

Consider an albuterol nebulizer treatment. Albuterol may help clear secretions and can open the child's airways to alleviate distress. In this case, the parent states that he has had to suction more frequently than usual and that he has already changed the tracheostomy tube that day. He states further that he thinks the child is getting sick and that her younger sister has had a cold for the last few days. This history makes an exacerbation of the child's chronic lung disease more likely and a mucous plug obstructing the tube less likely.

You decide to transport this child to her medical home hospital and continue the albuterol nebulizer treatment through her tracheostomy tube en route. You ask the caregiver to disconnect the feed through the gastrostomy tube to prepare for transport.

Bronchopulmonary dysplasia (BPD) is a chronic lung disease occurring in infants. It is characterized by stiff lungs and chronic lung disease. BPD is a worldwide problem with 5,000 to 10,000 new cases occurring each year and ranking with cystic fibrosis and asthma as one of the most common chronic lung disease in infants. BPD develops primarily in low birth weight infants who have respiratory distress syndrome (or RDS), a lung disease common in premature babies. Babies born prior to 32 weeks gestation may not have enough surfactant to keep these air sacks open. However, BPD development is not limited to RDS survivors, BPD may result from alveolar damage caused by lung disease, exposure to prolonged high oxygen concentrations, mechanical ventilation after birth (due to conditions such as neonatal pulmonary hypertension, pneumonia, or other infections or trauma to the lungs), all of which can cause harmful chemical reactions in the lungs.

A combination of fewer alveoli with a lack of surfactant can result in abnormally stiff lungs. This increases the work of breathing for affected infants who can quickly tire out. As they progressively weaken, carbon dioxide builds up in the lungs and blood. Respiratory infections can also worsen the inflammatory response in the lungs, leading to more fluid in the lungs and/or bronchospasm. Wheezing will result when tiny muscles in the bronchial tubes become more narrow and spasm. Other emergencies directly related to BPD include pulmonary edema, aspiration of food or stomach contents into the lungs, and apnea. Signs and symptoms of BPD can vary in severity depending on the infant's lung maturity. They may include tachypnea, retractions, paradoxical respirations, abnormal posturing, and wheezing.

BPD causes the most difficulties during the first year of life. Most deaths from BPD also occur during this first year. Problems after the first year become increasingly uncommon. The most common long-term lung complication of BPD is asthma. Approximately one half of the children with BPD will have asthma. Other less common complications resulting from BPD include apnea during infancy, gastro-esophageal reflux, pulmonary hypertension, high blood pressure, pulmonary edema, aspiration, subglottic stenosis, and tracheomalacia. Infants who have BPD are at risk for frequent hospitalizations because of their borderline respiratory reserve, hyperactive airway, and increased susceptibility to respiratory infection.

Chapter Review

Case Study ② page 219

This boy is in no distress. The PAT is normal. His vital signs are stable. He is totally dependent on this central venous catheter for his nutrition and hydration. Ask the caregiver how long the catheter site has been bleeding. Check the catheter for dislodgement or breakage. Apply direct pressure to the site to stop the bleeding. Ask the caregiver to disconnect the catheter if it is still connected. Prepare the child for transport, preferably to his medical home hospital, so that the catheter can be repaired or replaced.

A very common problem is dislodgement of a feeding catheter. This is especially true if the child is totally dependent on the gastrostomy tube (G-tube) for all of his nutrition and hydration. Also, the longer the tube is out, the more difficult its replacement is. Ask the family to bring the dislodged tube to the hospital and if they have a replacement tube, bring that as well. Not all hospitals will have the proper size tubes for children, so either call ahead to the local ED or bring the child to their home hospital.

Short gut syndrome results when a large section of the bowel has become necrotic and dies as a result of poor perfusion of the blood vessels. This phenomenon is more likely to occur in premature children, but can also occur in children who experience shock or hypoxemia to the bowel from infections, obstruction of the intestines, or trauma. These children often receive their nutrition through feeding catheters as this child did; however, if they have lost a significant amount of their bowel, they may need their nutrition (hyperalimentation and lipids) delivered through a central venous line. This boy no longer could receive all of his feeds through the gastrostomy tube and needed supplementation through his central venous catheter.

A young child who misses many hours of fluids may be tachycardic and have signs of dehydration, such as sticky mucous membranes and no tears, in the early stages of hypoperfusion. Interventions include oxygen supplementation, keeping the child warm, covering the stoma site with a dry gauze, and transporting the G-tube that fell out (along with any special adaptors) for sizing purposes.

Advanced Life Support

ALS interventions include a 20 cc/kg crystalloid fluid by peripherial IV bolus in a child who appears dehydrated with a G-tube out or dislodged or broken central venous line.

Case Study ③ page 224

Advanced Life Support

Assess airway, breathing, and circulation. You decide that this child needs assisted ventilations and begin to manually ventilate with a bag-mask device. As your partner is looking for an appropriate IV site, she notes that the child has swollen extremities. You then consider that this child is in congestive heart failure and opt not to start this child on IV fluids without advice from medical control. Because BP and perfusion are adequate, do not start a pressor drug. Transport immediately to the ED.

Down syndrome (DS) affects 1 in 800 births. This is lower than in the 1970s as a result of prenatal diagnosis and termination. Children with DS are at increased risk of medical complications. Some of the organ systems affected include: cardiovascular, sensory, endocrine, orthopedic, dental, gastrointestinal, neurologic developmental, and hematologic systems. People with DS are developmentally delayed.

Cardiovascular defects are the leading cause of neonatal death due to congenital abnormalities. When an infant is born with a severe cardiac anomaly, interventions are primarily directed towards home health care until definitive surgery can be performed or towards supportive treatment in the home of a child whose defect cannot be surgically repaired.

Suggested Readings

Textbooks

Adirim T, Smith E: *Special Children's Outreach and Prehospital Education (SCOPE)*. Sudbury, MA, Jones and Bartlett Publishers, 2005.

American Academy of Pediatrics and the American College of Emergency Physicians: *APLS: The Pediatric Emergency Medicine Resource,* 4th Edition. Sudbury, MA, Jones and Bartlett Publishers, 2004.

Articles

American Academy of Pediatrics, Committee on Children with Disabilities. Care coordination: Integrating health and related systems of care for children with special health care needs. *Pediatrics.* 1999; 104:978–981.

National Task Force on Children with Special Health Care Needs. EMS for children: Recommendations for coordinating care for children with special health care needs. *Annals Emerg Med.* 1997; 30:274–280.

Spaite DW, Conroy C, Karriker KJ, et al. Improving emergency medical services for children with special health care needs: Does training make a difference? *American Journal of Emergency Medicine.* Oct 2001; 19(6):474–478.

Spaite DW, Conroy C, Tibbitts M, et al. Use of emergency medical services by children with special health care needs. *Prehosp Emerg Care.* 2000; 4:19–23.

Spaite DW, Karriker KJ, Seng M, et al. Training paramedics: Emergency care for children with special health care needs. *Prehosp Emerg Care.* 2000; 4:178–185.

CD-ROM

Center for Pediatric Emergency Medicine (CPEM). Teaching resource for instructors in prehospital pediatrics (TRIPP), Version 2.0. New York: Center for Pediatric Emergency Medicine, 1998.

11

Sudden Infant Death Syndrome and Death of a Child

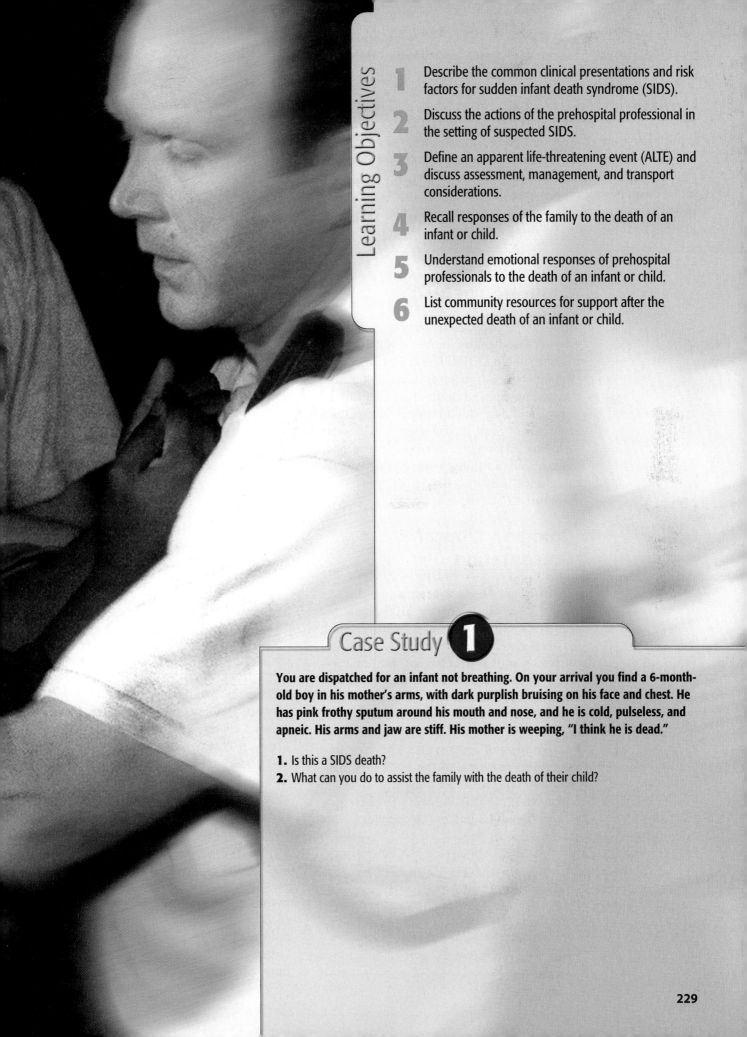

1   Describe the common clinical presentations and risk factors for sudden infant death syndrome (SIDS).

2   Discuss the actions of the prehospital professional in the setting of suspected SIDS.

3   Define an apparent life-threatening event (ALTE) and discuss assessment, management, and transport considerations.

4   Recall responses of the family to the death of an infant or child.

5   Understand emotional responses of prehospital professionals to the death of an infant or child.

6   List community resources for support after the unexpected death of an infant or child.

Case Study 1

You are dispatched for an infant not breathing. On your arrival you find a 6-month-old boy in his mother's arms, with dark purplish bruising on his face and chest. He has pink frothy sputum around his mouth and nose, and he is cold, pulseless, and apneic. His arms and jaw are stiff. His mother is weeping, "I think he is dead."

1. Is this a SIDS death?
2. What can you do to assist the family with the death of their child?

Introduction

SUDDEN INFANT DEATH syndrome (SIDS) and the death of a child are extremely difficult, emotional experiences for the prehospital professional. SIDS is the leading cause of infant death between 1 month and 1 year of age and the third leading cause of infant mortality in the United States. The causes of SIDS are not known.

The death of a child is an unparalleled family crisis and creates difficult emotional issues for the caregivers as well as for the prehospital professional. The infant may be in the care of a parent, child care provider, or babysitter at the time of death and may not be at home. Absence of one or both parents may complicate field management and interactions at the scene.

Definition of SIDS

SIDS is the unexpected death of an infant who is otherwise healthy. In 1989, the National Institute of Child Health and Human Development (NICHD) defined SIDS as, "the sudden and unexpected death of an infant under one year of age which remains unexplained after a thorough postmortem evaluation, including performance of a complete autopsy, examination of the death scene, and review of the clinical history." *Hence, SIDS cannot be diagnosed at the scene or in the ED.*

Common Clinical Presentation

When the prehospital professional arrives on the scene of a suspected SIDS death, the history is usually that of a healthy infant between 1 and 6 months of age who was put to sleep shortly after a feeding and then was found dead in bed. Often there is a history of a recent cold. The caregivers may have checked on the infant at intervals and found nothing out of the ordinary, and did not hear sounds of a struggle. The face and <u>dependent</u> portions of the body may have reddish-blue mottling, a condition called postmortem <u>lividity</u>. Lividity is caused by venous blood pooling in the dependent side

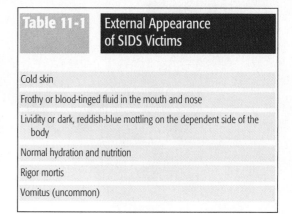

Table 11-1	External Appearance of SIDS Victims
Cold skin	
Frothy or blood-tinged fluid in the mouth and nose	
Lividity or dark, reddish-blue mottling on the dependent side of the body	
Normal hydration and nutrition	
Rigor mortis	
Vomitus (uncommon)	

of the body. There may be some blood-tinged discharge from the mouth.

Table 11-1 lists the signs of SIDS. Some signs differ, depending on how long the infant has been dead. Some cases of SIDS will not show any of these signs.

Epidemiology and Risk Factors

SIDS is the leading cause of death in infants between 1 month and 1 year of age. There are nearly 3,000 SIDS cases per year in the United States. It occurs most frequently between 2 and 4 months of age. Approximately 90% to 95% of all SIDS cases are babies less than 6 months of age. SIDS occurs more often in males (60%–70%) and more frequently in the winter months in all areas of the country.

Sometimes a sudden, unexpected infant death is not caused by SIDS, and the medical examiner identifies a specific illness or injury as the cause. This occurs in approximately 5% of suspected SIDS deaths. This group includes deaths caused by child maltreatment, as discussed in Chapter 12. On the scene, the prehospital professional cannot determine the

Tip

SIDS is the leading cause of infant death from age 1 month to 1 year.

Table 11-2	Risk Factors for SIDS

Formula feeding (possible)

Prematurity and low birth weight

Prone sleeping position and, to a lesser extent, side-sleeping

Soft, bulky blankets or comforters

Soft objects, such as pillows or stuffed animals, which trap air or gases in a baby's sleeping area

Soft sleeping surfaces

Tobacco smoke exposure (especially during pregnancy, but also after birth)

Young maternal age

The typical SIDS scenario is an apparently healthy baby, usually less than 6 months of age, who is found dead in his bed after having been seen alive a short time before.

true cause of death of an infant. Treat every caregiver as a grieving parent. *Never discuss child maltreatment as a possible cause of death while on scene.* Be sure, however, to note details of the death scene and record observations in the patient care report. To help identify deaths that may not be due to natural causes, document any observations related to the scene size-up, physical assessment, or focused history that seem atypical or inconsistent with SIDS. For example, dangerous or unclean home conditions, bruises or burn marks on the child's body, or changing or implausible stories are possible red flags for child maltreatment that require explicit documentation, as discussed in Chapter 12.

Although the causes of SIDS are unknown, there are a number of risk factors, which are noted in **Table 11-2**.

Summary of SIDS

SIDS is the most common cause of infant death. It is unpredictable and silent. The underlying cause is not known. The prehospital professional cannot "diagnose" SIDS in

Never discuss child maltreatment as a possible cause of death on the scene.

the field, and the emergency physician cannot diagnose SIDS in the ED. Determining the cause of death requires an autopsy. There are, however, common clinical signs and important risk factors that may be helpful in identifying probable SIDS cases.

Actions in Suspected SIDS

Clinical Interventions

The prehospital professional's first actions when SIDS is suspected must always be to assess and treat the baby. Immediately begin resuscitation, using standard treatment protocols, unless the infant meets local EMS system criteria for death in the field. In many SIDS cases, the baby has easily recognizable signs of death, and interventions or resuscitation are not indicated. If resuscitation is indicated, encourage the family to remain present during the resuscitative attempt, whenever possible.

The Transport Decision: Stay or Go?

After assessing the child's cardiopulmonary status, unless the patient meets local EMS system death in the field criteria, begin CPR if there is no detectable heart rate or other signs of life. If resuscitation is started and the child responds, transport as soon as medically appropriate, as discussed in Chapter 14.

If the infant is already dead upon the prehospital professional's arrival at the scene or the initial response to CPR is unsuccessful, it may be appropriate to leave the scene and allow the coroner or medical examiner to facilitate the death investigation. *The prehospital professional, however, should not leave the scene after a child has died until the appropriate authorities have arrived.* Notify medical oversight when there is uncertainty about treatment or transport. **Table 11-3** lists the pros

Table 11-3	Pros and Cons of Transporting Suspected SIDS Infants
Pros	**Cons**
ALS capability in ED	Caregiver concern about infant's body
Facilitation of autopsy	Disruption of scene investigation by medical examiner
More medical personnel to manage infant and caregivers	High costs in dollars, personnel, and equipment
Physician involvement in management	Possible violation of family's culture
Religious services	Removal of family from familiar setting
Social services for grief counseling	Transport liabilities, especially ambulance crashes and adverse bystander reactions

and cons of transporting suspected SIDS infants. Because the prehospital professional cannot distinguish a child with SIDS from any other child in cardiopulmonary arrest, use standard principles of treatment and transport for children in cardiopulmonary arrest, as discussed in Chapter 4.

In all cases of cardiopulmonary arrest, immediately begin resuscitation using standard treatment protocol, unless the infant meets local EMS criteria for death in the field.

Advanced Life Support

Value of Transport after Failed ALS Treatment in Cardiopulmonary Arrest
The value of immediate or delayed hospital transport when a child does not respond to resuscitation is controversial. The chances of neurologic survival of a child in the ED, after failed ALS in the field, are almost zero, unless rare extenuating circumstances (e.g., profound hypothermia, barbiturate overdose) are present.

Sometimes, the child will meet the EMS system's death-in-the-field criteria or resuscitation will not be successful, but grief counseling is not available at the scene. In this situation, consider transporting the baby to the hospital in a controlled transport mode (no lights or siren) with the caregiver, if possible. Encourage the caregiver to hold or touch the baby on scene. Before leaving the scene to transport a dead infant to an ED, give the

Encourage family presence during the attempted resuscitation.

name and address of the destination hospital verbally and in writing to family and friends. Simple verbal communications may not be "heard" by these stressed caregivers.

Support of Caregivers
The prehospital professional's emotional support of the caregivers is extremely important. When possible, have one person stay with the caregiver to provide information and support. Let family or caregivers stay with the child, and do not separate them even during attempted resuscitation and transport. *Be clear that the child is dead.* Do not use euphemisms, such as "your child has left us" or "she has gone to a better place." Avoid well intentioned but inappropriate remarks such as, "You can always have other children," "I know how you feel," or "You will get over this in time." **Table 11-4** suggests specific ways to communicate with caregivers when there is an unexpected death of a child.

Summary of Actions in Suspected SIDS

When faced with an infant in cardiopulmonary arrest, begin or continue CPR according to the local EMS system policies on death in the field. In some EMS systems, policy will permit withholding or discontin-

Table 11-4	Communicating About an Unexpected Death of a Child

Use the child's name.

Show **empathy** and express condolences.

Ask questions in a nonjudgmental manner. Never become hostile or angry.

Use a calm and directive voice.

Be clear with instructions and answers to questions.

Provide explanations to the caregivers about treatment and transport.

Repeat statements when necessary.

Reassure caregivers that there was nothing they could have done.

Allow the caregiver to accompany the baby if possible.

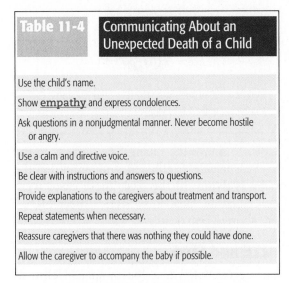

Table 11-5	Medical Examiner/Coroner and Local Health Department Responsibilities in Suspected SIDS Cases

Medical Examiner/ Coroner Responsibilities	Local Health Department Responsibilities
Performs death scene investigation	Provides information and counseling
Performs autopsy	Referral information for peer support
Notifies local health department	Provides information to state program
Notifies state program	Periodic follow-up
Signs death certificate	Community education (with peer group)
Notifies parents of cause of death	

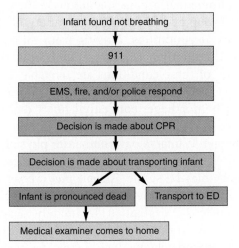

Figure 11-1 Flowchart of what to do in suspected SIDS cases.

Table 11-6	Key Questions in Focused History*

What happened?

Who found the infant and where?

What did the caregiver do?

Has the infant been moved?

What time was the infant last seen alive?

Had the infant been sick?

Was the infant receiving any medications?

*When asking these questions, use the infant's name rather than "the infant."

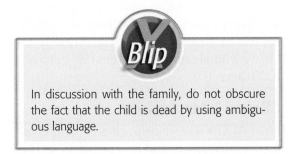

In discussion with the family, do not obscure the fact that the child is dead by using ambiguous language.

Information Collection

History

Get a focused history at the scene if the child is not transported to the ED. *Refrain from asking judgmental or leading questions.* **Table 11-6** gives examples of key questions to ask. Always ask the baby's name at the beginning of the interview and use her first name in all discussions with the caregiver.

Scene Size-up

Perform a scene size-up and note findings carefully and objectively. These are often important pieces of information for the medical examiner or coroner and medical experts who later review the entire case. Note the location of the infant on arrival at

uing resuscitation and focusing on the important tasks of talking to the family and helping them with their grief. **Figure 11-1** provides a typical sequence of events when there is a suspected SIDS case. **Table 11-5** lists the responsibilities of the medical examiner and local health department in a case of suspected SIDS.

Refrain from asking judgmental or leading questions that suggest that the caregiver may be at fault for the infant's death.

Ask the name of the child and use it in any discussions with the caregiver.

the scene (e.g., in the crib or bed, on the floor). If the infant has been moved, investigate the location where death occurred and document whether or not she was in her own crib, the nature of the sleeping surface, and whether she was sharing a crib or bed (and with whom). Also describe the covering blankets or comforter (soft, thick) and note whether the blanket was over the face.

Document the infant's position when placed down for sleep and when discovered (prone, side, or supine). Check for the presence of other objects in the area where the infant was found, especially pillows or other soft or bulky items. Note any unusual conditions such as high room temperature or odors. Look for street drugs and if possible, bring all medications to the ED.

Documentation

Document all findings in the history, patient assessment, treatment, and scene size-up completely and accurately on the patient care record. Failure to fully document can result in unnecessary investigations or significant emotional stress to the caregiver and prehospital professional.

Apparent Life-Threatening Events (ALTE)

Definition of ALTE

An apparent life-threatening event (ALTE) is an episode in which an infant demonstrates a significant behavioral or physical change that may reflect a serious physiologic problem. An ALTE is characterized by a transient episode of decreased muscle tone, change in color (pale or cyanotic), apnea, choking, or gagging. Often the caregiver provides a significant intervention (shaking, ventilation, or

CPR) to revive the infant. The witness to the event is usually frightened, and afraid that the baby is dying. In the past, these cases were described as "near-miss SIDS," "near SIDS," or "aborted crib death."

ALTE and SIDS

The term ALTE describes a special clinical syndrome that occurs in children in the same age group at risk for SIDS. A variety of diseases or conditions, ranging from minor to life-threatening, can cause such episodes. Many of these conditions are treatable, such as gastroesophageal reflux, sepsis, intracranial hemorrhage, congenital heart disease, metabolic disease, and seizures. As noted in Chapter 1, infants have immature physiology and signs and symptoms of serious illness or injury may be subtle. *Assume that every child with a report of an ALTE has a serious problem requiring ED evaluation.* Ultimately, despite extensive workup, no cause can be identified in approximately one-half of the cases.

The mortality rate of ALTE is unknown. Less than 7% of SIDS cases are preceded by ALTE. Due to this low association, terms such as "aborted crib death" or "near-miss SIDS" are inaccurate and inappropriate. These terms imply a misleading relationship between ALTE and SIDS.

Clinical Interventions

Most ALTEs resolve before arrival of prehospital professionals and it is common for the infants to appear normal on assessment (**Figure 11-2**). In this case, no immediate treatment is required and the additional assessment can be completed on scene. If the child appears unstable or needs urgent treatment as identified in the initial assessment, complete the additional assessment en route to the hospital. Always transport the baby, even if the complete assessment reveals no

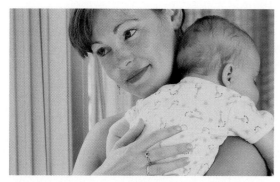

Figure 11-2 An ALTE is an episode in which an infant demonstrates a significant behavioral or physical change.

Consider every child with a reported ALTE to have a serious problem that requires evaluation in the emergency department.

"Near-miss SIDS" is not an accurate or appropriate term for ALTE.

abnormalities. Serious illnesses in newly borns and young infants are sometimes subtle and difficult to detect.

Summary of ALTE

ALTE is a special clinical condition of young infants involving a sudden and transient change in appearance, respiratory effort, or perfusion. Examples of ALTE presentations include sudden loss of muscle tone, cyanosis, or cessation of breathing. Half of the time, no cause is found despite hospital workup. An ALTE may be an indicator of serious occult illness or injury that may not be identified in the field. Perform a standard assessment and treat if there is a demonstrable physiologic or anatomic problem. In most cases, transport alone is the most important field intervention.

Responses to an Infant Death

Caregiver's Response

The prehospital professional is often the first responder on the scene following the discovery of the dead infant. Responses of the caregiver to the sudden and unexpected death of an infant are not predictable and may vary from numb silence to rage. Common reactions include denial, anger, hysteria, withdrawal, intense guilt, or no visible response. The caregiver may or may not accept that the infant is dead and that resuscitation is not possible. The caregiver may cling to the hope that the prehospital professional can do something to save the infant, even though the child is obviously dead.

The death of a child is likely the most stressful and tragic moment in the life of a parent or caregiver. It is not uncommon for caregivers in this situation to express strong preferences or make "demands" of the prehospital professional. Remember that this is that individual's last chance to fulfill their role of protecting and caring for the infant. Respond to them gently and professionally. The caregiver may:

- Ask repeated questions
- Request that you not start care or that you stop resuscitation efforts
- Request to be alone with the infant
- Want to know the cause of death
- Physically interfere with care
- Insist on continuation of care or that resuscitation efforts be started

When the caregiver or family expresses their preferences or asks difficult questions, use a calm and professional approach. Keep explanations simple. Follow EMS system protocol for death in the field, and maintain an empathetic and nonjudgmental attitude.

If there is no indication to attempt to resuscitate the infant, while awaiting the medical examiner or coroner at the scene, ask the family member or caregiver who to call to give them support (**Figure 11-3**). This may involve calling friends, relatives, clergy, or public agencies to help care for other

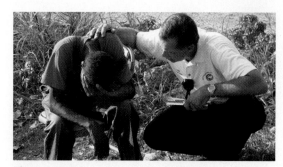

Figure 11-3 Caregivers can react to the death of a child in many ways, but all need support. Attempt to contact identified individuals who might give comfort.

Responses of the caregiver to the sudden and unexpected death of an infant are not predictable and may vary from numb silence to rage.

children at the home. If the scene is a child care setting, consider calling law enforcement to assist with other children and to contact the child's caregivers or the caregivers of other children present.

Prehospital Professional's Response

The prehospital professional has a difficult and sometimes agonizing role in the setting of unexpected infant or child death. After death is declared, comfort the parents. Never place blame on the parents or caregivers. Offering sensitive support to the family and gathering accurate information in a non-threatening manner helps surviving family members. This is often challenging because the prehospital professional may be struggling with overwhelming personal emotional responses related to the loss of a patient.

Talking to the family or caregivers can be difficult. There are techniques that may improve the quality of these interactions:

- Use the child's name. This acknowledges the child as an individual rather than a "patient" and the unique, intensely personal nature of this child's death.
- Try to find a quiet area to talk to the caregivers. Often the scene can become noisy with activity. Finding an area

where the caregiver can concentrate on your conversation will help to keep your message clear.

- Use concrete terms. The use of euphemisms to soften the news can make it harder for the caregiver to understand what has happened. "Your child has died" has a finite meaning, while "Your child is in a better place" has infinite possibilities (the hospital is a better place).
- It is okay to show emotion. Parents whose child has died often comment on how meaningful it was to them that a health care provider clearly cared. Expressing your emotions is appropriate in such tragic circumstances, so long as the focus remains on the family and child and you are able to fulfill your professional duties at the scene.
- Allow the caregiver a chance to touch or hold the child before transport. This may be the last time the caregiver has to be with the child. This may not be possible if the scene is related to a crime but is an important step in the grieving process.

Sometimes there are cultural or language differences between the prehospital professional and the caregiver. There may be unfamiliar rituals and behaviors in how death is regarded or how grief is expressed. This presents another important challenge. *Respect cultural diversity. This is necessary in order to effectively communicate.* When cultural or language differences arise, attempt to find an interpreter to explain and translate.

Responses of the prehospital professional to the sudden and unexpected death of an infant may include one or more of the following:

- Anger or blame
- Identification with the caregiver
- Withdrawal
- Avoidance of the caregiver
- Self-doubt (if resuscitation is attempted and the child does not recover)
- Sadness and depression

The prehospital professional may have unrealistic expectations of how the caregiver should behave and respond, or may believe that the caregiver was responsible for the

Table 11-7	Responses of Prehospital Professionals that Hinder Communication with Caregivers After an Unexpected Death

Having stereotyped expectations of how the caregiver should respond to the event

Judging a caregiver who did not initiate CPR

Distrusting a caregiver who has recognized the infant is dead and does not want resuscitation

Misunderstanding the mourning and grief behaviors of persons of different cultures or religious beliefs

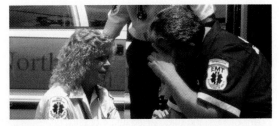

Figure 11-4 Stress is an unavoidable part of a prehospital professional's job. The death of a child can be agonizing.

Tip

The unexpected death of an infant or child is one of the most stressful experiences for the prehospital professional.

Table 11-8	Signs and Symptoms of Critical Incident Stress

Anger and irritability

Changes in eating habits

Changes in sleeping patterns

Depression

Excessive alcohol consumption

Inability to concentrate

Mood changes and emotional instability

Physical illness

Recurring dreams or frightening images

Withdrawal

baby's death. These feelings can become obstacles to communication, as outlined in **Table 11-7**.

Critical Incident Stress

Stress is an unavoidable part of the prehospital professional's job. The death of a child may be the most stressful situation in the prehospital professional's career (**Figure 11-4**). Acknowledging emotions is a key element in successfully coping with stress and maintaining a healthy mental attitude. **Table 11-8** lists the frequent signs and symptoms of stress.

There are many ways to decrease the impact of stress related to the death of an infant or child. Critical incident stress debriefing (CISD) may be an important technique for helping cope with the emotional toll of SIDS and unexpected infant or child death. Other techniques to help decrease stress include the following:

- Talk to field supervisors and experienced prehospital professionals to share feelings.
- Exercise, plan leisure time, and limit overtime hours. Maintain a well-balanced lifestyle outside of work.

Case Study ❷

You are dispatched to a coworker's home where a grandmother is weeping and largely incoherent. She leads you to a bedroom where a 3-month-old boy lies motionless in his crib, face down on a sheepskin. He is apneic, pulseless, has lividity on his chest and face, and is stiff. In between sobs, the grandmother tells you she put the baby to sleep 4 hours ago and found him this way when she checked on him 10 minutes ago. She asks you if he is dead.

1. What are your key medical actions?
2. How should you deal with the grandmother? The coworker?

Tip

Critical incident stress debriefing (CISD) may be an important technique for coping with the emotional toll of SIDS and unexpected infant or child death.

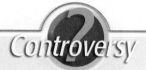

Controversy

Risk reduction and risk counseling are important community prevention activities. Further research must help define the appropriate educational role of the prehospital professional at the scene of an injury or death.

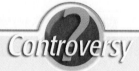

Controversy

The value and appropriate timing of CISD is not known. While the prehospital professional will suffer predictable stress after the death of a child in her care, how and when such intervention should occur has not been studied.

Tip

Prehospital professionals can play a key role in educating parents in the community on the ways to decrease the risk of SIDS.

- Get adequate rest and eat a balanced diet.
- Avoid excessive alcohol or drugs.
- Write a personal journal.
- Obtain religious or peer counseling.
- Request professional psychological assistance.

Community Resources

Community resources available to caregivers and to prehospital professionals to help them cope with the unexpected death of a child include the following:

- Local support groups
- Local public health departments
- National SIDS Alliance (1-800-221-SIDS)
- Professional counseling

Risk Reduction Activities and Risk Counseling

In addition to community resource groups, prehospital professionals can also play a key role in educating parents in the community on the ways to decrease the risk of SIDS. This includes distribution of the American Academy of Pediatrics "Back to Sleep" brochures and active support of their recommendation to place babies on their backs to

sleep. Although side-sleeping is several times safer than prone sleeping, the risk of SIDS for the side-sleeping position is still double the risk of the supine position. Prehospital professionals can participate in community risk reduction by advocating for firm, flat mattresses in safety-approved cribs, avoidance of soft or bulky blankets or comforters, and overheating in the infant's sleeping area.

Support of anti-smoking campaigns is also important. Recent research shows that the risk of SIDS doubles among babies exposed to cigarette smoke after birth, and triples for those exposed both during pregnancy and after birth. As for all infants, encouragement of breastfeeding is a useful action because formula feeding may be a risk factor for SIDS.

Prehospital professionals can also become involved in local or state child fatality review teams. These teams meet and discuss the community trends in infant and child deaths. They often review all sudden and unexpected deaths in children less than 2 years of age in order to improve the accuracy of SIDS as a diagnosis versus other natural causes and versus non-natural causes, especially child maltreatment.

Summary of Information Collection, Responses at the Scene, and Critical Incident Stress

The death of a child is an emotional event for everyone. When a baby's death is managed at the scene, there are many challenges to the prehospital professional. Use a supportive and nonjudgmental approach.

Expect complex caregiver responses that will vary between individuals and be impacted by cultural differences. Gather information and complete documentation on the scene that will help establish cause of death and identify possible risk factors in the environment. Recognize that a critical incident stress response is common for the prehospital professional and seek assistance if necessary. Consider involvement in community SIDS risk reduction campaigns.

Case Study 3

You are called to an apartment complex that is home to a large number of immigrant families. On arrival, there is a large, agitated group congregated at the doorway to the apartment, speaking in a language that you do not recognize. You enter the apartment to find a mother and father sitting on a couch, quietly weeping. They gesture toward a bassinet, where a stiff, cold 3-month-old infant with dependent lividity lays covered on a pile of blankets. Through a neighbor who speaks English, you explain that the baby is dead and ask if they would like to hold her. They decline, and seem offended by the proposal.

1. How do you react?
2. What steps do you take from this point?

Chapter Review

Case Study Answers

Case Study 1 page 229

The infant has many findings commonly associated with a SIDS death. Sleeping prone (indicated by the lividity on the chest and face), the pink frothy sputum, and the absence of traumatic injuries are the initial clues to a SIDS death. However, remember that SIDS is a diagnosis of exclusion made by a medical examiner or coroner at autopsy.

In this setting, provide a direct and calm explanation to the parent that the child is dead. Find out the child's name and use it. Do not ask questions in a way that suggests blame. Utilize a controlled and supportive dialogue with the parent. If the child is not transported, try to get grief counseling for the parent, contact the medical examiner or coroner from the scene, and consider critical incident stress debriefing for yourself and your partner. Gather family support resources.

Case Study 2 page 237

In most EMS systems, the child would meet death-in-the-field criteria and would not require any resuscitation attempt. If you are uncertain about whether resuscitation is indicated, begin CPR and call medical oversight to clarify treatment options.

The grandmother may need to be medically evaluated if she cannot be calmed down. Provide a calm and controlled environment. Do not blame.

Try to minimize radio communications if your coworker may be listening. If the employee is at work, have a supervisor contact the coworker and provide safe transportation to the scene. Contact other family, friends, or clergy if the situation warrants. Watch for symptoms consistent with that of critical incident stress and initiate CISD if indicated.

Case Study 3 page 239

Different cultures have different beliefs about death, afterlife, and the proper handling of a dead body. There may be rituals or taboos with which you are unfamiliar, as well as different ways of coping with loss. Since there is no medical intervention that will help this child, your focus must be on providing support to the survivors. Obtaining a professional interpreter, where available, is an important part of the scene management and the death investigation. Even through an English-speaking neighbor, you can inquire about family needs, who they might want you to contact, and any way that you might assist them at the scene. Remember that even with an interpreter present, concepts may be difficult to translate and the family may have a very different belief system with regard to illness, health care, and cause of death than you do. If you cannot communicate the rationale for your treatment or non-treatment to the family, transport may be necessary in order to mobilize an interpreter and necessary social support.

Suggested Readings

Textbooks

American Academy of Pediatrics and the American College of Emergency Physicians: *APLS: The Pediatric Emergency Medicine Resource,* 4th Edition. Sudbury, MA, Jones and Bartlett Publishers, 2004.

Hazinski M, Zaritsky A, Nadkarni V, et al: *PALS Provider Manual.* American Heart Association, 2002.

Horchler J, Rice R, Morris R: *SIDS & Infant Death Survival Guide: Information and comfort for grieving family and friends and professionals who seek to help them,* 3rd Edition. Hyattsville, MD, SIDS Educational Services, Inc., 2003.

Articles

Hall WL, Myers JH, Pepe PE, et al. Paramedics' perspective about on-scene termination of resuscitation efforts for pediatric patients. *Resuscitation.* Feb 2004; 60(2):175–187.

Kairys S. Distinguishing sudden infant death syndrome from child abuse fatalities. American Academy of Pediatrics. Committee on Child Abuse and Neglect. *Pediatrics.* Feb 2001; 107(2):437–41.

Kairys S. Distinguishing sudden infant death syndrome from child abuse fatalities. American Academy of Pediatrics. Committee on Child Abuse and Neglect. Addendum. *Pediatrics.* Sep 2001; 108(3):812.

Loyacono T. Family-centered prehospital care. *Emerg Med Serv.* June 2001; 30(6):64–7.

Schears R, Marco C, Iserson K. "Do not attempt resuscitation" in the out-of-hospital setting. *Ann Emerg Med.* July 2004; 44(1):68–69.

Stratton S, Taves A, Lewis R, et al. Apparent life-threatening events in infants: High risk in the out-of-hospital environment. *Ann Emerg Med.* June 2004; 43(6)711–717.

12

Child Maltreatment

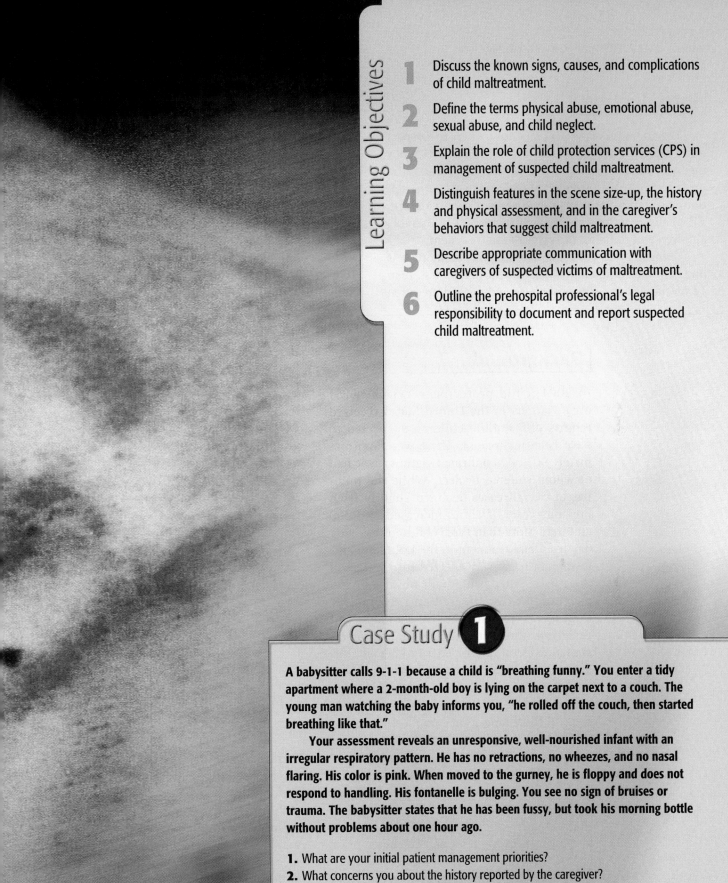

1 Discuss the known signs, causes, and complications of child maltreatment.

2 Define the terms physical abuse, emotional abuse, sexual abuse, and child neglect.

3 Explain the role of child protection services (CPS) in management of suspected child maltreatment.

4 Distinguish features in the scene size-up, the history and physical assessment, and in the caregiver's behaviors that suggest child maltreatment.

5 Describe appropriate communication with caregivers of suspected victims of maltreatment.

6 Outline the prehospital professional's legal responsibility to document and report suspected child maltreatment.

Case Study 1

A babysitter calls 9-1-1 because a child is "breathing funny." You enter a tidy apartment where a 2-month-old boy is lying on the carpet next to a couch. The young man watching the baby informs you, "he rolled off the couch, then started breathing like that."

Your assessment reveals an unresponsive, well-nourished infant with an irregular respiratory pattern. He has no retractions, no wheezes, and no nasal flaring. His color is pink. When moved to the gurney, he is floppy and does not respond to handling. His fontanelle is bulging. You see no sign of bruises or trauma. The babysitter states that he has been fussy, but took his morning bottle without problems about one hour ago.

1. What are your initial patient management priorities?
2. What concerns you about the history reported by the caregiver?

Introduction

PREHOSPITAL PROFESSIONALS MUST know when to suspect child maltreatment. While provision of emergency medical care is always the top priority, prehospital professionals also provide valuable scene documentation and reporting of suspected cases of maltreatment. All of these actions are critical to protect vulnerable children and to break the cycle of maltreatment.

Unfortunately, child maltreatment is common. It is one of the leading causes of death in infants less than 12 months of age. Physical abuse and neglect are often detectable, but sexual abuse, emotional abuse, and child neglect may not be clinically obvious. The prehospital professional's role in management of these conditions is more limited.

Some children who die from maltreatment are known to local child protection services, the legal organizations established in every community to monitor, manage, and prevent child maltreatment. These deaths are sometimes preventable. Abused or neglected children have a high probability of being maltreated again. Early recognition is important to prevent future injury or death.

Background

In 2001, child protective services (CPS) organizations in the United States received reports of 5 million children suspected to have been maltreated. There were approximately 903,000 confirmed victims, over half of whom suffered neglect. While the number of overall cases declined slightly from previous years, fatalities increased to 1,300 children. More than three children die every day from maltreatment in the US. Many survivors are negatively affected for the rest of their lives. After being both physically and psychologically affected, survivors may themselves become abusive or neglectful caregivers, thus perpetuating the intergenerational cycle of abuse. The number of children who suffer long-term effects from neglect is not as well documented, but is believed to be substantial. **Table 12-1** lists some of these long-term complications.

Younger children are at higher risk for fatal abuse and neglect than older children. About 85% of maltreated children who die are less than 6 years of age and over 40% are under 1 year of age. Approximately half of these deaths occur in children that are known to CPS agencies as current or prior clients.

Child maltreatment involves risk factors and lapses in child protection at the individual, family, community, and societal levels. No geographic, ethnic, or economic setting is free of child maltreatment. The

Table 12-1	Potential Complications of Maltreatment
Low self-esteem and underachievement	
Psychological disorders or psychiatric symptoms	
Abnormal growth and development	
Permanent physical or neurologic damage	
Poor school performance	
Teen promiscuity and pregnancy	
Social withdrawal	
Eating disorders	
Substance abuse	
Negative learned behavior	
Criminal behavior beginning in young adulthood	
Vulnerability to further abuse	
Suicidal tendencies	
Increased survivor health care costs to family and society	
Death	

incidence rates for sexual abuse are similar for urban, suburban, and rural communities. Children from low-income or single parent families, however, have more reported occurrences of neglect or physical maltreatment than children from higher-income families, and physically maltreated children are less likely to be identified in Caucasian, two parent families. The prehospital provider must consider maltreatment whenever circumstances suggest it, regardless of the family's socioeconomic status.

Table 12-2	Assessment Factors Associated with Maltreatment

Does the history change over time?

Was there a delay in seeking care, or was the closest treatment center bypassed?

Are there injuries of multiple ages?

Does the history fit the child's developmental ability?

Do the injuries fit the history?

Does the patient not seek comfort from the caregiver?

Does the caregiver inappropriately respond to the patients needs?

What are the other sibling's involvements with the patient and caregiver?

A perpetrator of child maltreatment can be any person who has care, custody, or control of the child. This can include the child's parents, relative, teacher, babysitter or child care staff person, institution staff person, bus driver, playground attendant, coach, religious leader, caregiver, or boyfriend or girlfriend of the caregiver. Inflicted traumatic brain injury (commonly known as shaken baby syndrome) may lead to seizures or apnea, but the person with the infant at the time of <u>decompensation</u> should not be assumed to be the perpetrator. *Often the caregiver with the child at the time of the 9-1-1 call or EMS arrival is not the one who hurt the child.* They may be unaware of the abuse, or be in denial and unable to believe that the child has been harmed. They may also be a victim of abuse or afraid of the abuser. Maltreatment happens for many different reasons. Often the perpetrators genuinely care for the child, but lack the resources or the parenting skills to deal with frustration and cope with anger. Rarely does the prehospital professional have sufficient information to determine with certainty that maltreatment has occurred. Information gathered in the field can, however, be critical in the eventual confirmation of maltreatment. **Table 12-2** lists factors that are suggestive of abuse. Particularly important is the documentation of the exact history given by the caregiver in cases of presumed injury. A

changing story is one of the most common hallmarks of maltreatment. Recognizing and reporting suspected child maltreatment is one of the most important ways the prehospital professional can prevent childhood injury.

Definition of Child Maltreatment

Child maltreatment is a general term that includes all types of abuse and neglect. Yearly, approximately 50% of substantiated maltreatment is classified as neglect, 25% is physical, and 12% is sexual abuse. The remaining types include emotional abuse, medical neglect, or combinations of any of them.

Physical Abuse

<u>Physical abuse</u> occurs when a person intentionally inflicts injury, or allows injury to be inflicted, to a child under 18 years of age or to a mentally disabled child under 21 years of age, which causes or results in risk of death, disfigurement, or distress.

Emotional Abuse

<u>Emotional abuse</u> occurs when there is an ongoing and consistent pattern of behavior that interferes with the normal psychological and social development of a child. This includes unreasonable, excessive, or aggressive demands on the child that are not age-appropriate, setting tasks that are beyond the physical ability of the child, or the caregiver not providing the nurturing, guidance, and/or psychological support critical for the

Tip

When adults with poor coping skills are faced with stressful situations, a cycle of child maltreatment may result.

growth and development of a healthy child. Verbal attacks such as belittling, insults, rejection, and constant criticism are a few patterns of emotional abuse.

Sexual Abuse

<u>Sexual abuse</u> occurs when an older child or adult engages in sexual activities with a dependent, developmentally immature child or adolescent for the older person's own sexual excitement or for the enjoyment of other persons (such as in child pornography or prostitution).

In most cases of sexual abuse, the perpetrator is an adult who knows the child and is often living under the same roof. A common misconception is that child sexual abuse is perpetrated by strangers. According to the 2002 report of the Administration of Children and Families, more than 80% of abuse is perpetrated by parents, 7% by another relative, and the remaining by someone the child knows or a stranger.

Sexual abuse usually does not occur as a single incident. It does not always involve violence and physical force, and commonly leaves no visible sign. The perpetrator may use the power of adult–child authority or the parent–child bond instead of force or violence. The child may be manipulated into thinking that "it's OK" and a normal behavior or that the child is "special" for making the perpetrator feel good. The child may also be made to feel deeply ashamed and powerless, or may even be kept silent by threats from the perpetrator. The insidious nature of this abuse makes it difficult to detect, unless the child discloses the information to a confidant or the prehospital professional.

Child Neglect

<u>Child neglect</u> occurs when a child's physical, mental, or emotional condition is harmed or endangered because the caregiver has failed to supply basic necessities or engages in child-rearing practices that are inadequate or dangerous. Child neglect may involve a caregiver's misuse of drugs or alcohol, or child abandonment. Neglect is the failure to act on

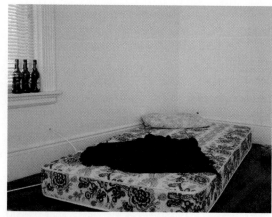

Figure 12-1 Child neglect occurs when a child's physical, mental, or emotional condition is harmed or endangered because the caregiver has failed to supply basic necessities or engages in child-rearing practices that are inadequate or dangerous.

behalf of a child, and is an act of omission. Neglect may not have visible signs, and it usually occurs over a period of time rather than as a discrete episode (**Figure 12-1**).

Neglect may be physical or emotional. <u>Physical neglect</u> is a failure to meet the requirements basic to a child's physical development and safety, such as supervision, housing, clothing, medical attention, and nutrition. Some social service agencies subdivide this category into more specific acts of omission, such as medical neglect, lack of proper supervision, or educational neglect. <u>Emotional neglect</u> is failure to provide the support or affection necessary to a child's psychological and social development.

Abuse versus Neglect

The difference between abuse and neglect is that abuse represents an action against a child, whereas neglect represents a lack of

Tip

Abuse represents an action against a child (commission). Neglect represents a lack of action for the child (omission).

action for the child. *Abuse is an act of commission; neglect is an act of omission.* In abuse, a physical or mental injury is inflicted on a child. In neglect, there is a failure to meet the basic needs of the child for adequate food, supervision, shelter, guidance, education, clothing, or medical care.

Summary of Background and Definition of Child Maltreatment

Child maltreatment occurs in all communities and in all socioeconomic strata. These conditions often involve repetition of dysfunctional behaviors through generations to create a cycle of maltreatment. Physical abuse is the most obvious form of maltreatment and can often be suspected during a physical assessment. The prehospital professional has a valuable role in the assessment, treatment, and reporting of child maltreatment in the community.

Child Protective Services (CPS)

The CPS agency is a legal community organization responsible for protection against child maltreatment. CPS has the legal authority to temporarily remove children at risk for injury or neglect from the home and to secure foster care placement. CPS is responsible for initial investigations of suspected maltreatment. They must make complicated and important decisions about the maltreatment accusations, at times remove children from home and place them into foster care, and provide services for abusive and neglectful families. **Table 12-3** lists the initial actions of the CPS when a report is filed. CPS may work in concert with law enforcement to investigate the facts and determine who is responsible for maltreating the child. Ultimately, the judicial system determines if an accused individual is "guilty." While emotions may run high when the prehospital professional suspects

Table 12-3	Initial CPS Actions

1. When a report of child abuse or neglect is received, either from a health professional or a law enforcement agency, the protocols of the receiving agency determine the timing and scope of the initial response.

2. The facts are reviewed to determine if a home visit is appropriate and, if so, which members of the team will be involved.

3. The CPS caseworker assesses risk to the child, the family's ability to provide safety, and supportive resources available to the family.

4. After the investigation and assessment, a reported incident is determined to be founded, unfounded, or unable to be determined because of lack of information.

child maltreatment, it is neither appropriate nor safe to confront caregivers with these concerns at the scene.

The prehospital professional can provide scene information that helps CPS determine safe placement of the patient. When maltreatment is suspected, always note the presence of other children in the home. If a determination is made that an environment may be unsafe, contact law enforcement or CPS to evaluate the safety of any other children who are present, based on local EMS protocol. When a patient is transported to a hospital, communicate any concerns of maltreatment to hospital staff, who are also mandated reporters.

Duties of the Prehospital Professional

The prehospital professional has an extremely important role at the scene. CPS and health professionals in the ED rely on the scene assessment and documentation of suspected child maltreatment. **Table 12-4** lists the prehospital professional's duties in suspected maltreatment cases.

Scene Assessment

First, ensure that the scene is safe for the child and for the prehospital professionals. Then, carefully document the scene conditions that might support suspicion of maltreatment (**Figure 12-2**). Record remarks or

Table 12-4	Duties of the Prehospital Professional in Suspected Maltreatment

Recognition of suspicious circumstances at the scene

Physical assessment of the child

Assessment of the history given by the caregiver

Communication with the caregiver and family

Careful documentation

Notation of other children living at the scene

Reporting of maltreatment concerns to the proper authority

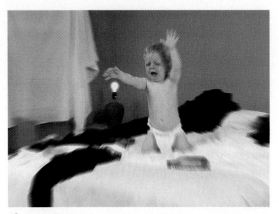

Figure 12-2 Document scene conditions that might support suspicion of maltreatment.

specific conversations with the caregiver and document specifics about the environment where injuries were reported to occur. For instance, note the approximate height of furniture an infant rolled off, the floor surface, or the location and condition of the sink or room where a child was burned.

Consider child maltreatment in every trauma call. Suspicious circumstances in the

Tip

Consider child abuse in every injury case, as well as in illness cases with suspicious circumstances in the environment, behavior of the child or caregiver, history, or physical exam.

environment, behavior of the child or caregiver, history, or physical exam may also raise concerns of abuse in responding to calls for unrelated complaints. Look for unsanitary or dangerous home conditions such as guns, drug paraphernalia, or other unsafe care situations.

Tip

Note and report the presence of other children in situations suggestive of maltreatment.

Blip

Judging or confronting caregivers or attempting to intervene in issues of dysfunctional parenting may interfere with patient care or a subsequent maltreatment investigation. The caregiver may in fact not know how their child was injured or by whom. Your interventions may put you at risk, and a confrontation does not help the child.

Initial Assessment

If the scene is safe, assess the child, as outlined in Chapters 1 and 2, and give appropriate medical care. If an infant with suspected maltreatment has an abnormal appearance (e.g., listlessness, inconsolability, weak cry) or altered level of consciousness (abnormal response to verbal or painful stimuli), but normal work of breathing and skin circulation, the child may have a brain injury.

One cause of traumatic inflicted brain injury is <u>shaken baby syndrome</u>. Shaken baby syndrome involves diffuse intracranial hemorrhage, usually from violent shaking of the child with or without impact. The signs, symptoms, and physical findings in shaken baby syndrome vary depending on the amount of trauma to the brain. These range from lethargy and irritability to seizures, coma, or death. <u>Petechiae</u>, or hand grip

Table 12-5	Focused History: Questions and Considerations in Evaluating Suspected Child Maltreatment
Question	**Considerations**
How did the injury occur?	Is the caregiver's explanation plausible? Do the physical conditions at the scene support the alleged mechanism of injury?
When did it happen?	Was there a long delay before 9-1-1 was notified? Does the injury appearance match the time frame?
Who witnessed the event?	Do all of the caregivers' or witnesses' stories match? Was there adequate supervision?
What is the child's medical history?	Are there preexisting psychosocial, developmental, or chronic problems?
Does the child have a physician?	When was the last visit? Does the physician know the child?

patterns on the arms or chest may also be found in shaken baby syndrome. The incidence of permanent neurological damage from shaken baby syndrome is high. Seizures, learning disabilities, blindness, and other handicaps are common. The fatality rate is 20% to 30%.

The Transport Decision: Stay or Go?

If the child with suspected maltreatment is physiologically unstable or has significant injuries, begin transport after the initial assessment and stabilization. If the scene is unsafe for the child or prehospital professional, call for law enforcement back-up and move to the ambulance to complete the assessment and initiate treatment. Transport every child with suspected maltreatment, even if the injuries are trivial.

Never leave a suspected victim of child maltreatment. Transport every child, even if the injuries are trivial.

Additional Assessment

Stay on scene for additional assessment only if the child is stable and the scene is safe. Take a careful history, using the questions

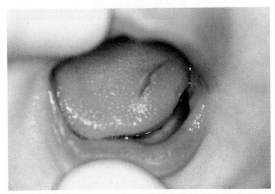

Figure 12-3 A caregiver's history of a child biting his tongue is not believable in an infant who has no teeth. This discrepant history suggests an inflicted injury.

suggested in **Table 12-5**. *The history is usually more important than the physical assessment.* Ask questions in a nonjudgmental way to maximize the quality of information and to avoid escalating the situation. Pay close attention to and document in detail the caregiver's description of the events leading to the call, noting inconsistencies or evasiveness. Consider the developmental capabilities of the child. Be concerned about inflicted trauma when the history does not account for the observed injuries (**Figure 12-3**), the caregiver's history changes over the course of the interview, or the mechanism of injury described is not plausible given the developmental level of the child. Note any unusual interactions between child and caregiver or other possible perpetrators. Although a child may appear wary or frightened of the perpetrator, at times a child may cling to or try to

Table 12-6	Distinguishing Fact from Common Fiction
History	**Fact**
"He fell off the couch, and then seized."	Fewer than 1 in 1000 falls of 4 feet (1.2 meters) or less result in serious injury.
"My one-month-old rolled off the bed."	Most infants cannot roll over until 3 to 4 months of age.
"He must have bruised himself."	Bruises are rare in infants who aren't yet pulling to a stand.
"I found him with his leg stuck in the crib slat."	Without an external force, either intentional or accidental, infants do not sustain fractures.

Table 12-7	"Red Flag" Caregiver Behaviors
Apathy	
Bizarre or strange conduct	
Little or no concern about the child	
Over-reaction to child misbehavior	
Not forthcoming with events surrounding injury	
Intoxication	
Over-reaction to child's condition	

appease an abusive caregiver to avoid further abusive behavior.

If the injury is described as an "accident," determine the mechanism. For example, if the caregiver reports that the child fell, determine the distance, the stopping surface, and the initial reactions of the child (**Table 12-6**). The information obtained at the scene may be more accurate than that obtained by the ED staff, CPS agency, and law enforcement.

Assessing the Caregiver's Behavior

Common characteristics among caregivers of maltreated children are drug use, poor self-concept, immaturity, lack of parenting knowledge, and lack of interpersonal skills. While none of these factors in and of themselves mean that an individual has abused the child, be alert for these "red flag" behaviors, as noted in **Table 12-7**. Conversely, an "appropriate" caregiver who does not show any of these characteristics may still be maltreating a child. In some cases a caregiver

may appear to be over-reacting to the child's condition, such as in cases of Munchausen Syndrome by Proxy, in which a caregiver may intentionally inflict illness or injury on a child to obtain attention for herself.

Never confront a caregiver with suspicions of maltreatment. Such an approach at the scene may delay care, endanger the child, and create a hostile and dangerous situation for the prehospital professional. Instead, note the presence of alcohol or drugs in the prehospital report and document any statements from the caregiver that reflect apparent misinformation, inconsistency, or evasiveness. Watch interactions among the caregivers and document them if they seem noteworthy. Be careful, however, to keep the tone of the report objective and neutral. Report what you see and hear, but avoid making judgments or interpreting intent in the written documentation. Particularly note any comments made by the child about how she was hurt. However, be aware that young children may attribute injury to an abstract perpetrator such as a monster or "bad man" rather than identifying the caregivers on whom they depend.

Focused Physical Exam

The prehospital professional may note suspicious findings in the focused physical exam of the child. Up to 90% of physical maltreatment victims will have some kind of skin injury. The detailed physical exam may reveal the suspicious patterns and physical findings of child abuse. In cases of suspected sexual abuse, defer a genital exam to providers with specialized training.

Bruises

Physical findings that suggest inflicted injury include the following:

- Bruises located on soft tissues, such as neck, back, thighs, genitalia, or buttocks
- Bruises on or behind ears
- Bruises in a child less than 9 months of age
- Facial bruises from slapping (**Figure 12-4**)

Differentiating bruises resulting from maltreatment versus normal wear and tear

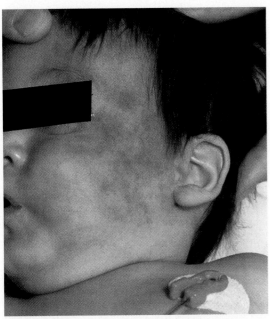

Figure 12-4 The face is a common target for physical abuse.

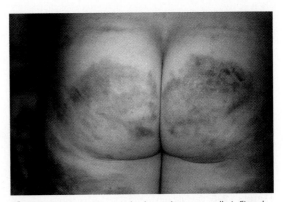

Figure 12-5 Bruises on the buttocks are usually inflicted injuries.

Tip

"Those who don't cruise rarely bruise." In a child who can't yet pull up to stand and walk while holding onto furniture (cruise), bruising or injury are rare. Most infants do not start "cruising" until they are about 9 months of age.

depends on appearance, location, and the developmental age of the child. Bruises over bony prominences such as the elbow, forehead, or below the knees are the common result of play injuries in children. However, bruises over soft tissues, such as the thighs, buttocks, cheeks, ears, or on the back are less common and should raise suspicions of inflicted injury (**Figure 12-5**).

ANY bruising in an infant who is not yet mobile may suggest inflicted injury. Most children are able to roll over by 4 months of age, and able to pull to stand and cruise by 9 months of age. A child who is not yet cruising should not have unexplained bruises or fractures. As children become older and increasingly mobile, bruises and lacerations from normal activity become more common.

Any bruise with an identifiable pattern is almost certain to have been inflicted. Common instruments are belts, cords, and hands. When an object hits the skin with high velocity, the edges leave an outline of petechiae. If a very thin object, such as a switch or a cord, hits the skin, parallel <u>petechial</u> lines form as an outline of the object.

It was previously thought that the time that a bruise was inflicted could be determined based on its appearance. This is now known to

be inaccurate. Bruises resolve at differing rates based on their location and the mechanism of injury, and bruises of different colors can result from injuries sustained in one event. Still, document the location and colors of all bruises to provide a complete description of the injuries sustained.

Burns

Inflicted burns are usually from immersion in hot water (scalds) or from forced contact between the child and a hot object. Adult skin can develop a full thickness burn from 2 seconds of exposure to 150° water—children may burn even faster. Accidental scald burns typically have varying depths and irregular borders, with a "flow" pattern evident. They are rarely symmetric (i.e., both hands or both feet), and occur infrequently in the pre-ambulatory child. In contrast, scalds from deliberately dipping a child in hot water are clearly <u>demarcated</u>, sparing <u>flexural creases</u> (such as the creases behind the knees or inside the elbows these areas are "protected" when the child reflexively tries to withdraw.) "Donut

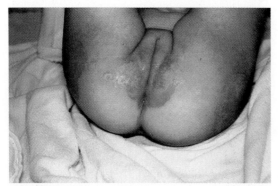

Figure 12-6 Donut burn.

burns" with sparing of the buttocks occur in children who have been dipped into hot water, but whose buttocks are pushed firmly down against the relatively cooler surface of the tub or sink (**Figure 12-6**). Children with inflicted burns may also have arm or leg bruises where they were restrained.

Pattern burns that are an even thickness throughout or are repeated are red flags for maltreatment. Remember that any <u>acute</u> burn is exquisitely painful, so consider administration of an analgesic as outlined in Chapter 6 as part of field management.

Fractures in children who are not yet ambulatory are also suspicious for maltreatment. While an infant who is being carried and is unintentionally dropped may sustain a fracture, it is not plausible that an infant who is only crawling or cruising could develop sufficient energy on their own to fracture a bone. Infant fractures of abuse have typical patterns on hospital radiographs. A history of <u>osteogenesis imperfecta</u> or problems causing decreased bone calcification may increase fracture occurrence in some children. Include these conditions in the documentation of the child's history.

Deceptive Skin Signs Masquerading as Abuse

Sometimes, normal physical findings suggest an inflicted injury. For example, "<u>Mongolian spots</u>" are birthmarks frequently seen in children of color (e.g., African American, Asian, Latino) that can be easily mistaken for

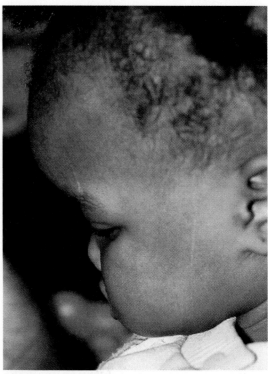

Figure 12-7 Mongolian spots are a defect in pigmentation and can be easily mistaken for bruises.

bruises (**Figure 12-7**). These birthmarks often take the form of large, flat patches of hyperpigmented skin, most commonly found on the low back or buttocks. Mongolian spots will blanch, bruises will not.

Certain disease states such as <u>leukemia</u>, <u>vasculitis</u>, <u>meningococcemia</u>, or bleeding disorders (i.e., <u>hemophilia</u>) can rarely produce skin findings that appear to be bruises. Infectious processes such as impetigo can appear to be burns, but will be much less painful. Insect bites in some children can cause redness and blistering. Distinguishing intentional injuries with certainty is sometimes impossible in the field.

Another benign skin finding that masquerades as abuse is the pattern of lesions produced by cultural rituals intended to treat illness. The most common of these patterns are associated with Asian practices called <u>cupping</u> (**Figure 12-8**) and <u>coin rubbing</u> (**Figure 12-9**). These superficial lesions have distinctive rounded edges. Caregivers of these children

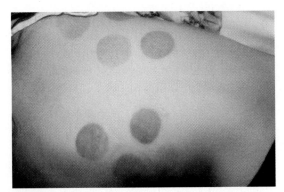

Figure 12-8 Cupping is the cultural practice of placing warm cups on the skin to pull out illness from the body. The red, flat, rounded skin lesions are often more intensely red at the borders.

can explain the purpose for such practices— information that can help distinguish inflicted injuries that are intended to help from inflicted injuries that are intended to harm.

Summary of Assessment in Suspected Maltreatment

The prehospital professional is in a unique position to recognize signs of possible child maltreatment. The initial principles of field care are the careful scene size-up, history taking, and careful physical assessment for physiologic abnormalities or anatomic patterns of inflicted injuries. Additional assessment and identification of "red flag" child

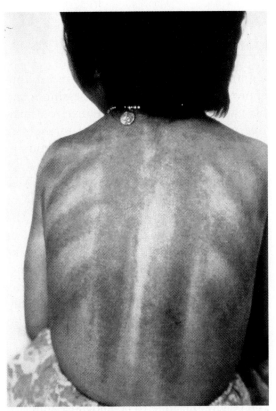

Figure 12-9 Rubbing hot coins, often on the back, produces rounded and oblong red, patchy, flat skin lesions.

and caregiver behaviors are sometimes extremely important to later maltreatment investigations. The diagnosis of child maltreatment is rarely possible in the field. All cases require a complete investigation by the community CPS agency.

Case Study 2

9-1-1 is called for a baby who "won't stop crying." You respond to a private home, where the mother of a 6-week-old infant tells you that the baby has been crying all day, and that she has no transportation to take her to the doctor. She explains that the baby seemed fine until this morning, and has not had a fever or other symptoms of illness. She makes no move to comfort the howling infant who is propped in an infant seat. You note that the baby is not moving her right leg, and that her crying increases when you manipulate it. During the physical exam, the mother says the child is acting more normally and declines transport.

1. What are the red flags for maltreatment?
2. What are your medical and legal responsibilities?

Communication with the Child and Caregivers

Communicate with the child in an age-appropriate manner. When assessing a stable child for whom there is concern of maltreatment, transport the child to the safe environment of the ED for full evaluation as soon as possible.

Communication with the caregiver in suspected maltreatment is a challenging task for the prehospital professional. Resist the impulse to "find out what really happened" or express anger at the caregiver. Do not make accusations or assume a judgmental tone. When confronted with suspicions of abuse, caregivers often respond defensively or angrily, whether or not they were the ones who inflicted the injuries.

Sometimes a caregiver may refuse to cooperate in further assessment, decline transport, or attempt to leave the scene with the child. If you believe the child to be in danger, immediately contact law enforcement for assistance. Never attempt to physically restrain a caregiver or to forcibly take possession of a child,

as this may put everyone in danger. If the scene is chaotic but not dangerous, consider contacting the medical oversight physician, who may be able to convince the caregiver to permit treatment and transport.

Medicolegal Duties

Documentation

When documenting the history and physical assessment on the ambulance record be thorough, but objective. Interjecting feelings or interpreting the facts may make the documentation inadmissible in court. For example, write, "palms show a 1-centimeter circular burn" instead of "cigarette burn to hand." Use objective, clear, specific terminology. Place in quotation marks and note in the records any statements from caregivers (e.g., father states that "child climbed into hot bathtub").

Duty to Report

In some states, prehospital professionals have a __legal mandate__ to report their suspicion of child maltreatment. In other states, the duty of the prehospital professional is to ensure that a report is filed. An agreement from the ED staff to report will usually suffice. States with mal-

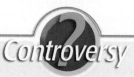

The on scene role of law enforcement in suspected child maltreatment is controversial. In most cases, it is prudent to transport a child to the ED for physician and CPS evaluation. If the scene is not safe or caretakers are refusing transport, the prehospital professional must call law enforcement for protection and assistance.

Never attempt to physically restrain a caregiver or to forcibly take possession of a child. Call law enforcement if the scene is unsafe.

Even in the face of probable maltreatment, remain nonjudgmental with the caregiver and maintain control of the scene and transport.

Document physical findings objectively. The facts will speak for themselves in court.

treatment laws may require health care providers to independently report suspected maltreatment to either law enforcement or CPS.

Although no law can forbid the filing of civil or criminal charges, most state laws protect the reporter of suspected child maltreatment from any decision or award in a lawsuit, if the report was made in good faith. *On the other hand, failure to report suspicion of child maltreatment may result in legal action against the mandated reporter.*

In small communities, especially when the prehospital professional knows the individuals involved, reporting suspected child maltreatment may have significant social implications. In many states, anonymous reports can be filed, and the identity of the person who reports maltreatment is protected. Remember that a report of suspected child maltreatment is not an attempt to harm or punish a family, but an attempt to help the child.

Summary of Communication and Medicolegal Duties

When child maltreatment is suspected, the prehospital professional faces a challenging and potentially explosive situation. Communication with the child may be difficult or limited, and interactions with the caregiver may be frustrating and sometimes hostile. A professional, nonjudgmental approach is necessary. Document conditions in the environment, the child's and caregiver's behaviors, the history, and relevant physical findings that may suggest maltreatment. The prehospital professional has a moral and legal duty to report suspected cases of maltreatment to the proper authorities.

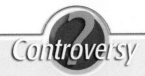

Controversy

It is the duty of the prehospital professional to ensure that someone submits a CPS report when abuse is suspected. Depending on state law, this duty may be legal or it may be ethical. In some jurisdictions, a single report from hospital personnel is sufficient, while in others the prehospital professionals must file their own report.

Case Study 3

9-1-1 is called by a babysitter because a child has been burned. On arrival at the scene, the EMS crew finds a teenage girl holding a sobbing 2-year-old boy. The teenager states that the child has been fussy and crying for the two hours in her care. On changing the child's diaper, the sitter noted what looked like burns on the buttocks, and on her mother's advice called 9-1-1.

The child is alert but upset and is not easily consolable by the babysitter. There are areas of denuded skin on the buttocks covered with diaper rash cream, with one unpopped blister near the sacrum. The centers of both buttocks, as well as the gluteal cleft, do not appear to be injured. Extremity exam shows no bruises or other abnormalities.

1. Is this injury caused from abuse?
2. What interventions are indicated?

Chapter Review

Case Study Answers

Case Study **1** page 243

The sudden onset of a decreased level of consciousness and bulging fontanelle after a report of a short fall are all hallmarks of traumatic inflicted brain injury (shaken baby syndrome). This child is too young to roll spontaneously, and a short fall onto a carpeted surface should not cause significant injury.

Carefully document the scene, the comments of the caregiver, and the reported events leading to the injury.

Immediate transportation is critical. One common complication of inflicted head injury is respiratory failure or apnea as a result of elevated intracranial pressure and compression of the medulla (respiratory center in the brain stem). Be prepared to provide respiratory support. Ensure that the ED staff will make a report to the CPS agency, or file a report yourself.

Case Study **2** page 253

While caregiver behavior cannot definitively indicate child maltreatment, it is concerning that the mother does not attempt to comfort her child. Her lack of resources and a lack of explanation for the apparent injury raises concerns about maltreatment.

Lower extremity fractures can be very difficult to assess in a newly born or young infant without radiographs, and are common inflicted injuries. A child of this age could not sustain such an injury without a significant observed mechanism (for example, a fall from arms or involvement in a motor vehicle crash). If the prehospital provider has reason to suspect maltreatment, and the caregiver refuses transport, law enforcement involvement may be necessary.

The child is physiologically stable, but transport her to the ED as soon as possible. Do not confront the mother with your suspicions.

Case Study **3** page 255

This child has stigmata of an inflicted scald injury. The sparing of creases and the central buttocks may indicate the child was forcibly held in hot water. There is no way for the prehospital professional to know who inflicted the injury, nor is establishing responsibility part of their role.

Provide analgesia if possible. Large burns can lead to significant fluid losses, so evaluate carefully for dehydration. Document the scene size-up, the child's and caregiver's behaviors, and the history. Transport this child to an ED for burn care as well as an evaluation for inflicted injury. Treatment at a burn center may ultimately be necessary.

Suggested Readings

Textbooks

American Academy of Pediatrics and the American College of Emergency Physicians: *APLS: The Pediatric Emergency Medicine Resource,* 4th Edition. Sudbury, MA, Jones and Bartlett Publishers, 2004.

Hazinski M, Zaritsky A, Nadkarni V, et al: *PALS Provider Manual.* American Heart Association, 2002.

Reece R, Ludwig S: *Child Abuse: Medical Diagnosis and Management,* 2nd Edition. Lippincott, Williams & Wilkins.

Articles

Johnson CF. Child maltreatment 2002: Recognition, reporting and risk. *Pediatr Int.* 2002; 44:554–60.

Kairys S. Distinguishing sudden infant death syndrome from child abuse fatalities. American Academy of Pediatrics. Committee on Child Abuse and Neglect. *Pediatrics.* Feb 2001; 107(2):437–41.

Kempe CH. The battered child syndrome. *JAMA.* 1962; 181:17–24.

Krug EG, Dahlberg LL, Mercy JA, Zwi AB, Lozano RE. World report on violence and health. Geneva, World Health Organization, 2002.

Website

Krug EG, Dahlberg LL, Mercy JA, Zwi AB, Lozano RE. World report on violence and health. Geneva, World Health Organization, 2002. Available in pdf format at: *http://www.who.int/ violence_injury_prevention/violence/world_report/en/FullWRVH.pdf.* Last accessed: February 13, 2004.

CD-ROM

American Academy of Pediatrics: Visual Diagnosis of Child Abuse. American Academy of Pediatrics, Elk Grove Village, IL, 2001.

Lauridson J, Levin A, Parrish R, Wicks A. Shaken Baby Syndrome: A visual overview. Version 2.0 National Center on Shaken Baby Syndrome, 2003.

13

Medicolegal and Ethical Considerations

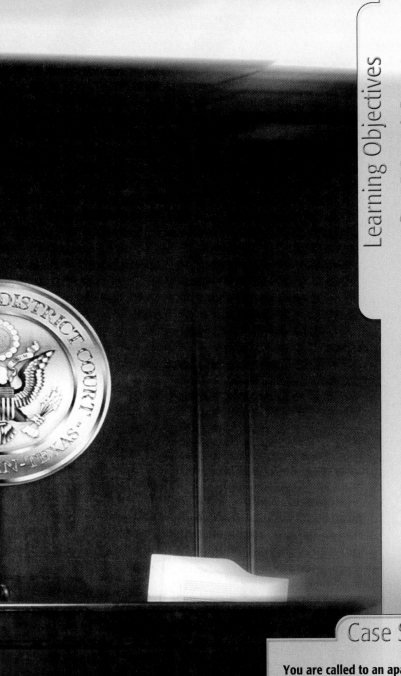

Case Study 1

You are called to an apartment where you find a 3-year-old girl in mild respiratory distress. She is interactive and consolable, but has bilateral wheezes and a pulse oximeter reading of 94%. She is home alone with a 16-year-old babysitter who tells you that the child's parents will not return for several hours and did not leave information about their destination or contact information.

1. Can the babysitter give you legally valid consent to treat the child?
2. Can you legally provide care and transport this child?

Introduction

THE PREHOSPITAL PROFESSIONAL will frequently encounter ethical and legal issues while caring for children. These may include the inability to obtain the legal guardian's permission to treat a child, refusal of consent by parents or older children, challenges to confidentiality, issues related to truth telling, and the identification of possible child maltreatment. This chapter discusses these issues and emphasizes the importance of protocols and policies for prehospital professionals to address common pediatric ethical and legal concerns.

Consent

The requirement to obtain <u>informed consent</u> from a patient or legal guardian before delivering medical care is a central feature of American health care law and ethics. A legally mature individual may not be touched, treated, or transported without her consent. <u>Minors</u> (children under 18 years of age), however, present a special problem because they do not have the legal authority to give or refuse consent. Therefore, in most states, a parent or legal guardian must give permission before a minor can be medically treated or transported (**Figure 13-1**). In situations where a minor has a medical condition that represents a threat to life or health and a legal guardian is not readily available to provide consent, prehospital professionals can assess the child, provide necessary medical treatment, and transport the child. The legal basis for taking action in an emergency when consent is not available is known as the <u>emergency exception rule</u>.

The emergency exception rule is also known as the doctrine of <u>implied consent</u>.

When a legal guardian is not readily available to provide consent for a minor, the prehospital professional must provide medically necessary treatment and transport.

For minors, this doctrine means that the prehospital professional can presume consent and proceed with appropriate treatment and transport if all of the following four conditions are met:

1. The child is suffering from an emergent condition that places her life or health in danger.
2. The child's legal guardian is unavailable or unable to provide consent for treatment or transport.
3. Treatment or transport cannot be safely delayed until consent can be obtained.
4. The prehospital professional administers only treatment for emergency conditions that pose an immediate threat to the child.

This emergency exception rule is based on the principle that if the legal guardian knew the severity of the emergency, she would consent to medical treatment of the child. Any time a minor is treated without consent, the burden of proof falls on the prehospital professional to justify that the emergency actions were necessary. The prehospital professional must fully and clearly document on the prehospital record the nature of the medical emergency, attempts to contact the legal guardian, and the reasons the minor required immediate treatment and/or transport.

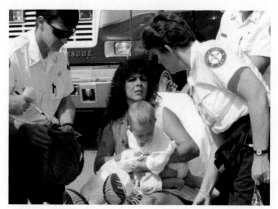

Figure 13-1 In most states, a parent or legal guardian must give permission before a minor can be transported.

If possible, contact on-line medical control for assistance when consent is unclear or unavailable. If the guardian is unavailable and/or cannot be notified, provide information about the destination ED to the most responsible person on scene (in writing whenever possible), with instructions to pass the information on to the minor's legal guardian. *As a general rule, when the prehospital professional's authority to act is in doubt, always do what is in the best interest of the minor.*

When the prehospital professional's authority to act is in doubt, always do what is in the best interest of the minor.

Refusal of Care or Transport

Guardian Refusal

A special situation occurs when the prehospital professional is faced with a legal guardian who refuses to give permission for medical treatment or transport of a child with an acute illness or injury. As long as a child's legal guardian is alert, oriented, and mentally competent, she has the right to refuse medical care for the child. However, the guardian must act in the best interest of the child.

When a guardian refuses to allow provision of care or transport to a child whose life or health might be threatened, an important legal and ethical issue arises. In such circumstances, first notify medical control for guidance. The medical control physician may speak directly to the legal guardian in attempt to convince the guardian to allow treatment and transport. If medical control agrees that the child's condition requires immediate treatment in order to prevent serious harm, yet the legal guardian continues to refuse consent for care, it may be necessary to notify law enforcement and enlist their assistance in placing the child in <u>temporary protective custody</u>. Likewise, when a legal guardian appears to be intoxicated or otherwise impaired, involvement of law enforcement officers may be necessary to place a minor in temporary protective custody. If necessary, have medical control speak to law enforcement officers to explain the need for treatment and transport. Local EMS pediatric policies should guide the prehospital professional's procedure in such situations.

While temporary protective custody may allow the prehospital professional to transport a minor to a medical facility for purposes of medical evaluation, it does not give the prehospital professional the right to treat a minor for medical conditions that are not serious or life-threatening. *A prehospital professional can provide medical treatment without consent only when the child has a medical condition that poses a risk of death or serious harm, when immediate specific treatment is necessary to prevent that harm, and when only those specific treatments are provided.* Discuss these situations with medical control before initiating treatment, whenever possible. Sometimes an intermediate solution is possible. Document everything fully and clearly about the medical condition of the child, the need for emergency care, and the basis for overriding the wishes of the legal guardian.

Every case of unclear consent or refusal needs careful scene management, notification of medical control if available, and full and accurate documentation in the prehospital record.

Never confront the caregiver with accusations, moral judgments, or threats when difficult circumstances develop at the scene. This approach will only aggravate the situation and will not help the child. Try to establish whether the caregiver refuses all care and transport, or only certain aspects of care. For example, some caregivers may prefer that prehospital professionals not initiate therapy, but will permit the child to be transported to the hospital. If the child can be safely transported

Tip

Get police assistance when an impaired or intoxicated guardian refuses care or transport of an ill or injured child.

Blip

Never confront the caregiver with accusations, moral judgments, or threats.

Table 13-1	Characteristics of Emancipated or Mature Minors
Emancipated Minor	
Married	
Pregnant	
Has a child	
Active-duty status in the armed service	
15 years or older, economically self-supporting, and living apart from parents	
Mature Minor	
14 years or older and declared a mature minor by state Superior Court	
AND patient is not on a psychiatric hold	
AND patient demonstrates competency to refuse	

without initiating care, respect the caregiver's wishes concerning care. It may be appropriate for the caregiver of a child with terminal illness or significant disabilities to restrict certain kinds of care for their child. Discuss these difficult situations with medical control.

Child Refusal

There are two situations in which a minor has the legal authority to refuse care and make decisions regarding her health care. First, state law designates certain minors as "emancipated" and grants these <u>emancipated minors</u> the right to make decisions, including health care decisions. Children who are legally emancipated may give consent for medical treatment and transport. They may also refuse medical care and/or transport. While emancipated minor laws vary from state to state, most states recognize minors to be emancipated if they are married, pregnant, have a child, are economically self-supporting and not living at home, or are on active-duty status in the armed services.

A second situation in which a minor might have legal status to make decisions arises when a court has declared an individual a <u>mature minor</u>. This is different than an emancipated minor. In most states, mature minors are over 14 years of age and have been formally declared adults by the court. **Table 13-1** lists the legal circumstances in which pediatric patients can provide or refuse consent for medical care and transport in most states. *Since*

these laws vary, the prehospital professional should be familiar with the specifics of emancipated and mature minor laws in the state in which care is being provided.

If a child is not an emancipated or a mature minor, then she has no legal capacity either to give consent or to refuse medical care. Regardless of whether a child has the legal authority to provide or withhold consent, it is always prudent to try to get the child's agreement or "assent" to treat and transport. This approach respects the personal dignity and self-determination of the child/patient and minimizes confrontation. A willingness to provide the child with some control and some choices may allow for a compromise that will help prehospital professionals to achieve a safe transfer. Reserve force or restraint to transport a child only for those situations in which all efforts to negotiate respectfully with the child have failed and the child is at risk of serious harm if she is not transported.

Caregivers Who Disagree

One rare, but confusing situation, arises when the prehospital professional is confronted by caregivers who disagree about whether to consent to treatment and transport of a sick or injured child. In these cases, establish whether one or both caregivers are legal decision-makers for the child. If both caregivers have legal authority, the prehospital professional may need to negotiate a plan that is acceptable to both. Focus on the child's needs and the common

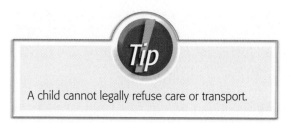

A child cannot legally refuse care or transport.

desire to assist the child, while deflecting attention from the disagreement. Medical control may need to be involved to assist the prehospital professional in determining the proper course of action and to determine the need for law enforcement.

Summary of Consent

Laws strictly protect the right of adult patients to accept or reject medical care. Interpreting these consent laws for children in a prehospital setting, however, can pose special problems. The prehospital professional faces a difficult situation in cases where the caregiver refuses to consent or where consent to provide care and transport for a child cannot be readily obtained. Every case requires careful scene management, notification of medical control if available, and accurate documentation in the prehospital record. EMS systems should provide clear policies, procedures, and protocols based on state law to guide the prehospital professional and/or medical control. Local EMS policy on consent should clearly define the following:

- Who can refuse ambulance transport according to state law
- The process for field evaluation, consultation, and documentation

- The method for enlisting police and medical control when the patient or guardian is dangerous and refuses transport, or when a child has a life-threatening problem and the guardian is refusing transport

Respect for Cultural or Religious Differences

Cultural differences and religious beliefs may present exceptionally difficult situations. While the care of the patient is always of primary concern, the prehospital professional must attempt to respect requests from the family or patient regarding preferences that may originate from their religious or cultural beliefs, especially when these do not interfere significantly with the provision of treatment to the child. The prehospital professional must always remain nonjudgmental about requests that stem from cultural or religious beliefs, acknowledge the importance of these requests to the family, and attempt to accommodate them when possible. When the prehospital professional cannot accommodate requests that are based on cultural or religious beliefs because they would put a child at risk of serious harm, the reasons the requests cannot be accommodated must be respectfully explained. Medical control and police may need to be involved if parents refuse to consent to necessary care and the child is at risk of harm.

Language barriers may also present a challenge as the prehospital professional attempts to communicate with a child's caregiver. The prehospital professional should be familiar with what resources are available

Case Study 2

You are called to attend to a homeless 15-year-old whose friends called because he wasn't feeling well and wasn't acting normally. You find the young man lying on the sidewalk, complaining of a headache. When you attempt to assess him, he starts cussing, pushes you away aggressively, and demands to be left alone.

1. What rights does the teenager have to refuse care and transport?
2. What methods of persuasion can you use?

> The prehospital professional must always remain nonjudgmental about cultural or religious beliefs, acknowledge their importance to the family, and attempt to accommodate them when possible.

locally to provide translation in a timely manner. Miscommunications can have a significant impact on a child's care, especially if the prehospital professional is unable to obtain information about a child's underlying medical conditions, allergies, current medications, or other factors relevant to field care. If professional translation services are available, use these rather than family members or bystanders. If translation services are not available, a family member or neighbor may be asked to assist with translation, with the understanding that the information transferred may be inaccurate or incomplete, especially with regard to medical terminology.

Prehospital DNR Orders

The caregivers of some terminally ill children, usually in consultation with their primary physician, may decide on limitations to treatments and interventions. These decisions usually arise from the child's underlying condition and the desire to avoid futile or burdensome interventions if the child develops a life-threatening condition. Prehospital professionals, in responding to a call about a sick child, may be confronted with a <u>Do Not Resuscitate</u>, or DNR, order. A DNR order must be signed by a physician to be valid (**Figure 13-2**). These orders inform health care providers that CPR or resuscitation should not be initiated in the event of a cardiopulmonary arrest. Some local EMS regions do not recognize DNR orders for children. *Prehospital professionals must know the limits of the DNR law governing their area of coverage and develop protocols for dealing with them.*

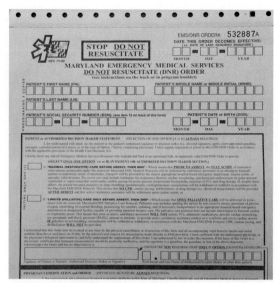

Figure 13-2 DNR order.

Regardless of the nature of the local DNR law or prehospital policy, a legal guardian may always revoke a DNR order written on behalf of a child. When faced with a valid DNR order written for a child and a legal guardian requesting that the child be resuscitated, always follow the legal guardian's wishes. Even in the face of a valid DNR order, clarify with the legal guardian what kinds of interventions she considers to be acceptable and which she does not. For example, oxygen delivery and transport may be acceptable and expected for some children with DNR orders.

Resuscitation

Sometimes resuscitation attempts are ineffective for children in cardiopulmonary arrest, and occasionally such attempts are unnecessary, as discussed in Chapter 11. Resuscitation policy should define circumstances when cardiopulmonary resuscitation must be initiated, when it may be withheld, and when it may be stopped. For pediatric cases, the policy must take a medically conservative approach, but allow appropriate withholding of resuscitation to focus on grief management and family interactions.

Local resuscitation policy may allow prehospital professionals to withhold or stop resuscitation when a child is clearly dead, as defined by specific criteria. This may be emotionally difficult for the prehospital provider, and all crew members must be in agreement with the decision to stop or to forego a resuscitation attempt. Likewise, it may be difficult emotionally for family members if prehospital professionals do not attempt resuscitation. *In cases where family members of the child are clearly distressed by the decision to forego resuscitation, consider providing resuscitative efforts as a gesture to the family that every effort has been made to save their child.* In such cases, the child can be treated with BLS measures only and transported to the emergency department, where physicians can formally pronounce the child dead and terminate resuscitation.

Suspected Sudden Infant Death Syndrome (SIDS)

The actions of the prehospital professional are especially important to caregivers of SIDS victims and may have a big influence on grief responses and psychological and social adjustments (see Chapter 11). EMS systems should have, as part of educational and training requirements for field personnel, a formal training program for SIDS. Local EMS policies should clearly establish the responsibility of the prehospital professional at death scenes regarding care of the body, notification of the coroner or medical examiner, and interaction with caregivers.

Confidentiality

Medical information is private. Carelessly or inadvertently revealing identifiable information is an ethical and legal risk that prehospital professionals face, because they frequently care for individuals in a public environment. *It is essential to remain aware of the potentially*

Tip

Prehospital professionals must be aware of the potentially sensitive nature of identifiable information and take every possible precaution to protect confidentiality.

sensitive nature of identifiable information and to take every possible precaution to protect confidentiality. Conduct all sensitive discussions, when possible, in a setting where bystanders cannot overhear. Avoid using last names, if at all possible, at the scene. Do not share private information with concerned bystanders (other than those legally responsible for the patient). Finally, since EMS radio communication systems may be monitored by other individuals in the community, avoid names unless absolutely essential to the receiving hospital. If a name is important, use a telephone at the scene rather than the radio.

Telling the Truth in Difficult Situations

Prehospital professionals should deal as honestly as possible with children and their caregivers. It is not unusual for caregivers to ask about the condition of a child or request information about a child's "chances of survival." In such situations, refrain from speculating, but respond instead with honest reassurance. For example, the statement "We'll take the best possible care of your child," provides an honest and reassuring response without speculating about uncertain outcomes.

Case Study 3

You respond to the scene of a motor vehicle crash where you find a 10-year-old child with facial bruising, a tense, tender abdomen, and an obviously deformed left thigh. The child appears scared and begins to cry. The adult woman who had been driving the car has obvious head injuries and lacks a pulse. Another team begins work on the adult while you tend to the child. As you stabilize the child for transport, she asks you if her mother is okay.

1. Would it be appropriate to tell the child her mother is okay in order to enable a safe and efficient transport?
2. How should you respond to this child's question?

The prehospital professional may also face situations in which multiple patients have sustained injuries, and the parent or child requests information about others involved in the incident. It may be appropriate to deflect such questions, especially when the other party has suffered severe injuries or has died. The best tact may be to offer an honest statement of reassurance such as, "I need to focus on taking the best care of you right now. My partners are doing their best to take care of the others." While there is an ethical obligation to be honest, it may be appropriate to delay sharing particularly distressing information until a patient has been transported safely, and other sources of emotional support are available.

Physician On Scene

Out-of-hospital care is under the authority of EMS medical control. Unless specifically authorized by medical control or the medical director of the EMS agency, prehospital professionals cannot carry out orders from other physicians, even the patient's private physician. This policy is sometimes controversial. *Medical control may either allow the*

on-scene physician to assist prehospital professionals or transfer total authority to the on-scene physician. If the on-scene physician takes responsibility for treatment, she must be available to accompany the child to the ED.

Hospital Destination

The hospital destination policy for children must define the following components:

1. Field triage criteria (which patients with what conditions go where)
2. Designated receiving hospitals
3. Specialized pediatric centers

The appropriate ED for a sick or injured child may differ from the ED appropriate for an adult with a similar condition. Some EMS systems may identify specialized pediatric centers (e.g., general trauma centers with pediatric capability, pediatric critical care centers, or pediatric trauma centers) as primary receiving facilities for certain pediatric patients. In some cases, a child may meet multiple conflicting triage criteria (e.g., should a severely burned child be transported to a regional children's hospital or a non-pediatric hospital with a regional burn center?). The destination policy must either provide guidance on where such patients should be transported or specify that medical control will make all complex triage decisions. The prehospital professional must transport the child to the ED preferred by the legal guardian unless hospital destination policy requires an alternative facility.

Child Maltreatment and Sexual Assault

Education of prehospital professionals in identifying possible maltreatment is an essential component of initial education and continuing medical education in pediatrics (see Chapter 12). A policy and procedure for reporting suspected cases of maltreatment and for appropriate patient transport to an ED are important components of every EMS system. The prehospital professional must ensure that victims of

If the on-scene physician takes authority for care, she must usually go along with the child to the ED.

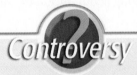

The role of the child's private physician in on-scene care is controversial. The prehospital professional must abide by local EMS system policy, but the precise limitations in providing assistance to an on-scene physician are sometimes unclear. Always act in the best interests of the child when the policy is confusing.

Never confront the caregiver or others with accusations, moral judgments, threats, or suspicions.

maltreatment and sexual assault victims are initially evaluated in a careful, compassionate, and respectful way. Transport these patients to an ED staffed by clinicians experienced in working with child victims of maltreatment and sexual assault and equipped with the appropriate <u>ancillary</u> and follow-up services. Never confront the caregiver or others with accusations, moral judgments, threats, or suspicions. Although these situations are emotionally difficult, the immediate goal must always be to provide necessary treatment and ensure the safe transport of the child.

Pediatric Policies and Procedures

EMS systems should provide clear guidelines for common problems related to ethical and legal issues involving children. In addition, on-line medical control provides the prehospital professional with the ability to obtain real time consultation regarding particularly difficult situations, such as: the inability to obtain consent, refusal of consent by a child or guardian, presence of a physician on scene, resuscitation decisions, and suspected child maltreatment or sexual assault.

EMS Operational Systems

Operations are the administrative backbone of the EMS system. They include the <u>policies</u>, <u>procedures</u>, and <u>protocols</u> that define the <u>medical responsibility</u> and <u>legal authority</u> of the prehospital professionals and medical director within the EMS system. These written directives assist the prehospital professional in knowing what to do in complicated out-of-hospital situations.

Protocols outline specific clinical treatment guidelines for common illness and injury conditions.

Protocols, Policies, and Procedures

The goal of <u>operations</u> is to manage day-to-day field care with standards established by the EMS system. Performance standards are promulgated in education and training, as well as in the protocols, policies, and procedures that guide practice in the EMS system. Since the needs of children differ from those of adults, pediatric-specific protocols, policies, and procedures are necessary tools for a comprehensive EMS system.

Protocols define explicit field treatments or the order and type of medical interventions for specific illness and injury conditions. They give the appropriate pharmacologic options, including drug doses, routes of delivery, and methods of administration. Most EMS systems have out-of-hospital pediatric advanced life support (ALS), illness, and trauma treatment protocols (**Figure 13-3**).

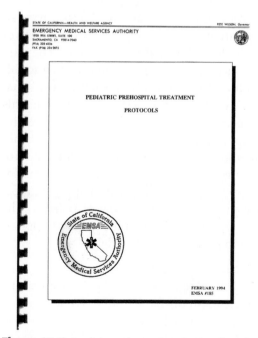

Figure 13-3 A policies and procedures book outlines EMS field treatments for children.

Table 13-2	Examples of Pediatric Treatment Protocols
Airway obstruction	
Allergic reaction/anaphylaxis	
Altered level of consciousness	
Bradycardia	
Burns	
Cardiopulmonary arrest	
Hypoperfusion or shock	
Neonatal resuscitation	
Seizures	
Respiratory distress	
Tachycardia	
Toxic exposures	
Trauma	

Appropriate treatment protocols for out-of-hospital basic life support (BLS) personnel, as well as for first responders, are also important, but are not yet widely available. **Table 13-2** lists some common EMS pediatric treatment protocols.

Policies and procedures reflect the <u>medicolegal</u> expectations of the community for out-of-hospital care, quality management, and system accountability. These forms of regulation consist of clear, written directives to guide prehospital professionals. They are intended to help with decision-making in difficult or legally-sensitive pediatric field situations such as those discussed earlier in this chapter. Policies usually explain how the prehospital professional should handle certain situations, rather than medical treatment. Procedures describe the sequence of actions for the prehospital professional in applying medical protocols or medicological policies. The field policies with the most frequent application to pediatric care include:

- Consent for care or transport
- Refusal to consent for care or transport
- Death in the field
- Triage guidelines
- Hospital destination
- Child maltreatment

Tip

Policies and procedures reflect the medicolegal expectations of the community for out-of-hospital care, quality management, and system accountability.

State statutes and the state EMS authority usually set basic requirements for local EMS systems, provide guidelines for quality management, accountability and enforcement, and establish EMT scope of practice. Local policies, procedures, and protocols may be very different from one EMS system to the next. Mutual aid agreements between bordering geographic areas are especially useful because resources, equipment, and personnel for specialized care of children are not distributed evenly. Indeed, specialized trauma care and critical care centers for children are usually only available at major hospitals in large urban areas. In some states, no specialized centers exist for children at all.

Medical Control for Pediatrics

<u>Medical control</u>, medical direction, or medical oversight, is the mechanism by which physicians, mobile intensive care nurses, and EMS officials supervise field practice. Medical control includes direct and indirect methods.

On-line (Direct) Medical Control

On-line or <u>direct medical control</u> refers to any communication between the prehospital professional and medical control by telephone or radio. This form of control is required by some local EMS systems for many or all cases involving children under 18 years of age (**Figure 13-4**) because decisions about pediatric ALS treatment (e.g., IVs, drug routes, and doses), triage, scene control, and transport are often difficult. **Table 13-3** lists some examples of problems in pediatric field practice that often require on-line physician input or direct medical control.

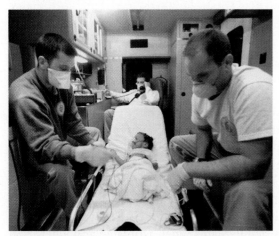

Figure 13-4 Direct medical control can be extremely helpful when the prehospital professional confronts medical and legal problems with children.

Table 13-3	Possible Pediatric Issues Needing Direct Medical Control
Pediatric Issue	**Possible Scenario**
Type of field treatment	IV or rectal diazepam for status epilepticus
Hospital destination	Appropriate ED for infant trauma patient
Specialized scene control	Hazardous materials exposure in school
Transport	Requirement for ED care after minor poisoning

Table 13-4	Indirect Medical Control

Examples of Prospective Control

Pediatric BLS and ALS ambulance equipment/drugs

Pediatric out-of-hospital treatment protocols

Skills training
   Airway foreign body removal
   Endotracheal intubation
   IO needle insertion
   Rectal diazepam

Pediatric-specific policies
   Hospital destination
   Triage
   Transport
   Refusal of care
   Suspected SIDS
   Maltreatment

Examples of Retrospective Control

Review of compliance with treatment, triage, and transport policies

Review of success, failure, and complications of pediatric procedures and patient outcomes

Epidemiologic data on types of pediatric illness and injury

Review of ED or hospital capabilities for the care of children

Off-line (Indirect) Medical Control

Off-line or <u>indirect medical control</u> involves both prospective and retrospective guidance. Prospective indirect control consists of planning for expected educational and operational requirements within the prehospital professional's scope of practice. Retrospective indirect control involves review of individual and overall system performance against expectations or standards of care to provide accountability. **Table 13-4** lists common examples of how indirect control creates and monitors different types of policies, procedures, and protocols for children.

Summary of Rationale for Protocols, Policies, and Procedures

Pediatric-specific guidelines—as defined in protocols, policies, and procedures—help set standards for care of children. Medical control is especially important in the delivery of out-of-hospital services to families and children because of the unusual circumstances that often arise medically and legally.

Chapter Review

Case Study Answers

Case Study **1** page 259

Although a babysitter (even an adult babysitter) cannot provide valid consent to treat, the emergency exception rule allows you to treat and transport this child who is in respiratory distress. She suffers from an emergent condition that places her at risk, her legal guardian is unavailable, and it would be unsafe to delay treatment. If the babysitter has a phone number for the parents, call them, apprise them of the situation, and ask permission to provide necessary treatment and transport. If there is no way to reach the parents, you should provide treatment for the child's wheezing and respiratory distress with oxygen and a bronchodilator and transport her to an appropriate facility. Finally, make sure this 16-year-old babysitter is safe, and leave a note with her to give to the child's caregivers that explains what happened and where you have transported the child.

Case Study **2** page 263

Unless you can persuade the child to allow you to deliver care, this will be a difficult situation. As a homeless adolescent, most states would consider this child to be a ward of the state, not an emancipated minor. However, despite the fact that he cannot legally refuse treatment and transport, every effort must be made to show respect, involve him in decisions, and avoid the use of force. If he persists in his refusal to be evaluated, contact medical control. If his "combativeness" appears to be the result of a medical condition that impairs judgment (i.e., meningitis, a head injury, intoxication), call law enforcement to provide assistance in restraining the adolescent sufficiently to allow a safe assessment and transport.

As a practical matter, respect the boy's dignity but be firm that transport to an ED is necessary. Try to establish rapport and do not be judgmental. If a friend or counselor is available, try to get assistance in persuading the teenager to agree to care and transport.

Case Study **3** page 265

Carefully consider your answer to this child's concerned question. On the one hand, avoid being dishonest. Since you do not know whether her mother will survive, you should not assure the child that her mother will be okay. On the other hand, it would be appropriate to withhold your concerns and suspicions about the mother's condition until the child has been transported safely, more is known about the mother's condition, and there are resources (like a social worker) available to assist the child in receiving what may be terrible news. One honest answer might be, "I know you are worried about your mother. My partners are taking good care of her. I need to take good care of you, and I'm going to take you to the hospital. Once we get there, we'll try to find out more about your mother."

Suggested Readings

Textbooks

Bledsoe B, Porter R, Cherry R: *Essentials of Paramedic Care.* New Jersey, Prentice Hall, 2003.

Dieckmann RA: *Pediatric Emergency Care Systems: Planning and Management.* Baltimore, MD, Williams and Wilkins, 1992.

Hazinski M, Zaritsky A, Nadkarni V, et al: *PALS Provider Manual.* American Heart Association, 2002.

Schneid T: *Legal Liabilities in Emergency Medical Service,* 1st Edition. Taylor & Francis Group, 2001.

Selbst S, Korin J. The medical record. In: *Preventing Malpractice Lawsuits in Pediatric Emergency Medicine.* Dallas, TX, American College of Emergency Physicians, 1999; 46–53.

Articles

Larkin G. Essential ethics for EMS: Cardinal virtues and core principles. *Emerg Med Clin North Am.* Nov 2002; 20(4):887–911.

Schears R, Marco C, Iserson K. "Do not attempt resuscitation" in the out-of-hospital setting. *Ann Emerg Med.* July 2004; 44(1):68–69.

Selbst S. Medical legal issues in prehospital pediatric emergency care. *Pediatr Emerg Care.* 1998; 4(4):276–78.

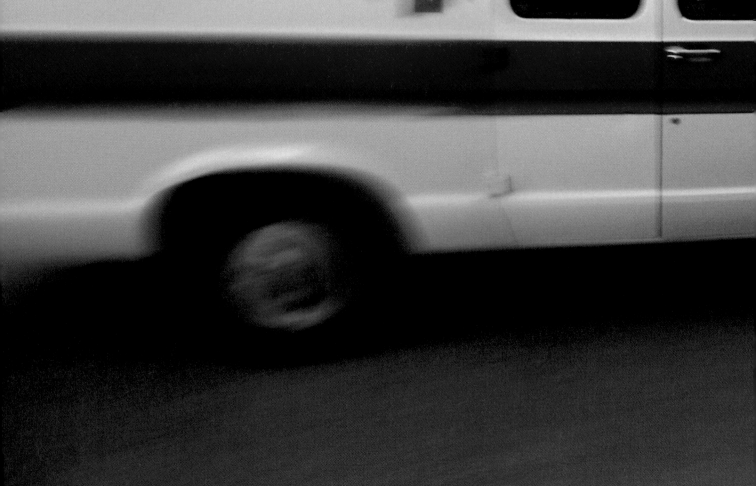

Transportation Considerations

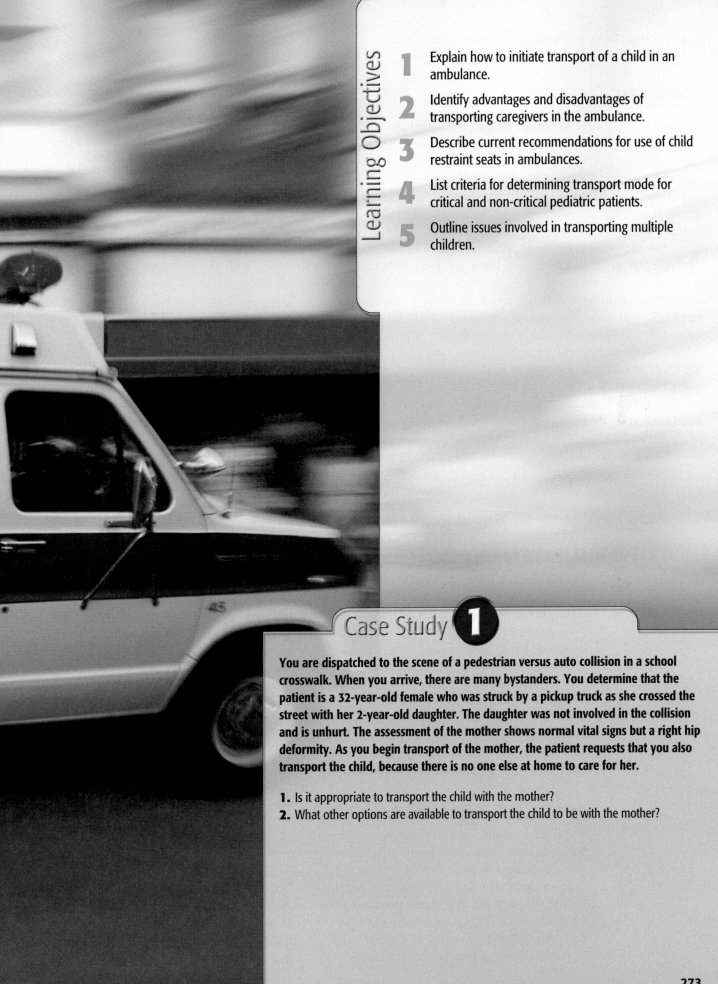

Case Study **1**

You are dispatched to the scene of a pedestrian versus auto collision in a school crosswalk. When you arrive, there are many bystanders. You determine that the patient is a 32-year-old female who was struck by a pickup truck as she crossed the street with her 2-year-old daughter. The daughter was not involved in the collision and is unhurt. The assessment of the mother shows normal vital signs but a right hip deformity. As you begin transport of the mother, the patient requests that you also transport the child, because there is no one else at home to care for her.

1. Is it appropriate to transport the child with the mother?
2. What other options are available to transport the child to be with the mother?

Pediatric Transport

AT SOME POINT on every pediatric run the prehospital professional must decide when and how to transport the child. Whether to stay or go requires an immediate decision after the initial assessment and initial resuscitation, as outlined in Chapter 1. *How* to transport is the next question, at the point when the prehospital professional is ready to go. There are many predictable considerations, but each case presents an individual set of issues. The prehospital professional must know the local EMS protocols for safe transport of children, the local motor vehicle laws addressing child occupants in vehicles, and the EMS regulations that govern the treatment of children en route. Most importantly, the prehospital professional must also meet the sometimes urgent and changing medical needs of the patient while considering the operational issues around transport.

The decision process about whether to stay or go is addressed in detail in Chapter 1, and depends on multiple factors. In a BLS system, early transport is appropriate if the scene is unsafe for the child, caregiver, or prehospital professional, or if the child has any of the following:

- A serious mechanism of injury
- A history compatible with serious illness
- A physiological abnormality noted on initial assessment
- A potentially serious anatomic abnormality
- Significant pain

In an ALS system with more extensive treatment options in the field, the transport decision is often complicated. Major factors to consider include:

- Type of clinical problem (injury versus illness)
- Expected benefits of ALS treatment in the field
- Local EMS system treatment and transport policies
- The ALS provider's comfort level

The operational considerations in transporting a child are sometimes complex. Some EMS systems do not have clear policies and protocols that define pediatric transport practices at all. National guidelines about safe transport of children in ambulances are still in evolution.

How to Begin Transport

Is the Child the Patient?

Why a child is being transported is the first factor in determining *how* to transport. Is the child the patient or is the child with a caregiver who needs ambulance transport? *Children who are not patients and only need transport because they must accompany the patient are best transported in a vehicle other than an ambulance.* There are too few positions available to secure a child properly and there may be risk of injury in transporting any patient in an ambulance. Ambulances are not for transporting children who are not patients.

When a Sick Child Is the Patient

If the child requires airway, breathing, or circulatory support more than simple oxygen delivery or nebulized bronchodilators, or if the child requires ALS monitoring or treatment, secure him to the stretcher in a supine position. This is a position that will best and most safely allow the prehospital professional to perform ongoing assessment and treatment en route.

When the Child Is the Patient but Not Sick

Often the initial assessment reveals that the child has only minimal or mild illness and is not seriously injured. In these cases, there are numerous options on how to transport that will protect the child's safety, permit appropriate monitoring, and provide comfort. Many children, especially in the infant and preschool-age groups and CSHCN, who are strapped supine to a stretcher, will become distressed from the effects of restraint, stranger anxiety, fear, and pain. When possible, attempt to transport children who are only mildly ill or injured in an upright position, in order to minimize the emotional distress and discomfort from a stiff stretcher.

Summary of How to Begin Transport

Avoid transporting a child who is not a patient in an ambulance. Determine another safe means to care for the child or arrange transport by another vehicle. When a child is the

Tip

Except in the case of mild illness or injury, transport a sick child secured on a stretcher in a supine position. This provides the safest and most effective position for ongoing assessment, monitoring, and treatment.

Blip

Avoid transporting a child who is not a patient in an ambulance.

patient, consider carefully how to position him to maximize effectiveness of interventions, to allow appropriate monitoring, and to preserve comfort. If the child has any immediate or anticipated requirements for interventions other than oxygen delivery or simple wound care, secure the child to a stretcher in a supine position. When a child is well or only mildly ill or injured, attempt to transport the child in an upright position that will allow observation and promote comfort.

Taking Caregivers in the Ambulance

Taking parents or caregivers in an ambulance is usually regulated by local EMS protocols. Usually the caregiver can decrease the anxiety of the child during the transport, especially the infant, preschool child, or CSHCN, who are more likely to experience emotional distress when transported without familiar caregivers. Dealing with emotional distress of children is an important principle in prehospital pediatric care and represents a key ingredient in quality care. The effect of the presence of family or caregiver on the effectiveness and comfort level of the prehospital professional is not known, but in other settings has been associated with higher provider satisfaction in pediatric care delivery (**Figure 14-1**).

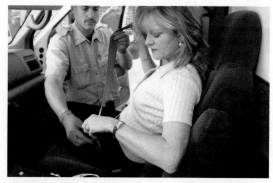

Figure 14-1 Allowing a parent to accompany a child may reduce the child's anxiety, but make sure all occupants are safe.

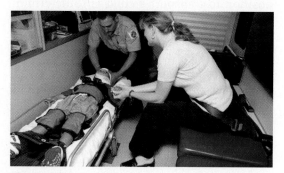

Figure 14-2 If caregivers are allowed to ride in the ambulance with the child, make sure all equipment and personnel are securely fastened.

On the other hand, extra ambulance occupants can get in the way if urgent care or resuscitation is required. Also, some prehospital professionals may feel less confident or comfortable when a caregiver is present in an ambulance during a resuscitation or when an advanced procedure such as endotracheal intubation is being performed.

If local EMS policy allows caregiver transport with the child, it should specify where the child and caregiver should be positioned during the transport. One common place for a caregiver during transport is in the front seat of the ambulance. As with any passenger, make sure the caregiver fastens his seat belt correctly and remains seated. Another place to seat a caregiver is in the rear of the ambulance. This will allow a child to visualize the caregiver and may provide some emotional consolation. Always have the caregiver wear a seat belt. If the caregiver is positioned on the bench seat, make sure any additional personnel are belted and all equipment is stowed or secured (**Figure 14-2**).

Child Restraint Systems in Ambulances

Dangers Facing Children During Transport

There are several factors that can decrease the possibility of additional injury to a child during ambulance transport. These factors include how the child is secured, the environment of the ambulance, and whether the crew is secured.

The first step in deciding how or in what position to transport a child is to determine what assessment, monitoring and treatment skills or procedures will be necessary during transport. *If the patient is stable and weighs less than 40 pounds and no interventions are anticipated, then transport the infant or child in an upright position using a car seat or child restraint system (CRS).* This consists of a car seat secured with a restraint device in the ambulance. Secure children over 40 pounds (approximately 18 kg) to the ambulance stretcher in a seated position using the existing straps altered to meet the size requirements of the child. Some circumstances make this standard approach impossible, such as transporting a child on a backboard. If the child requires a backboard, or if no other safe position is possible, transport the child in the supine position.

If EMS policy allows a CRS in the ambulance, decide where to place the device in the ambulance. Car seats are designed to restrain a child during a front end or rear end collision. They provide only moderate lateral stability.

Tip

If EMS policy allows, transport stable children weighing under 40 pounds with a child restraint system (CRS) when possible. This consists of a car seat secured with a restraint device in the ambulance.

Blip

Never secure car seats sideways to a bench seat in the ambulance, as there is not sufficient lateral stability.

This means that securing these seats sideways to a bench seat is potentially unstable. This limits the choices about where to position the CRS in the rear of an ambulance to the cot or the seat at the head of the stretcher.

Choosing a CRS

There are many types of car seats for the ambulance. Some seats are convertible to fit children of differing ages and weights. They are usually recognizable by the multiple slots to adjust the shoulder harness along the back of the device. Others will only work with one size of child. Infant seats are often limited to infants less than 20 pounds and are designed to fit in a rear-facing position. Some seats are manufactured specifi-

Case Study ❷

You are called to the scene of a vehicle crash involving two automobiles that collided at moderate speed in a downtown intersection. There are three patients, one who is the restrained driver of the vehicle that struck another vehicle broadside. The other patients are the restrained driver of the second vehicle and an 11-month-old boy, who was fully restrained in a rear-facing car seat on the opposite side of the point of collision. The two drivers have minor wounds and no significant physiologic abnormalities. Assessment of the child reveals a crying infant with no signs of injury.

1. Should the child be transported?
2. Should the child be transported in his own car seat or an ambulance car seat?

cally for ambulances; however, there are limitations for height and weight. Other specialty seats include the side-facing car bed and other vest and harness devices.

A CRS should be cleaned and maintained. Pads that are removable and surfaces that can be wiped down are preferable. Check with the manufacturer to see what cleaning materials are acceptable for the seat. If there is a dedicated ambulance CRS, check with your EMS policy as well as the manufacturer to make sure there have been no safety recalls.

Using Car Seats after a Collision

If the ambulance does not have a CRS and a stable child requires transport, an important dilemma arises when the child's own car seat is available. If local EMS policy permits using a personal car seat, be sure that it is fully intact. If the device shows any signs of damage, do not use it in the ambulance.

Securing a Car Seat to the Stretcher

Transport children weighing under 40 pounds in a rear-facing position unless medical attention is indicated. This is easily accomplished using the ambulance stretcher. Place a car seat that is size appropriate for the child on the cot and move the straps to position them as shown in **Figure 14-3**. Push down and in on the seat, and secure the straps tightly (**Figure 14-4**). The seat should have less than 1 inch of slack when pulled at the top of the seat (**Figure 14-5**).

Younger children weighing under 20 pounds may require slight modifications to the method of securing the seat. Choose an appropriate seat for an infant. When the infant is secured in the seat, support his head in the seat in a slightly reclined position. This may require a pad placed under the front edge of the seat to change the angle to 45 degrees. Then secure the seat as above.

Blip

If a child's personal car seat shows any signs of damage, do not use it in the ambulance.

Always transport smaller children in a rear-facing position unless a supine position is required. An alternate means of transporting these infants includes a side facing car bed, which can be secured to the cot.

Securing the Child in the Seat

Once the child seat has been secured, place the child into the seat and secure according to the seat manufacturer's instructions. There are several universal considerations when securing the straps. Place the straps over the shoulders (**Figure 14-6**). The chest clip should then be moved up to the level of the armpits (**Figure 14-7**). Next, adjust the belts according to the instructions for the seat. Check to make

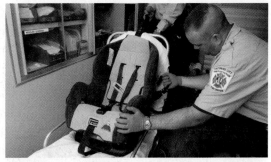

Figure 14-3 Place the car seat on the stretcher and use one belt from the horizontal member and one from the vertical member of the stretcher to secure it.

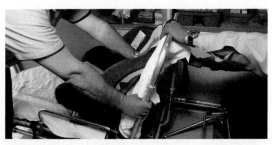

Figure 14-4 Place the car seat padding securely in place to minimize any movement when it has been secured.

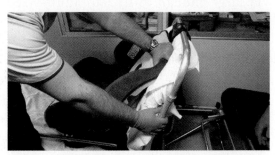

Figure 14-5 When the car seat is secured, there should be less than 1 inch of movement when tested.

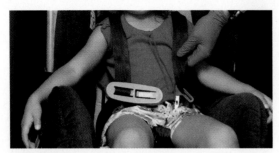

Figure 14-6 To secure a child in a car seat, place the shoulder straps over the child.

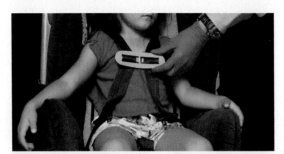

Figure 14-7 Move the chest clip up to the level of the armpits and secure the shoulder straps.

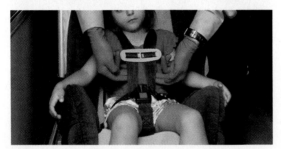

Figure 14-8 Check for excessive movement after the child is secured but before transporting to the hospital.

sure the child does not have excessive movement when secured (**Figure 14-8**).

Securing Older Children to the Stretcher

Children weighing over 40 pounds have outgrown most car seats. However, they are not yet large enough to fit into adult-sized restraint systems. Booster seats help make the restraint system meet the needs of the smaller child. For stable children who are to be transported without treatment, but not on a stretcher, use a booster seat. To secure the child to the stretcher, adjust the stretcher straps to meet the size of the patient. Move the belt to rest at the armpit level across the chest. Fit a second belt on the upper part of the thighs just below the pelvis. Arrange these belts so that the position on the cot is

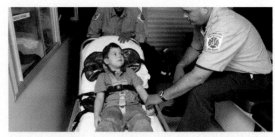

Figure 14-9 Cot straps should be placed allowing the straps to be stabilized using the cross members of the cot.

Tip

Crash tests of ambulances have shown that unrestrained passengers in the patient compartment present a risk to the patient during a collision by being launched and landing on the patient.

secured by a cross member limiting the movement along the rail (**Figure 14-9**).

During an ambulance crash children can move up the stretcher. Use shoulder straps to minimize this effect. There are some difficulties with these straps, however. Ultimately the straps should be secured similarly to those used in a car seat, adjusted low and over the shoulders. Ideally, the straps should enter through the padding and be secured to the frame of the stretcher at the height of the shoulders. Unfortunately, this is not possible with most of today's stretchers.

Other Dangers in Transporting Children

Placing the child in an appropriate transporting device is the first means of creating a safe mode of transport. It is important to recognize that crew members and flying debris can create a significant hazard to the patient during a collision. When transporting a child, secure or store all loose equipment before leaving the scene. Monitors, portable oxygen containers, equipment bags, and all other loose pieces can create missile-like objects that have been shown to be potentially dangerous to crew members and patients. Keep crew members secured in a seat belted position throughout the transport. Crash testing of ambulances has shown that unrestrained passengers in the patient compartment present a risk to the patient during a collision by being launched and landing on the patient.

Summary of Child Restraint Systems

Whenever possible, use a size-appropriate child restraint system to transport a stable child in an upright position. This is the preferred position for transport. There are important guidelines for proper use of car seats for children of different weights as well as how to secure the devices to the ambulance to maximize safety during transport. If local EMS policy allows use of the child's own car seat in the ambulance, be sure it is not damaged and that it is properly secured to the ambulance. Also, if EMS policy allows, encourage presence of the caregiver in the ambulance to provide comfort and solace to the child, and to improve ongoing assessment.

Transport Mode

Emotions can run high in pediatric calls, and prehospital professionals may feel a strong desire to transport quickly to the emergency department. However, lights and sirens transport, especially through crowded urban areas in the daytime, is fraught with risk to ambulance occupants and innocent bystanders. A way to minimize the dangers of transport to ambulance occupants and the public is to determine the best mode of transport prior to moving, based upon the type call, the presenting illness or injury, and the degree of physiological instability of the patient. The child with the highest priority for rapid transport is the critically injured child who needs

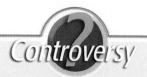

blood products and/or operative interventions. This child always requires a time-sensitive response and lights and sirens transport mode. Children with illness and any physiological abnormality are also important candidates for lights and sirens mode.

Multiple Patients

If there are multiple pediatric patients, extra transportation units may be required to transport the children safely. There are limited locations to secure a car seat or to be able to adjust the adult straps to fit the child in the patient compartment of the ambulance.

Summary of Transport Mode and Multiple Patients

Children are often the source of great provider stress. Transport mode is best determined prior to beginning transport. While lights and sirens are the fastest method, this mode is more dangerous and is best reserved for unstable trauma cases and physiologically unstable illness cases. When there is more than one child at the scene, activate additional units in order to avoid logistical problems with securing different sized car seats to the ambulance.

Case Study 3

You arrive at the scene of a 3-year-old girl who has just experienced a grand mal seizure. She had a high fever last night. The child has never seized before. The primary assessment shows a child with lethargy who is poorly interactive with her mother, no increased work of breathing, and hot pale skin. Vital signs show a heart rate of 150 beats/min, respiratory rate of 36 breaths/min and blood pressure of 84 mm Hg/palp. She weighs 33 lb (15 kg).

1. Should this child be transported in a car seat?
2. Should the mother be transported with the child?

Chapter Review

Case Study Answers

Case Study **1** page 273

This case demonstrates an important dilemma. While family centered care is highly desirable, this must take place without placing the patient, family member, accompanying child, or provider at increased risk. Whenever possible, arrange alternative safe care and/or transportation for the child so that attention of the medical providers can be centered on the patient. This includes care by or transportation with a competent adult, ensuring that appropriate child restraints are available and in use. Additional potential options for transporting the child could include a supervisor's, auxiliary, or child service's transportation vehicle. Transporting the child in the front seat of the ambulance or in the rear seat of a police car or other emergency vehicle is dangerous.

Parent and child separation, however, may cause undue distress to the mildly injured parent. In that case, if your system allows and enables the transport of the child in the ambulance, follow proper procedures to secure the child in the appropriate restraint system and in the correct position. This method of transportation must include enough participants to meet the child's as well as the patient's needs, and ensure that observation or immediate needs of either one doesn't detract from those of the other. This is an option that is often unavailable due to space or personnel resource limitations.

Case Study **2** page 276

Assessment of infants after a collision is very difficult in the best of environments. The significant mechanism of this incident necessitates assessment during the transport process and medical evaluation of the infant at the appropriate emergency department. The question then is how to best transport the child. If a careful inspection of the child yields no physiological or anatomical abnormality requiring further stabilization or intervention, and the child is appropriately visible to the provider when secured in the car seat, this method is appropriate. If a detailed inspection of the child's car seat does not yield evidence of fracture or abnormality, it is an appropriate seat for the child's weight, and EMS policy allows, then use this seat and secure in the usual rear-facing position in the emergency vehicle, unless the ambulance has its own CRS or local EMS policy forbids this practice. If there is any question as to the appropriateness or the structural integrity of the child's car seat, then use another more appropriate car seat.

Case Study **3** page 279

This is a case where the patient will need appropriate positioning, airway and vascular access, monitoring, and perhaps intervention during the transport process. "Stabilization" in a car seat affords none of those requirements and therefore should not be used. This is a child who should be restrained in a standard fashion on the ambulance stretcher, with attention to airway positioning, vascular access, and appropriate observation. Here, accompaniment of the parent can often be advantageous to both the parent and child. While the medical team can attend to the physiological needs of the child, they cannot meet their emotional needs. Be sensitive to the parent's need to offer support to their child as well as the mother's ability to keep the child calm. The parent may also be able to provide additional history and assist in reassessments. The parent cannot be allowed to carry the child during transport, either on their lap while seated or with the parent and child secured together to a stretcher.

Local protocol will often dictate when a parent can accompany their child, and specific requirements for this process. These protocols should include preferred parental seating location and safety instructions for the parent prior to transport. Parents must be instructed that the primary role of the providers is to care for the sick child, and that precious attention cannot be diverted from that task. Having the parent sit in the front is one way to include them in the environment, while allowing some separation for the providers.

Providers may express concern that parents will critique their techniques or skills during the transport or that the providers will be nervous when confronted with this environment. Parents, however, generally report very positively about the experience and comment mostly on the caring nature of the providers, not their technical capabilities.

Suggested Readings

Textbook

Bledsoe B, Porter R, Cherry R: *Essentials of Paramedic Care.* Upper Saddle River, NJ, Prentice Hall, 2003.

Articles

Becker LR. Relative risk of injury and death in ambulances and other emergency vehicles. *Accid Anal Prev.* 2003; 35(6):941–948.

Bledsoe BE. Emergency EMS Mythology, Part 4. Lights and sirens save a significant amount of travel time and save lives. *Emerg Med Serv.* 2003; 32(6):72–73.

Bull MJ. Crash protection for children in ambulances. *Annu Proc Assoc Adv Automot Med.* 2001; 45:353–367.

Kahn CA. Characteristics of fatal ambulance crashes in the United States: An 11 year retrospective analysis. *Prehosp Emerg Care.* 2001; 5(3):261–269.

Warren J. Guidelines for the inter- and intrahospital transport of critically ill patients. *Crit Care Med.* 2004; 32(1):256–262.

Making a Difference: What Can We Do?

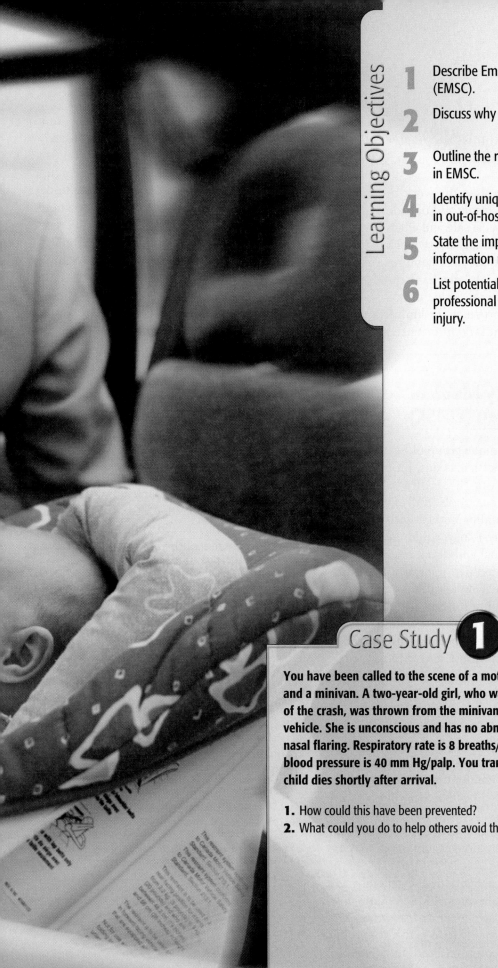

Learning Objectives

1 Describe Emergency Medical Services for Children (EMSC).

2 Discuss why injuries are not accidents.

3 Outline the role of the child's "medical home" in EMSC.

4 Identify unique quality and safety issues for children in out-of-hospital care.

5 State the importance of data collection and information management in EMSC.

6 List potential community roles for the prehospital professional in prevention of childhood illness and injury.

Case Study 1

You have been called to the scene of a motor vehicle crash between a compact car and a minivan. A two-year-old girl, who was not wearing her seat belt at the time of the crash, was thrown from the minivan and lies approximately 15 feet from the vehicle. She is unconscious and has no abnormal airway sounds, retractions, or nasal flaring. Respiratory rate is 8 breaths/min, heart rate is 50 beats/min, and blood pressure is 40 mm Hg/palp. You transport the child to the nearest ED, but the child dies shortly after arrival.

1. How could this have been prevented?
2. What could you do to help others avoid this type of tragedy?

Introduction

"Life affords no greater responsibility, no greater privilege, than the raising of the next generation." —C. Everett Koop

Emergency care for children involves the work of many health care professionals, both inside and outside of the community's hospitals. To provide safe and effective emergency care, these professionals must work together as a team to develop and implement comprehensive clinical services and oversight mechanisms designed specifically for children suffering acute illness and injury. Professionals must also recognize the limitations of an emergency care system largely oriented toward treatment *after* an illness or injury occurs, and embrace the essential role of prevention. Of all community activities that can improve children's overall health and well-being, prevention of acute injury and illness is by far the most cost-effective. Making a difference means practicing prevention both as part of day-to-day work duties and as part of volunteer roles as community leaders and health advocates. Making a difference entails professionals getting involved in injury and illness prevention in many new ways. This includes understanding and supporting the prevention and safety programs conducted through Emergency Medical Services for Children (EMSC) and prevention programs within local EMS systems.

Emergency Medical Services for Children (EMSC)

Children are a unique group of EMS patients. They have special needs and problems that are different from those of adults. They require equipment, tools, and medications designed for smaller bodies with different anatomy and physiology. Children also have different emotional and developmental needs that require a modified approach to assessment and treatment. While children under 18 years of age account for only 10% to 20% of out-of-hospital transports, evaluating, treating, triaging, and transporting this group can create significant stress and multiple challenges for prehospital professionals.

Emergency Medical Services for Children (EMSC) is a federal program initiated over twenty years ago to ensure high quality care of children within the EMS system. With federal grant funds and sustained EMSC program support, EMS communities across the country have developed pediatric-specific policies, procedures and protocols to assist prehospital professionals in pediatric care at the local level. These pediatric considerations may be outlined in a state or local "EMSC Plan," or in pediatric components within a general EMS plan. For example, most EMS systems now have pediatric triage, treatment, and transport policies. Most systems have pediatric-specific equipment and supplies, and allow special pediatric procedures, such as <u>intraosseous</u> infusions and rectal <u>diazepam</u> administration. In addition, most EMS systems also have specialized operational policies that address unique pediatric legal considerations, such as a pediatric refusal policy that recognizes the legal issues surrounding consent and provision of care to unaccompanied minors.

The umbrella of EMSC is broad and includes out-of-hospital and in-hospital care within both general hospitals and specialized pediatric hospitals. Because there are relatively few specialized pediatric centers (<u>**pediatric critical care centers**</u> and <u>**pediatric trauma centers**</u>), most children (over 90%) receive emergency care in general hospitals. Hence, <u>**universal standards for pediatric emergency care**</u> in all EDs within an EMS system, urban and rural, general and specialized, are an important part of EMSC development in the new millennium.

The <u>EMS-EMSC Continuum</u> (**Figure 15-1**) is the planned and organized interface between the clinical services of the EMS system itself, other out-of-hospital emergency care resources, the community's primary child health services, and the in-hospital system. The five major

The umbrella of EMSC is broad and includes general hospitals and specialized pediatric hospitals.

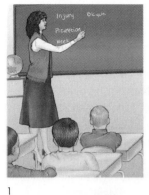

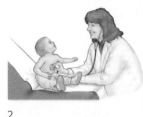

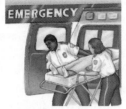

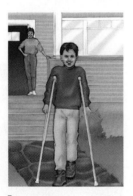

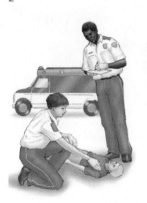

Figure 15-1 EMS-EMSC Continuum: (1) Prevention; (2) Primary care and the medical home; (3) Out-of-hospital care; (4) Hospital care; (5) Rehabilitation.

Tip

Standards for pediatric emergency care in EDs, urban and rural, general and specialized, are an important part of EMSC development in the new millennium.

phases in the continuum include: (1) prevention; (2) primary care and the child's "medical home"; (3) out-of-hospital care; (4) hospital care; and (5) rehabilitation. The prehospital professional has an opportunity to support children's emergency care throughout all phases of the continuum.

Summary of EMSC

EMSC began as a federal grant program to improve out-of-hospital pediatric services, within the community EMS system. Over two decades, the prolific work in the field has forged a broad concept of EMSC as a continuum of multiple clinical services in the community that are coordinated and child-specific. The essential phases of the "EMS-EMSC Continuum" include prevention, the medical home, out-of-hospital care, in-hospital care, and rehabilitation.

Injury and Illness Prevention

Many ill and injured children die in every community each year, despite receiving optimal medical care. There is a scientific discipline that is even more effective at saving lives than optimal medical care: injury and illness prevention. *Prevention is an essential feature of all EMS systems.* Prehospital professionals have the opportunity to affect the health and safety of their own children and every child in their community.

Prevention is the first phase of the EMS-EMSC Continuum. While prevention does apply to both illness and injury, out-of-hospital services have concentrated primarily on injury control. **Table 15-1** lists the eight identified elements of injury control; these elements make injury control an objective and scientific effort. For the prehospital professional, injury control involves understanding how and why injuries occur, knowing

Table 15-1	Elements of Injury Control
1. Recognize injury as a disease process.	
2. Maintain a reliable database.	
3. Identify problem injuries and high-risk groups.	
4. Identify the factors in injury causation.	
5. Practice appropriate injury **assessment**.	
6. Formulate injury prevention strategies.	
7. Select efficient, practical injury prevention strategies.	
8. Reevaluate selected injury prevention strategies for the desired effects.	

Case Study 2

You are dispatched to a local elementary school for a 7-year-old boy with a history of diabetes who has altered level of consciousness (ALOC). On your arrival the child is confused, pale and diaphoretic. He has no increased work of breathing, and the skin is pink. His heart rate is 120 beats/min, respiratory rate is 24 breaths/min and the BP is 94/62 mm Hg. The school nurse has measured his serum glucose at 40 mg/dL and administered oral glucose. You establish an intravenous line and administer intravenous 50% dextrose at 1 mL/kg. The child becomes coherent, answers questions appropriately, and his vital signs return to normal. His repeat glucose a few minutes later is 120 mg/dL. The child's mother arrives and states that the child has a new insulin pump and that they have been struggling to regulate his insulin. She asks that you contact the child's pediatrician, rather than taking the child to the emergency department. When you do this, the pediatrician states that she will see the child in the clinic now. The child is medically stable.

1. What are your options in the care and transport of this child?

how to identify the risks in the environment, and doing something in the community to stop injuries from happening.

Injuries Are Not Accidents

When injury patterns are carefully studied, it is clear that injuries, like illnesses, vary with the seasons, can occur in epidemics, and often have local trends and demographic distributions. In other words, injuries are largely predictable, whether they are unintentional (such as drowning) or intentional (such as handgun assaults). Whether they are intentional or unintentional, injuries are often predictable and are therefore potentially preventable.

Webster's Dictionary defines the word accident as, "an unforeseen and unplanned event or circumstance." True accidents that cause injuries are rare. Even apparently random events, such as lightning strikes or tornados, have predictable features and can be anticipated. For example, homes may be equipped with lightning rods and their foundations reinforced for earthquake stability. "Injuries are not accidents" has become a common slogan by injury professionals. The slogan reflects our current scientific understanding of how injuries really happen. *Almost all injuries are predictable and potentially preventable.* Injury prevention experts refer to automobile accidents as "crashes" rather than "accidents," because crashes almost always have predictable and

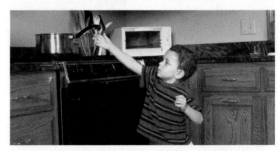

Figure 15-2 Components of an injury event: the host, the agent, and the environment. The child is the host, the heat from the boiling water is the agent, and the dangerously placed handle is the environment for a burn injury.

Injuries are not accidents. They are usually predictable and preventable.

preventable features. For example, crash injuries commonly occur because of persons driving while intoxicated, speeding, or because of improper use of child restraints. By identifying these predictable factors that cause or contribute to injuries, we can eliminate the "set-up" for future injury events.

Components of an Injury Event

Part of understanding how injuries occur involves looking at the three components of an injury event: the host, the agent, and the environment (**Figure 15-2**).

The <u>host</u> is the person who is the recipient of the injury. An injury occurs when potentially destructive energy is too much for the host to tolerate. Human hosts have different levels of tolerance. Children, because of their unique <u>anatomic</u> and <u>physiologic</u> features, are particularly vulnerable to high energy transfers. Their smaller body size means they are more likely to be injured over a larger percentage of body surface and are, therefore, at higher risk for multiple trauma.

The <u>agent</u> is a form of energy. The major agents of injury are kinetic, thermal, chemical, electrical, and radiation energy. Most injuries are associated with these types of energy. Kinetic energy is the most common injury agent in circumstances that involve prehospital professionals. For example, falls, auto-passenger injuries, pedestrian versus auto, and bicyclist versus auto events all involve a human as the host and kinetic energy as the agent. Burns, in contrast, involve thermal, chemical, or electrical energy.

The <u>environment</u> is the setting where the agent meets the host. The environment causes or influences the injury event. Some examples are an unfenced swimming pool, a poorly maintained road, or an open upper-story window without a protective barrier. Any of these factors may provide the environment for an injury event to occur that might involve a young child as a host and kinetic energy as the agent.

Looking at injury events, the prehospital professional can consider what component(s) of an injury can be modified to prevent future occurrences (**Figure 15-3**). Modifying the host's behavior to prevent drowning or head injury, for example, may involve education in swimming skills or driving techniques. Modifying the agent may include providing bicycle helmets (**Figure 15-4**) or installing soft stopping surfaces in playgrounds to reduce the effect of kinetic energy on vulnerable brain tissue. Modifying the environment may include fencing of swimming pools or setting up window bars.

Phases of Injury

Just as there are three components in every injury event, there are also three separate

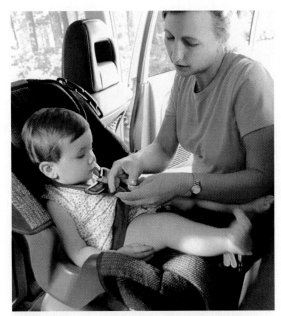

Figure 15-3 EMS professionals can become involved directly in injury prevention by attending a child safety seat technician training and then by providing a child safety seat checkpoint program.

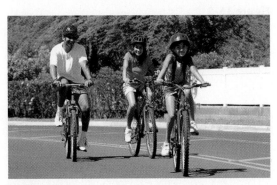

Figure 15-4 When worn correctly, bicycle helmets significantly reduce the complications and incidence of death from closed-head injuries. Prehospital professionals have an important community role in teaching simple injury control strategies.

phases of every injury that need to be considered when devising control strategies: the pre-event period; the event itself; and the post-event period (**Figure 15-5**).

Pre-event factors are conditions in the host, the agent, or the environment that make an injury more or less likely to occur. For example, riding a bicycle with a helmet is a pre-event factor that might significantly decrease the probability of injury. Event factors are conditions that increase or decrease the effect of the agent on the host. An event factor that would decrease the risk of injury in a vehicle crash would be lower speed of the

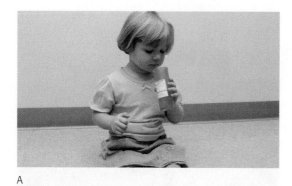

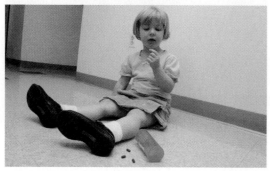

B

Figure 15-5 The first two phases of an injury: (A) The pre-event period. An unlocked medicine cabinet invites an adventurous toddler. (B) The event itself. A toddler will put anything into her mouth, including dangerous medications.

Prevention is an essential feature of all EMS systems and represents an opportunity for prehospital professionals to profoundly affect the health and well-being of their own children and every child in their community.

automobile at the time of the crash. Post-event factors are conditions that increase or decrease the effect of the agent on the host after the injury event. An example of a post-event factor that would affect the outcome in a severely head-injured child might be on-scene airway management by the prehospital professional.

Traditionally, out-of-hospital care has focused almost exclusively on the post-event period, or medical care and transport after the injury has occurred. Prehospital professionals must now recognize their potential to influence the pre-event and event phases of injury by acting as community educators

Table 15-2	Modifiable Factors in Different Phases of an Injury
Phase	**Examples of Modifiable Factors**
Pre-event	Maintaining child restraint seats
	Installing proper fencing around pools
	Ensuring that smoke detectors work in homes
	Wearing bicycle helmets
Event	Properly using child restraint seats
	Deployment of front and side airbags
Post-event	Performing pediatric airway management skills
	Proper spinal stabilization
	Choice of an appropriate transport destination for an injured child

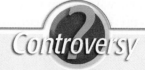

Until recently, prehospital professionals were not taught injury or illness prevention. While adding prevention to the prehospital professional's scope of practice has exciting potential, the role of EMS in injury prevention has not yet been fully explored.

and advocates. **Table 15-2** provides examples of injury control strategies aimed at modifiable factors in different phases of injury. The prehospital professional can have an important role in all of these prevention strategies.

Summary of Prevention and Injury Control

Injury and illness prevention is a key feature of EMSC, and it is the first phase of the EMS-EMSC Continuum. Injuries are not "accidents" and are almost always predictable. Prehospital professionals have a unique role in community injury control. They are at the scene and able to assess accurately the principle components in an injury or illness event. This includes assessing the child or host, the energy type or agent of injury, and the environment as well as understanding the pre-event, event, and post-event phases of injury to assist with injury reduction activities in the community.

The "Medical Home"

The second vital link in the EMS-EMSC Continuum is the child's primary care provider, or <u>medical home</u>. The American Academy of Pediatrics (AAP) defines a medical home as the child's primary source of medical care. Creating an effective medical home requires that infants, children, and teens have accessible, continuous, comprehensive, family-centered, coordinated, compassionate, and culturally effective services in a geographically close location. The child and family need to know the primary care provider and develop a partnership of mutual responsibility and trust. This is especially important for children with special needs (Chapter 10) who often require specialized medical care. Trained pediatricians and family physicians create the medical home. They should not only manage and facilitate ongoing pediatric primary care, but also have a linkage to the EMS system in case a child requires emergency services beyond what is offered by the office or clinic. In some offices, there are written protocols and procedures that define how to identify an emergency requiring EMS services, when to summon 9-1-1, and what to do immediately in a medical emergency. The providers in the medical home should have an accurate understanding of the pediatric capabilities of the prehospital professional and EMS system, know the closest hospital for pediatric care, and know the local EMS system's policies and procedures regarding triage, transport, and treatment of children by prehospital professionals.

The Prehospital Professional and the Medical Home

Traditionally, prehospital professionals have had little contact with primary care physicians who provide the medical home, although both are part of the community settings in the EMS-EMSC Continuum. There are many opportunities for collaboration between the physicians and providers in the child's medical home and the prehospital professionals in the EMS system. Under some conditions, with the permission of a parent or guardian, the primary provider can offer valuable history and infor-

Tip

Communication and teamwork are essential features in the linkages between all components of the EMS-EMSC Continuum.

mation to the prehospital professional. This may be especially important in evaluating and treating children with special health care needs. This information may be communicated in the form of a written care plan or via a telephone consult on scene. This does not require the prehospital professional to delay care or transport of a critically ill or injured child, but can take place as part of an EMS system optional procedure for history gathering in stable patients. Sometimes the primary physician can deliver emergency care on scene with the prehospital professionals, and accompany the child to the ED. *Effectively treating a child with the assistance of prehospital professionals requires that the primary physician understand the local scope of practice, drugs, equipment and supplies available for children within the local EMS system.* The prehospital professionals should have a "physician on scene" policy that defines the relative roles and responsibilities of the parties in such circumstances.

When possible, with children with special needs, communication from the medical home is especially important and should include the Emergency Information Form, as described in Chapter 8 (**Figure 15-6**). Communication and teamwork are essential features in the linkages between all components of the EMS-EMSC Continuum.

Summary of the Medical Home

The medical home is the child's primary medical provider, usually a pediatrician or family physician, sometimes in concert with other medical practitioners. The medical home is the source of key information and decision making for the child. When appropriate, utilize the expertise of the primary provider in

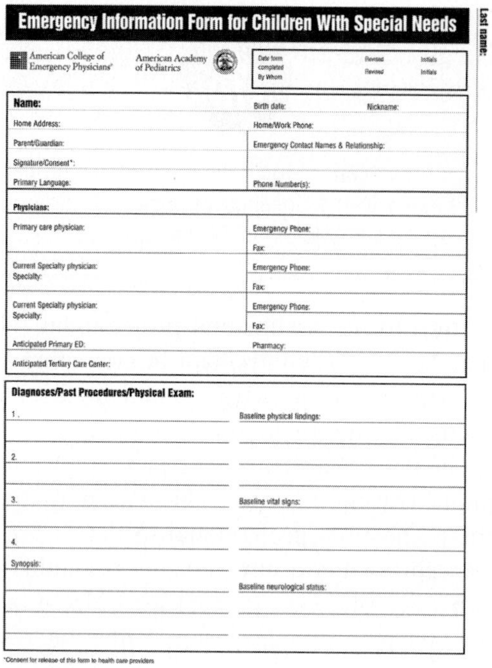

Emergency Information Form for Children With Special Needs

Last name:

American College of Emergency Physicians® American Academy of Pediatrics

Date form completed By Whom | Revised | Initials | Revised | Initials

Name: | Birth date: | Nickname:

Home Address: | Home/Work Phone:

Parent/Guardian: | Emergency Contact Names & Relationship:

Signature/Consent*:

Primary Language: | Phone Number(s):

Physicians:

Primary care physician: | Emergency Phone: | Fax:

Current Specialty physician: Specialty: | Emergency Phone: | Fax:

Current Specialty physician: Specialty: | Emergency Phone: | Fax:

Anticipated Primary ED: | Pharmacy:

Anticipated Tertiary Care Center:

Diagnoses/Past Procedures/Physical Exam:

1. | Baseline physical findings:

2.

3. | Baseline vital signs:

4.

Synopsis: | Baseline neurological status:

*Consent for release of this form to health care providers

Figure 15-6 Emergency Information Form.

information gathering and in decision making about emergency care. Always ask caregivers of a child with special needs if they have an Emergency Information Form. From their position, primary care physicians should be aware of the pediatric capabilities and scope of practice of the prehospital professionals and local hospitals and about the services of the other components of the EMS-EMSC Continuum.

Quality and Safety in EMSC

Quality assurance (QA) and quality improvement (QI) have long been recognized as methods of ensuring efficiency, decreasing waste, and increasing customer satisfaction in industrial settings. Over the last few decades, the concept of continuous quality improvement has been adopted by the health care industry as well. The ingredients of health care quality now defined in health institutions include: *patient-centered care, efficiency, effectiveness, timeliness, equity,* and *safety.* All of these domains are relevant to pediatric out-of-hospital care:

- *Patient-centered care* is "respectful of and responsive to individual patient preferences, needs, and values."
- *Efficiency* avoids waste, including waste of equipment, supplies, ideas, and energy.
- *Effectiveness* entails treatment grounded in the best scientific evidence that links clinical practice to improved patient outcome. To date, there has been limited research on the effectiveness of prehospital interventions for children. A commitment to participating in clinical research studies is an important element of an EMS program.
- *Timeliness* has always been a primary goal of EMS systems, where treatment and transport delays have long been linked to adverse outcomes for cardiac and trauma patients.
- *Equity* implies providing the same level of care to all patients and families, regardless of socioeconomic status, race or ethnic background, disability, or language barriers.

Safety is a paramount concern for every health care professional, and certainly for the prehospital professional who faces unique risks in the out-of-hospital setting. Medical error and safety in the prehospital environment are issues now receiving increasing attention. Error rates—in terms of medication dosing and administration, performance of critical procedures, and misdiagnosis—are higher in children than in adults. This discrepancy is probably related to the limited number of pediatric calls and limited opportunities to reinforce pediatric knowledge and skills in the field. EMS efforts to improve pediatric patient safety might include competency-based pediatric training modules; use of length-based tapes or medical software to assist in equipment sizing and medication dosing; the development and dissemination of guidelines of care for common or critical pediatric emergencies; and routine run reviews to identify factors that contribute to adverse outcomes related to field care. The emerging availability of computer-based decision support systems that prehospital professionals can access by vehicle desktop computers or personal digital assistants (**Figure 15-7**) may help to reduce pediatric errors.

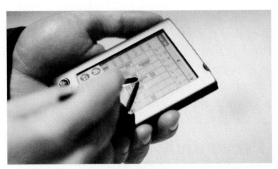

Figure 15-7 Pediatric medical decision support software systems will soon be available for prehospital professionals on vehicle computers and PDAs.

Data and Information Management

To improve systems of care, providers must have substantive knowledge of how the system currently works. This requires collection and analysis of data on system performance both at baseline and after a process or procedure has been introduced or modified. Change for the sake of change does not necessarily represent improvement! Therefore, before any quality improvement initiative is undertaken, the following three questions should be answered:

1. What are we trying to accomplish?
2. What changes can we make that will result in improvement?
3. How will we know that a change is an improvement?

A Prehospital QI Case Study

Consider the following hypothetical scenario: An ED physician contacts the manager of your EMS agency with concerns about two children who were transported over the past month after scene endotracheal intubations following apparent febrile seizures. Both had been treated in the field with IV diazepam, suffered brief respiratory depression, received endotracheal intubations, and were extubated shortly after arrival in the ED. A query of your agency's electronic database reveals a total of 10 children over the past year with a diagnosis of seizure who were intubated in the field after treatment with IV diazepam. Knowing that most febrile seizures are brief and self-limited, you are concerned that the potential complications of intu-

bation likely outweigh the benefits of diazepam therapy. You bring this to the QI committee for review. They ask the following questions:

Question #1: What are we trying to accomplish?

Answer #1: We want to decrease the incidence of children experiencing respiratory depression and intubation due to benzodiazepine treatment for seizures.

Question #2: What changes can we make that will result in improvement?

Answer #2: Possible changes might include: education of ALS personnel on indications for benzodiazepine administration in children with seizures; adding computer-based decision support software or length-based resuscitation tapes to each drug box to promote accurate dosing of benzodiazepines; switch from IV to rectal diazepam administration for prolonged seizures; teaching the technique of nasal airway placement and bag-mask ventilation.

Question #3: How will we know if a change is an improvement?

Answer #3: Our intubation rate for children with seizures will drop, without an associated increase of children with low oxygen saturation on arrival to the ED.

Together with your medical control physician, you develop a new protocol for assessing and managing seizures in children, provide in-service training with your ALS personnel, and develop a data sheet to be filled out after every seizure call. After six months, you find that your intubation rate for children with febrile seizures has been cut by 75%.

This data-driven approach is based on examining the status quo and looking for opportunities to improve prehospital practice.

Importance of Data Collection and Information Management in EMSC

Injury prevention begins with an understanding of the community's injury problems. Data are an injury prevention program's best guide. Data, when correctly collected, integrated, and interpreted, becomes useful information. A properly maintained injury database can be analyzed to identify patterns of preventable injury in a community, which then can be used to generate financial and political support for focused prevention programs. These data also allow an evaluation of the effectiveness of targeted programs in reducing the frequency and severity of injuries.

Elements of an injury database that will be useful in EMS system management include the type, severity, and frequency of fatal and non-fatal injuries; persons at risk; geographic location; time of day and year; and contributing factors such as alcohol, weather, and lack of (or improper use of) protective devices. Analysis of these data can help set the agenda for program planning and evaluation. For example, the data indicate that a community is experiencing a high rate of injury among unrestrained young children in car crashes. An injury prevention effort must then examine why the injured children are not restrained. The problem may be an issue of education or accessibility. Perhaps the problem is a community cultural belief that a baby is always safest in a mother's arms. Understanding the basis of the problem is critical in determining the best intervention strategy.

Summary of Quality, Safety, Data Collection, and Information Management

Quality improvement is now a key feature of EMSC. There are many opportunities to evaluate clinical practice with children and to implement system improvements to reduce error. Appropriate data collection is key to improvement. There are many types of EMS data that pertain to children. Simply collecting data is not enough. In order for data to be useful, it needs to be accurately collected and then reviewed with a problem orientation. When data are effectively managed, the essential information can be used for focused education and program development.

Prevention: The Prehospital Professional's Role

Prehospital professionals can have a valuable role in community illness and injury prevention. *They can have a greater impact in reducing illness and injury through prevention than they can through treatment.* However, to be effective in this new role, prehospital professionals need education and training. Recognizing how injuries can be avoided is the first step in developing prevention activities in the community.

Role On Scene

Prevention actions of the prehospital professional begin during the "scene size-up" and include: (1) ensuring scene safety, and (2) performing an <u>environmental assessment</u>. Ensuring scene safety involves prevention of injury and illness to the prehospital professional herself and to other medical and law enforcement personnel. This includes identification of possible communicable diseases in the child that can be transmitted to unwary scene personnel unless proper body substance precautions are observed. Ensuring scene safety also may prevent an injury to the child herself or to her caregiver.

Performing an environmental assessment adds a crucial piece to the overall picture at the scene. ED providers cannot do an

Data, when correctly collected, integrated, and interpreted, becomes useful information.

Prehospital professionals can have a greater impact in reducing the incidence and impact of illness and injury through prevention than through treatment.

environmental assessment. Observation and documentation of the physical and interpersonal environment by the prehospital professional may provide the basis for important prevention actions. Such actions may include providing information directly to the caregiver on safety hazards in the home.

Another type of environmental assessment involves observing and noting any evidence of possible maltreatment by the caregiver, and then communicating these concerns to the ED physician. This preventive action may be lifesaving to the child, as explained in Chapter 12.

Role in Safe Transport

Another important aspect of childhood injury prevention for the prehospital professional is safe vehicular transport. *Most serious and fatal vehicular injuries occur to occupants in the rear seat and to occupants who are improperly restrained.* This pertains to ambulance transport as well as automobile transport. The key step for safety of the prehospital professional AND the patient is the simplest: Wear a seat belt and secure the pediatric patient in a proper restraint device for the entire transport.

For a child who requires spinal stabilization, use a stabilization device secured to the ambulance gurney to package the child safely, as described in Chapter 14. If the child is critically ill, treat and transport the child in a <u>supine</u>, secured position on a gurney. This position will allow rapid management and monitoring of the child's airway, breathing, and circulation. For a child with mild-to-moderate illness or injury not requiring spinal stabilization or a supine position, use an age-appropriate and locally approved approach to restraint, as promulgated by the EMS system.

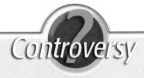

The safety of child transport in personal restraint seats is unknown. Always follow local EMS protocol.

For some children with respiratory problems, an upright position of comfort is important, as explained in Chapter 3. The child with cardiopulmonary or neurological disabilities may require a specialized child seat to breathe effectively, as described in Chapter 4.

Consider the use of family's child restraint seats for pediatric transport, but remember that seats are only approved for traditional passenger vehicles. Many EMS programs advocate for the transport of children involved in motor vehicle crashes in their own child safety seats. *The National Highway and Traffic Safety Association (NHTSA), however, recommends that a child restraint seat involved in a crash be replaced before the child is transported again.* This is a controversial issue that requires more data collection and interpretation.

In addition to passengers, unsecured items/equipment move like unsecured people in the back of an ambulance, especially with lights and sirens transport. If the transport requires additional equipment for special patient care, such as a drug box or a medication pump, then secure the items prior to transport. There is always the potential for an ambulance crash, or even just a hard stop, and preparation and prevention will avert damage and injury.

Role in the Community

Detailed and accurate observations at the scene may serve to start or support community-wide strategies for injury and illness control. For example, in Europe and Australia prehospital professionals played a key role in recognizing the relationship between sleep position and <u>sudden infant death syndrome (SIDS)</u>. Scene observations were part of the scientific studies that confirmed the increased risk of SIDS in babies who slept <u>prone</u> and assisted in the campaign that has decreased SIDS <u>mortality</u>. Chapter 11 discusses SIDS in more detail.

Prehospital professionals can help in the understanding of community injury and illness patterns by documenting the mechanism and scene circumstances of an acute event in the prehospital record and by assisting in other local data collection efforts. **Table 15-3** lists some specific community injury prevention

Table 15-3	Examples of Common Injuries and Possible Prevention Strategies
Injury	**Prevention**
Vehicle trauma	Infant and child restraint seats Seat belts and air bags Pedestrian safety programs Motorcycle helmets
Cycling	Bicycle helmets Bicycle paths separate from vehicle traffic
Recreation	Appropriate safety padding and apparel Cyclist/skateboard/skater safety programs Soft, energy-absorbent playground surfaces
Drowning	Four-sided locked pool enclosures Pool alarms Immediate adult supervision Caretaker CPR training Swimming lessons Pool/beach safety instruction Personal flotation device
Poisoning and household	Proper storage of chemicals and medications Child safety packaging
Burns	Proper maintenance and monitoring of electrical appliances and cords Fire/smoke detectors Proper placement of cookware on stove top
Other	Discouragement of infant walker use Gated stairways Babysitter first aid training Child care worker first aid training

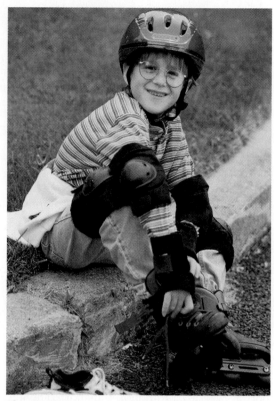

Figure 15-8 Prehospital professionals have the opportunity to teach prevention.

activities that prehospital professionals might consider in their expanded roles as community advocates, public educators, and teachers.

Summary of Roles in Prevention

The prehospital professional has many opportunities to teach and practice prevention, on the job and as a community member (**Figure 15-8**). Recognition of scene safety issues, documentation of suspicious home circumstances, and recording of injury mechanisms are fundamental information for EMS systems. Error reduction through careful equipment sizing and drug dosing prevents adverse outcomes as a result of medical care delivered in the field. Best practice for ensuring proper child restraint in an ambulance has not been defined. Fulfilling the dual agendas of ensuring the child passenger's safety in the event of an ambu-

Tip

Wear your seat belt and secure all portable items in the ambulance.

Tip

Scene observations were part of the scientific studies that confirmed the increased risk of SIDS in babies who slept prone.

lance crash and permitting ongoing monitoring and treatment continues to represent a challenge for EMS professionals. Last, there are many opportunities as a community member to advocate for injury control in the voluntary role of a concerned health provider.

Call to Action: Advocacy for EMSC

Advocates can support EMSC on and off the ambulance. There are numerous roles for the prehospital professional in both the clinical and operational aspects of EMSC and there are endless problems to undertake in every community. National and state EMSC programs offer many excellent models and templates for system improvement, and often provide funding to support new programs for children. New pediatric-specific software is now available to support bedside clinical care of children. In addition, many funding agencies, public and private, have resources to support children's services and enhancements in pediatric emergency care in the community. Advocacy for EMSC includes looking creatively for sources of support outside traditional EMS to help or strengthen pediatric services.

Possible roles to advance children's issues within EMS may involve participation on EMSC committees and advocating on a day-to-day basis for training, equipment, policies, procedures, and protocols that pertain exclusively to children. Other roles may include serving as a volunteer educator at school, developing school first aid services, becoming a CPR trainer, or joining community programs on injury control and children's health issues. National associations such as the American Academy of Pediatrics, American College of Emergency Physicians, and the Emergency Nurses Association, as well as local fire departments and prehospital organizations sponsor programs for pediatric illness and injury prevention, but these visionary programs require advocacy and participation for success.

There is unprecedented potential for exciting improvements in saving lives, decreasing pain and suffering, preventing injury and illness, and facilitating the complex interface of out-of-hospital pediatric care with community and in-hospital services. Preserving the health and safety of our children demands constant advocacy and vigilance from all prehospital professionals—to sustain quality pediatric services in our EMS sytems now, and to continue the evolution of EMSC tomorrow.

Case Study 3

You arrive on the scene and find a toddler who is actively seizing. He is in the care of a frantic teenaged babysitter who states that the child has been seizing ever since she called 9-1-1 about 10 minutes ago. She does not know the child's exact age, his weight, or whether he has a history of seizures. The child has a heart rate of 150 beats/min, respiratory rate of 26 breaths/min, and is having a generalized tonic-clonic seizure. His lips are blue. Based on your seizure protocol, he is a candidate for treatment with a benzodiazepine.

1. What tools can help you more effectively and safely care for this child?

Chapter Review

Case Study Answers

Case Study ❶ page 283

Factors that may have helped prevent or modify the injuries include: car safety education in schools and communities, especially use of seat belts and child restraint seats, reduced vehicle speed, and better traffic signs for drivers.

For the prehospital professional, the key prevention steps in this case are to do the scene size-up, document the important scene conditions, provide appropriate on-scene care, and rapidly transport the child. Documenting the mechanism and informing hospital professionals of the preventable aspects of the injury (unrestrained child) has many benefits. It is highly unlikely that any type of medical care would have changed this child's outcome. Hence, while the prehospital professional's interventions *after* an injury event are few and futile in such cases, there are many useful preventive interventions *before* the event.

Careful documentation of the circumstances of injury will also contribute to vital data collection and help define patterns of injury within the community. The prehospital professional can become a community advocate for injury prevention, helping to educate parents and policymakers about known risks and identifying and promoting solutions to the important public health problems of childhood injury.

Case Study ❷ page 286

This child's primary care physician plays an active role in managing his chronic illness, and is likely best qualified to make an adjustment in his insulin regimen. Given the child's medically stable status after treatment, contact with medical control to discuss transport destination is reasonable. Effective out-of-hospital care is a phase of the EMS-EMSC continuum and requires not only appropriate equipment and education of prehospital personnel, but also teamwork, knowledge of community resources, and expert communication. Transport of this child to his "medical home" if allowed by local EMS policies, may have advantages that must be weighed against potential risks of further physiologic compromise.

Case Study ❸ page 295

A computer-based decision support software program or length-based tool can assist the prehospital professional in choosing the appropriately sized oxygen delivery device and the correct sized intravenous catheter as well as the correct dosages of medications. Having pediatric equipment well organized and accessible will facilitate the search for the correct size equipment and safeguard the care of the child.

It can be difficult to concentrate on math calculations during the treatment of a critically ill or injured child. Using computer software tools or length-based tapes may elevate critical thinking, reduce cognitive load, and allow the prehospital professional to focus on assessment, prioritization, medical interventions, and transport.

Suggested Reading

Textbooks

Barss P, Smith G, Baker S, Mohan D: *Injury Prevention: An international perspective,* 1st Edition. Oxford University Press, 1998.

Seidel J, Knapp J: *Childhood Emergencies in the Office, Hospital, and Community: Organizing systems of care,* 2nd Edition. Chicago, American Academy of Pediatrics Committee on Pediatric Emergency Medicine, 2000.

Articles

American Academy of Pediatrics. Medical home initiatives for children with special needs project advisory committee: The medical home. *Pediatrics.* 2002; 110(1):184–186.

Gausche M. Out-of-hospital care of pediatric patients. *Pediatr Clin North Am.* Dec 1999; 46(6):1305–27.

Horowitz L. Mental health aspects of emergency medical services for children: Summary of a consensus conference. *J Pediatr Psychol.* Dec 2001; 26(8):491–502.

Sia C. The medical home: Closing the circle of care. In Seidel JS and Henderson DP, editors: *Emergency Medical Services for Children: A report to the nation.* Washington DC, National Center for Education in Maternal and Child Health, 1991.

Procedure 1: Field Reporting

Introduction

Gathering and organizing pertinent information about children to report to other prehospital professionals, medical oversight, and the receiving ED requires pediatric terms. Clear, concise communication helps ensure an orderly flow of out-of-hospital tasks: describing children and their clinical problems accurately to medical oversight personnel; informing the receiving ED personnel about incoming patients; and making an effective transfer of information about the patient's assessment and care. Each EMS region has unique requirements for field reporting to medical oversight and to the receiving ED. The patient criteria requiring field reporting are variable in different EMS systems. Sometimes the reporting is not by radio, but via telephone or another form of real-time communication. Many local EMS agencies have reporting or communications protocols that specifically address on-line medical oversight and ED notification requirements for *children*.

In addition to the spoken presentation format for field reporting, pediatric-specific documentation is also essential for later review and analysis. Each EMS agency has its own reporting form on which the prehospital professional must record clinical facts, as well as the necessary information for billing and for detailed incident or system analysis.

Indication

Use good field reporting procedure in any radio, telephone, facsimile (fax), personal, or other communication with medical oversight, the receiving ED, or other prehospital providers regarding on scene or inbound pediatric emergency patients. Good reporting technique is also indicated for chart documentation.

Contraindication

The only relative contraindication to appropriate field reporting is the child with a physiologic abnormality requiring constant hands-on care. This situation may make it difficult for the prehospital professional to communicate fully with a receiving ED or medical oversight while on the way to the ED. In most cases, a coworker, such as a partner, can assist with notifying the ED that a distressed child is on the way, although complete reporting of patient assessment, treatment, and response to treatment may not be possible. There are no contraindications to accurate reporting through chart documentation.

Equipment

Equipment requirements vary depending on the EMS system. Equipment may include telecommunications equipment, computerized real-time data transmission, or video. The patient care record is essential, as are other assessment worksheets in some EMS systems.

Rationale

A logical and descriptive format for presentation of key information about ill or injured children is essential for everyday field practice. It promotes the cost-efficient use of communications equipment and personnel time. Proper field reporting also integrates efforts from all emergency care professionals—prehospital professionals, nurses, and doctors—and helps ensure that vital data are transmitted completely and concisely. Pediatric-specific reporting techniques will assist appropriate age-related modifications in assessment, treatment, triage, and transport.

Preparation

1. The prehospital professional should prepare for and practice field reporting about children.

2. It is helpful to have a field reporting format that is agreed on by the EMS agency, medical oversight, and the ambulance providers. The desired format can be printed on small pads as a checklist. This may help in the flow and understanding of patient information during situations when the prehospital professional has multiple tasks and when the environment or equipment make communicating difficult.

3. Such notes may be useful not only during transport, but also when transferring care at the ED.

Do not give long field reports when there is a distressed child in the ambulance.

Possible Complications

Using incorrect, deceptive, or unclear terminology, or failing to distinguish the pediatric report from the more frequent adult-oriented report, may confuse medical oversight and delay preparation by the receiving ED.

Avoid focusing on vital signs.

Do not contact the receiving ED or medical oversight until you are prepared to give accurate patient information.

Procedure

1-1 Field Reporting

① State child's age, gender, and estimated body weight. Using the patient's name is generally not pertinent to treatment, triage, or transport, so do not use names in the field report. Emergency medical channels are easily monitored, and omitting the patient's name protects her identity and medical confidentiality.

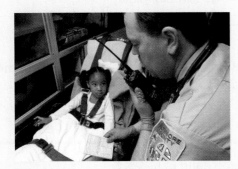

② Give the child's chief complaint.

③ Provide in one sentence the mechanism of injury or history of illness, and state pertinent past medical history (usually none or brief).

④ Summarize the assessment and establish the level of severity and urgency for treatment using the Pediatric Assessment Triangle (PAT). Address all three elements of the triangle, using appropriate descriptive words and terms, as listed in **Table P1-1**.

⑤ Report any abnormalities in the ABCDEs. Avoid focusing on vital signs.

⑥ State treatment and response, using the PAT.

⑦ Estimate time of arrival and state the proposed receiving ED.

⑧ Request agreement from medical oversight with interventions and request additional orders as per local EMS protocol.

⑨ Repeat medical oversight orders to confirm understanding. **Table P1-2** is a sample pediatric reporting template.

Report the patient's assessment using the PAT.

Table P1-1　Examples of Pediatric-Specific Terminology for PAT

Appearance (use TICLS mnemonic to recall individual features)

Tone

Active, vigorous, good muscle tone
Limp, listless, motionless, will not sit or walk

Interactiveness

Alert, interactive, attentive, playful
Restless, agitated, screaming

Consolability

Consolable or distractible by caregiver, comfortable
Cannot be consoled

Look/Gaze

Fixes gaze, maintains good eye contact
Will not engage or make eye contact

Speech/Cry

Strong cry, normal speech
Weak cry, cannot speak

Work of breathing

Apneic

Abnormal positioning (sniffing position, tripoding)

Abnormal airway sounds (snoring, stridor, wheezing, grunting)

Retractions (supraclavicular, intercostal, subxiphoid)

Nasal flaring

Circulation to skin

Pink, good color

Mottled, dusky

Pale

Cyanotic

Table P1-2　Sample Pediatric Reporting Template

We are [on scene] or [en route to (name of ED)] with a [state age in days, weeks, months, or years as appropriate] [state boy or girl] patient weighing [state approximate body weight in kilograms].

CC	The patient's chief complaint is [state chief complaint in one or two words].	
HPI	State brief history of present illness/injury.	
PMH	State brief, pertinent, medical history (note: usually there is none).	
PAT	Appearance	Describe the patient's appearance using descriptive terms.*
	Work of breathing	Describe the work of breathing using descriptive terms.
	Circulation to skin	Describe the circulation to skin using descriptive terms.
Initial ABCDEs assessment	Summarize key findings from the ABCDEs. Avoid emphasis on vital signs.	
TX	Report the treatment and the patient's response. Use these elements as the basis for ongoing assessment: the PAT, the ABCDEs, repeating vital signs in children over 3 years of age, and reassessing of positive anatomic findings in distressed children who have received the focused and detailed exams.	
ETA	Our ETA to [state receiving ED] is _____ minutes. Do you have any advice or questions? [Request additional orders as per local protocol at this point.]	

*See Table P1-1 for examples of pediatric-specific descriptive terminology.

Procedure 2: Length-Based Equipment Sizing and Drug Dosing

Introduction

Selecting the appropriately sized piece of equipment or drug dose is often challenging during pediatric resuscitations. Errors are common, and may be dangerous or life-threatening. Several types of devices are useful for determining the correct equipment sizes and drug doses. The pediatric length-based resuscitation tape is a simple and effective tool to measure body lengths and to determine approximate weights. Knowledge of the child's body length and approximate weight is the basis to calculate appropriate equipment sizes and drug doses.

Indication
Children requiring equipment, medication, or fluids, weighing from 3 to 34 kg body weight

Contraindications
Premature infant weighing less than 3 kg
Child older than 10 to 12 years of age or weighing more than 34 kg body weight (use adult equipment and drug dosages)

Equipment
Pediatric resuscitation tape
Pediatric decision support software on a computer or PDA

Computerized methodologies that use length and weight for instantaneous equipment sizing and drug dosing may include pediatric-specific software on a computer or hand-held personal digital assistant (PDA). Software has the advantage of including essential resuscitation information such as algorithms, drug doses, and equipment sizes for a wide range of clinical problems. Computerized calculation of drug and/or fluid doses facilitates precise equipment sizing and drug dosing.

Rationale

Treatment of infants and children in the out-of-hospital setting is difficult because children of different ages require different sizes of equipment, doses of medications, and volumes of fluids. Mistakes are common when selecting appropriate equipment and medications in critical pediatric emergencies without the benefit of an accurate weight. Pediatric resuscitation equipment for drug and fluid calculations use weight or length as a valid marker of size-specific equipment and medication needs. These devices are portable, easy to use, and applicable to all out-of-hospital equipment and medications.

Computerized Calculations

Indication
Children requiring equipment, medication, or fluids

Contraindications
None

Equipment

Length-based resuscitation tape
Computerized software specific to pediatric resuscitation

Possible Complications

None

Preparation

Length-Based Resuscitation Tape
1. Place the patient in a supine position.
2. Extend the patient's legs.

Tip

Store the length-based resuscitation tape in a place that is easily accessible, such as the pediatric equipment kit.

Computerized Technology

1. Knowledge of the particular software application for the PDA or computer.
2. After entering the patient's data (weight, length, and/or age), the device will provide equipment information, and drug and fluid calculations specific to the clinical problem.

Tip

Practice using the computerized applications prior to resuscitation events to allow easy use during resuscitation.

Procedure

2-1 Length-Based Resuscitation Tape

1 Measure child's length—from head to heel—with the tape (with the red portion at the head). Note and say weight in kilograms that corresponds to the child's measured length at the heel. If the child is longer than the tape, use adult equipment and medication doses. From the tape, identify appropriate equipment sizes. From the tape, identify appropriate medication doses.

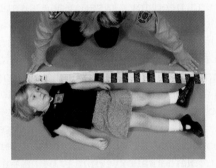

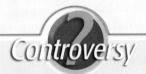

Controversy

There are several different brands of length-based pediatric resuscitation tapes; these have not been compared for speed, accuracy, or safety.

Blip

Measuring to the child's toes (instead of heel) will add a number of kg to the estimated weight and may result in equipment sizes that are too large or excessive drug doses.

Procedure

2-2 Pediatric Resuscitation Software

1 Enter the child's length into the software program, then select the clinical condition or type of resuscitation. The software will calculate the equipment size and drug dose for the child's size and present the information in a flow algorithm.

Procedure 3: Oxygen Delivery

Introduction

Hypoxia in the infant or child causes cardiopulmonary distress and may lead to organ failure. Careful assessment of the child's cardiopulmonary status includes standard physical assessment techniques and pulse oximetry. A normal room air pulse oximetry reading is 95% or greater. A pulse oximetry value of less than 95% on room air is an indication for supplemental oxygen. A value less than 90% with the child on 100% oxygen is also an indication for ventilatory support. Acute hypoxia is usually easy to treat. Rapid intervention may slow or reverse cardiopulmonary distress or failure and avoid the need for ventilatory support. While respiratory disease is usually the cause of hypoxia in children, other conditions such as hypovolemic shock, severe poisonings, or seizures may also produce hypoxia from ischemia or inadequate ventilation.

There are different procedures for giving oxygen to children that vary the amount of actual oxygen supplementation. Use an oxygen delivery technique that matches the child's clinical condition, age, and need for oxygen. For example, give oxygen by nasal cannula or simple mask to the child in no or mild distress who has an open airway. Give oxygen via a nonrebreathing mask or bag-mask device to the child with moderate to severe respiratory distress. Rarely, a critical child requires endotracheal intubation for positive pressure ventilation and oxygen administration. When supplemental oxygen does not improve the child's condition, consider other complicating factors, such as a pulmonary disorder (such as pneumonia), a circulatory disorder (such as hypovolemic shock), or, rarely, a toxicologic disorder (such as carbon monoxide poisoning).

Be creative in delivering oxygen to young children. Under some circumstances, giving blow-by oxygen may avoid agitating the child and increasing his distress. In the newly born be careful about oxygen delivery, because it is unnecessary if the child has a normal pulse oximetry and supplemental oxygen may be harmful to the immature brain.

Indications

Respiratory distress
Pulse oximetry less than 95% on room air
Respiratory failure
Partial upper airway obstruction
Partial lower airway obstruction
Worsening of chronic lung disease
Status epilepticus
Overdose
Shock from any cause
Multiple trauma
Any condition possibly causing decreased oxygen delivery to tissues
Smoke inhalation
Carbon monoxide poisoning

Contraindications

There are few absolute contraindications to oxygen delivery to a child who may be hypoxic. There are, however, rare relative contraindications to certain oxygen delivery techniques that do not match the child's clinical condition. For example, oxygen delivery by a nonrebreathing mask may be relatively contraindicated in a child with a mild worsening of chronic lung disease (e.g., **cystic fibrosis**, bronchopulmonary **dysplasia**) who depends on hypoxia for ventilatory drive. Oxygen has proper doses and routes of administration for maximum benefit, minimum toxicity, optimal feasibility, and reasonable cost.

Rationale

A child's immature anatomy and physiology make respiratory distress and failure common pediatric emergencies. When apnea or hypoventilation occurs, hypoxia develops quickly. Therefore, give oxygen to any child with clinical signs of cardiopulmonary distress or failure, or with a history suggesting possible abnormalities in gas exchange. *Children seldom have a condition where excess oxygen turns off their respiratory drive, so it is better to overtreat with oxygen than to undertreat.*

The appropriate oxygen delivery technique is based on the child's condition, age, and need for oxygen.

Preparation

1. Connect the pressure regulator and flow meter to the oxygen source. Turn on the tank.
2. Match the correct oxygen delivery device with the patient assessment (child's condition, age, and need for oxygen; **Table P3-1**).

Equipment

Infant and pediatric nasal cannula
Pediatric mask sizes
Pediatric nonrebreathing mask
Oxygen connecting tubing
Oxygen source

Possible Complications

Injury, if the pressurized tank is punctured or a valve breaks off

Potential for fire, because oxygen supports combustion

Respiratory arrest if high concentrations of oxygen are given to the child with chronic lung disease (rare)

Agitation and worsening of hypoxia, if delivery technique is overly aggressive

Hypothermia in an infant under 6 months of age with an endotracheal tube in place, who receives cool, unhumidified oxygen for more than 30 minutes

In newly borns with normal pulse, brain injury may occur because of unnecessary supplemental oxygen

Table P3-1	Oxygen Delivery Technique and Patient Assessment			
Device	**Flow Rate**	**Concentration Delivered**	**Considerations**	
Nasal cannula	1 to 6 L/min	Up to 44%	Low-flow system Least restrictive Slowly start flow of oxygen after cannula is secured to avoid frightening child May help to tape cannula to child's cheeks Use in infants who are obligatory nose breathers or if there is difficulty in obtaining a correctly sized mask	
Simple mask	6 to 10 L/min	35% to 60%	Low-flow system Infant, pediatric, and adult sized masks are available Use minimum flow rate to flush the mask	
Nonrebreathing mask	12 to 15 L/min	60% to 90%	High-flow system Consists of face mask and reservoir bag with a valve on the exhalation mask port to prevent drawing in room air during inhalation and a valve between the reservoir bag and mask to prevent exhalation of air into the reservoir bag Use in spontaneously breathing patients who require highest concentration of oxygen available (children with respiratory distress and shock) Make sure the flow rate keeps the reservoir bag inflated With a snug fit, delivers highest oxygen concentration available by mask Pediatric and adult masks are available Partial rebreather masks are indicated in neonates and infants who cannot overcome valve resistance	
Blow-by	6 to 10 L/min	Depends on flow rate and proximity to face	Indicated for infant or young child requiring oxygen who will not tolerate mask on the face Start oxygen flow through simple mask, corrugated tubing, or oxygen tubing threaded through the bottom of a cup Hold the delivery device as close to the child's nose and mouth as tolerated	

Reprinted with permission from: Emergency Nurses Association. Respiratory distress and failure. Adapted from *Emergency Nursing Pediatric Course, Provider Manual.* Park Ridge, IL; 1999.

Do not give oxygen to a newly born who is not hypoxic. It may cause brain injury in immature patients.

An oxygen mask may frighten a child.

Do not force the child to lie down because it may increase the child's anxiety and agitation.

Procedure

3-1 Oxygen Delivery

1 Explain to the child and family why oxygen is needed and how the device works. Use developmentally appropriate language. **Table P3-2** suggests methods to ease anxiety in the child who does not want to cooperate with oxygen delivery. For blow-by oxygen using a paper cup, punch a hole in the bottom of the cup and insert the tubing through the hole. Placing stickers on the cup or drawing smiley faces may decrease the child's anxiety.

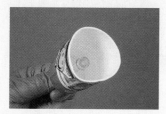

2 Allow the child to remain in a position of comfort, which may be sitting on the caregiver's lap. In the ambulance, the child must be safely restrained.

3 To apply a mask, select the correct size. The mask should extend from the bridge of the nose to the cleft of the chin. Avoid placing pressure on the eyes.

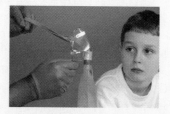

4 Place the mask over the child's head, starting from the nose downward. Squeeze the nose clip and adjust the head strap.

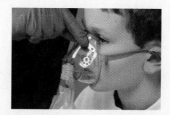

5 To apply a nasal cannula, curve the plastic prongs back into the nostrils. Loop the tubing around the ears.

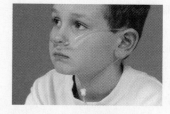

6 For blow-by oxygen, instruct the caregiver to hold the tubing or paper cup close to the child's face to maximize oxygen delivery.

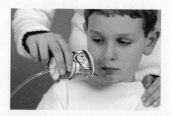

Table P3-2	Methods to Gain Child's Cooperation for Oxygen Delivery

Allow the child to hold the mask prior to placing it on his face.

Allow the child to feel the flow of oxygen prior to placing the mask on his face.

Describe the mask in appealing terms, such as a space mask or Santa Claus beard.

If the child struggles, consider using the blow-by technique to avoid agitation and increasing the oxygen demands. Placing stickers or drawing smiley faces on the cup may decrease the child's anxiety.

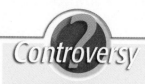

Controversy

The amount of oxygen to give routinely to children with chronic lung disease is unknown and probably differs for each individual. In some children, oxygen delivery may have the unexpected effect of worsening hypoxia. If the child has a history and assessment suggesting acute hypoxia and increased work of breathing, give oxygen but be ready to assist ventilation with a bag-mask device.

Procedure 4: Suctioning

Introduction

Children of all ages are prone to airway obstruction from secretions, vomitus, pus, blood, edema, and foreign bodies. In newly borns, airway obstruction from amniotic fluid, meconium, and blood is a common and potentially critical problem that is usually treatable with suction alone. In infancy and childhood, conditions such as closed head injury or status epilepticus may cause the loss of airway protective reflexes, and put the child at risk for loss of airway patency from aspiration or airway obstruction. Children needing endotracheal intubation often have diseases or trauma associated with fluid in the endotracheal tube, airways, or air sacs; this fluid must be removed to ensure adequate oxygenation and ventilation. Children with tracheostomy tubes may get fluids or foreign bodies in the tubes, which must be evacuated.

Indications
All newly borns
Infants or children with fluids or foreign bodies in the **nasopharynx** or **oropharynx**
Intubated patients with fluids or foreign bodies in the tubes
Patients with tracheostomy tubes with fluids or foreign bodies in the tubes

Contraindications
Children with complete airway obstruction and suspected airway foreign body, prior to seeing the airway with laryngoscopy
Intubated children with increased intracranial pressure and approaching herniation

Equipment
Bulb syringes, one- and two-piece types
Endotracheal tube suction catheters, sizes 8 to 12 French
Feeding tubes, size 5 or 7 for small infants
Large-bore rigid suction catheter

Rationale

Suctioning is a basic technique to maintain an open airway. Children have tiny airways that are easily obstructed. The type of suction device and suctioning procedure to use depends on the child's age and clinical problem (**Table P4-1**). Bulb syringes remove thin secretions from newly borns or infants, but do not permit deep suctioning. Suction catheters remove thin secretions from the mouth, nose, or throat, and are useful in all age groups. Suction catheters are also necessary for endotracheal tube suctioning. Large-bore rigid suction catheters are useful in infants and children (not newly borns) to remove thick secretions, vomitus, pus, blood, or particulate matter from the mouth.

Table P4-1	Suction Technique Based on Age and Type of Obstructing Material
Newly borns	Bulb syringe or suction catheter
Infants and children with thin secretions	Bulb syringe or suction catheter
Newly borns, infants, and children with endotracheal tube	Suction catheter
Infants and children with thick secretions or particulate matter	Large-bore suction catheter

Preparation

1. Select an appropriate suction device based on clinical condition or type of obstruction and age. If there is no functioning negative pressure or suction source (vacuum outlet, battery-powered or electric portable suction, or hand-powered portable suction), use a bulb syringe for thin secretions.
2. Make sure the suction device is operational.
3. Determine correct catheter size with the pediatric resuscitation tape. The suction catheter should be smaller than the nostril.
4. Open catheter package.
5. Connect suction tubing or rigid suction catheter to connecting tubing and suction source.
6. Set suction force to maximum (80–120 mm Hg).
7. Maintain sterile technique.

Possible Complications

Injury to the mouth, airway, or lung
Gagging, vomiting
Aspiration of stomach contents
Hypoxia from prolonged suctioning
Pushing foreign body into trachea with suction device
Increased intracranial pressure

Procedure

4-1 Oro/Nasopharyngeal Suctioning with Bulb Syringe

1 Squeeze the bulb away from the infant to remove air. Suction the mouth, then the nose.

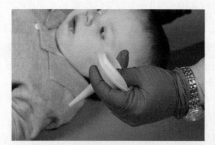

2 Open the mouth and insert the syringe tip at the side of the mouth, and then advance the syringe to remove thin secretions. Avoid inserting the syringe tip into the deeper soft tissues at the back of the mouth. Do not use a two-piece bulb syringe in the mouth because it may come apart.

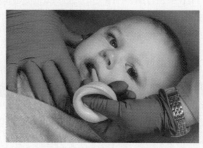

3 Lift the nostril slightly and suction the nose. Insert the syringe tip straight back into the nostril or at a right angle to the face.

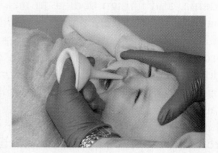

Procedure

4-2 Oro/Nasopharyngeal Suctioning with Suction Catheter

1 Suction the mouth, then the nose. Open the mouth and advance until the tip touches secretions.

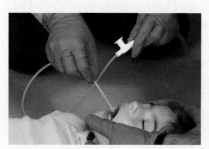

2 Block the side port and begin suctioning. Do not do deep suctioning beyond what is in direct vision. Remove catheter with twisting motion.

3 Insert the catheter into the nostril.

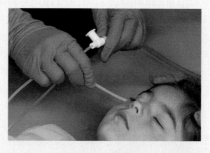

4 Block the side port to begin suctioning when the tip touches secretions. Remove the catheter with a twisting motion. Never suction longer than 5 seconds.

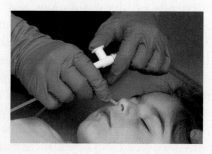

Tip

In suspected foreign body aspiration, look at the airway prior to suctioning.

Blip

Do not suction beyond your direct vision to avoid causing gagging, vomiting, and possible aspiration.

Tip

Suction for less than 5 seconds, but use enough time to remove secretions.

Procedure

4-3 Tracheal Tube Suctioning with Suction Catheter

① Ask partner to pre-oxygenate the patient 5 to 6 times with a bag-mask device using 100% oxygen.

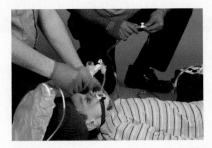

② With thumb off the side port, insert suction catheter through endotracheal tube and down the trachea until resistance is met.

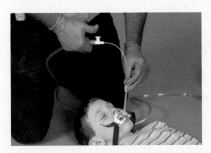

③ Apply suction off and on by placing thumb over the side port while withdrawing and twisting catheter (maximum 5 seconds).

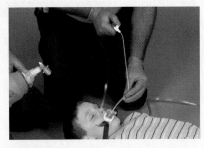

④ Irrigate catheter with normal saline.

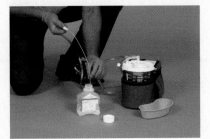

⑤ Ask partner to hyperoxygenate 5 to 6 times. Repeat, as necessary.

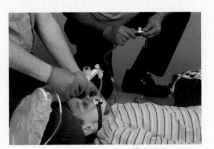

Procedure

4-4 Oropharyngeal Suctioning with Large-bore Rigid Suction Catheter

① Open the mouth and advance catheter until it touches secretions.

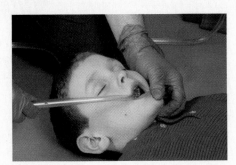

② Close the side port or turn on suction to begin suctioning. Remove the catheter with a twisting motion. Do not suction more than 5 seconds.

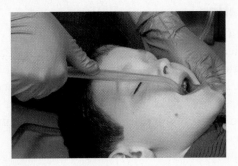

Procedure 5: Airway Adjuncts

Introduction

An oropharyngeal (OP) or nasopharyngeal (NP) airway **adjunct** is often helpful to maintain an open airway for optimal ventilation. Sizing is important, as improperly-sized OP or NP airways may cause further obstruction. The prehospital professional must know when to use an OP or NP airway adjunct, how to determine the proper size, and how to insert the adjunct safely and effectively.

Indications
Respiratory insufficiency
Airway obstruction
Seizures

Contraindications
OP airway
Conscious patient with gag reflex
Unconscious patient who may have ingested a caustic or petroleum product
NP airway
Age less than 1 year
Nasal obstruction
Possible basilar skull fracture
Major **nasofacial** trauma

Equipment
Nasopharyngeal airways
Oropharyngeal airways

Rationale

Opening the airway of a small infant or child by positioning alone, with the head-tilt/chin-lift maneuvers or jaw thrust, may not keep the tongue from obstructing the airway. Adequate ventilation often requires placement of airway adjuncts. They are easy to insert and may markedly improve airway patency. Adjuncts may immediately improve the child's spontaneous ventilation. In addition, they may allow more effective bag-mask ventilation, reduce gastric inflation, and avert the need for endotracheal intubation.

Preparation

1. Position patient's airway:
   Medical patient
   - Perform the head-tilt/chin-lift maneuver to open the airway. Avoid **hyperextension** of the neck because it may cause airway obstruction.
   - Use a towel under the shoulders of an infant or small child to get neutral airway position.
   Trauma patient
   - Use the modified jaw thrust maneuver with in-line spinal stabilization to open the airway.

2. Select the properly sized adjunct:
   OP Airway
   - Use resuscitation tape or refer to resuscitation software (see Procedure 2) OR
   - Measure the device on the patient:
     ○ Place OP airway next to face with the **flange** at the level of the central **incisors**, and the bite block segment parallel to the hard **palate**.
     ○ The tip of the appropriate-sized OP airway should reach the angle of the jaw.
   NP Airway
   - Use resuscitation tape or refer to resuscitation software (see Procedure 2) OR
   - Measure the device on the patient:
     ○ The outside diameter of the NP airway should be less than the diameter of the nostril.
     ○ Place the NP airway next to the face and measure from the tip of the nose to the **tragus** of the ear.
     ○ Adjust movable flange (if present) up or down to get appropriate length.

> **Tip**
>
> An NP airway is useful in maintaining an open airway during an active seizure.

Procedure

5-1 OP Airway Insertion

1 Depress tongue with a tongue blade (if available). Place OP airway down into mouth until flange rests against lips.

2 If a tongue blade is not available, point the OP airway tip toward the roof of the mouth and depress the tongue with the curved part of the OP airway (do not scrape the palate).

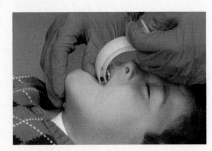

3 Insert OP airway until flange is against lips; gently rotate 180 degrees into position. Flange should be resting against lips.

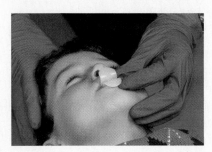

Procedure

5-2 NP Airway Insertion

1 Lubricate NP airway.

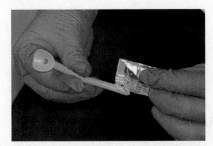

2 Insert with **bevel** toward **septum** (center of nose).

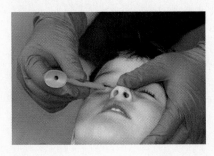

3 Advance tip along floor of nasal cavity.

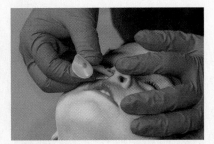

4 If using the right nostril, advance until flange is seated against outside of nostril. The tip should be in the nasopharynx.

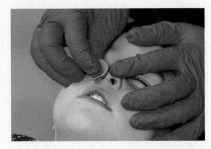

5 If using the left nostril, begin inserting the airway with the curvature upward until resistance is felt (about 2 cm), and then rotate the device 180 degrees and advance until flange is against outside of nostril.

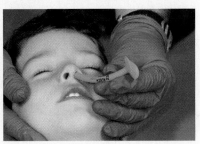

Possible Complications

OP Airway

If OP airway is too small, the tongue may get pushed back into the pharynx, obstructing the airway

If OP airway is too large, it may obstruct the larynx

Pharyngeal bleeding

Laryngospasm

Vomiting

NP Airway

Adenoidal tissue laceration

Pharyngeal bleeding

Obstruction of tube with fluids or soft tissues, causing airway obstruction

If an NP airway is too long, vagal stimulation or esophageal entry with gastric distention may occur

Laryngospasm

Vomiting

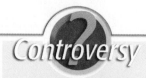

Controversy

The use of airway adjuncts in facial trauma is controversial. If the child has an open fracture of the craniofacial bones, the device could penetrate into the brain and cause further brain injury or hemorrhage. The devices must be used cautiously or not at all in the setting of severe bone injury.

Blip

Never attempt to insert an OP airway in a conscious child.

Blip

Do not insert an OP airway that is too small, or it will push the tongue back and obstruct the airway.

Procedure 6: Foreign Body Obstruction

Introduction

Foreign body obstruction of the airway is a common cause of hypoxic brain injury and death in toddlers and preschool children, who place objects in their mouths as part of the exploratory behavior normal for patients in these age groups. The infant or child with a completely obstructed airway poses the ultimate medical challenge because a moment's delay can be devastating or fatal. When treating a patient with foreign body obstruction, it is important to begin with basic maneuvers to clear the airway, but sometimes more advanced techniques are necessary.

Indications
Complete airway obstruction
Severe partial airway obstruction and respiratory failure

Contraindication
Partial airway obstruction with maintenance of the airway

Equipment
Laryngoscope and straight blades (Miller sizes 1 and 2)
Pediatric Magill forceps
Bag-mask devices (infant and pediatric)

Rationale

In the setting of complete airway obstruction, prehospital professionals can make the difference between life and death. Immediate removal of an airway foreign body can often be achieved using basic life support (BLS) procedures, yet every year many children suffer grave injury and death because of failure to use basic clearance maneuvers. Sometimes, the foreign body is deeper in the airway or embedded in tissue, so that basic maneuvers are unsuccessful. In such cases, using Magill forceps and direct laryngoscopy may be the best option for removal.

Preparation

1. Attempt BLS maneuvers first (see Procedure 6-1).
2. Move to advanced life support (ALS) maneuvers if BLS maneuvers fail.

3. Attach appropriately-sized straight blade to laryngoscope handle.
4. Ensure light is working on laryngoscope blade.

Possible Complications

Hypoxia
Foreign body is pushed farther into airway
Laryngeal and tracheal injury
Teeth and mouth injury

Blip

Do not perform blind finger sweeps, which may push the foreign body further into the airway.

Procedure

6-1 BLS Maneuvers

1 Open airway with the head-tilt/chin-lift or modified jaw thrust maneuver. Attempt to ventilate.

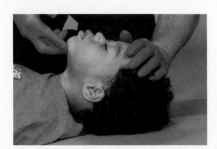

2 Use obstructed airway maneuvers appropriate for age. Younger than 1 year: Give 5 back blows with the infant in a prone position, then 5 chest thrusts with the infant in a supine position. Reassess, repeat. Older than 1 year: Give 5 abdominal thrusts with the child supine.

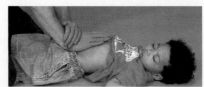

3 If the foreign body is visible, remove it. Do not use blind finger sweeps.

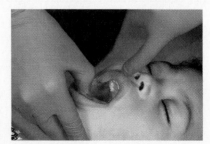

Procedure

6-2 Laryngoscopy and Magill Forceps

1 Grasp laryngoscope handle. Hold laryngoscope in left hand. Use trigger-finger technique.

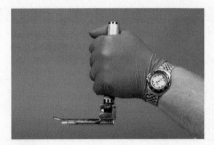

2 Open mouth by using thumb pressure on chin. Insert pediatric straight laryngoscope blade into mouth.

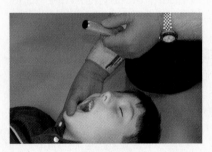

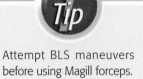

Attempt BLS maneuvers before using Magill forceps.

3 Lift tongue with blade. Exert gentle traction upward along the axis of the laryngoscope handle at a 45-degree angle. Do not use teeth or gums for leverage. Advance blade. Watch the tip until foreign body is visible. Do not go past vocal cords. Use suction to improve visibility and maintain airway.

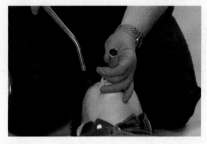

4 Grasp closed Magill forceps in right hand, palm down. Insert Magill forceps into mouth, tips closed. Open forceps and move tips around foreign body. Grasp foreign body and remove while looking directly at it. Look at the airway and make sure it is clear of foreign bodies or debris. Remove laryngoscope blade. After removal of foreign body, reassess respiratory status. Use suction if needed. Attempt to ventilate if the child does not breathe spontaneously. Return to BLS maneuvers if no foreign body is seen by direct laryngoscopy.

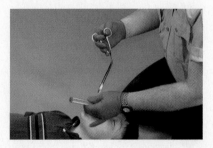

Suctioning may push the foreign body farther into the airway, so look at the airway before suctioning.

Repeat BLS procedures if no foreign body is seen by direct laryngoscopy.

Controversy

There is no universal procedure to maintain airway patency after removal of an airway foreign body. Each case is unique. Endotracheal intubation may not be necessary if the child is breathing effectively without stridor at rest.

Procedure 7: Bronchodilator Therapy

Introduction

Wheezing from bronchospasm is one of the most common out-of-hospital pediatric problems. Children who are wheezing are usually in acute respiratory distress and are often anxious, agitated, and uncooperative. The prehospital professional must use a developmentally appropriate approach with both the child and the caregiver when giving general noninvasive respiratory care and using bronchodilator medications. The caregiver can help by holding, soothing, and supporting a scared child. One way to give aerosolized bronchodilators is with an oxygen-powered nebulizer. Another way is the metered dose inhaler (MDI), although this inhalation technique has not been studied in the out-of-hospital setting. If the child is uncooperative or unable to use inhaled bronchodilator therapy, subcutaneous (SQ) drug delivery is another possibility.

Indication
Wheezing

Contraindication
Known sensitivity to bronchodilator drugs

Equipment
Inhalation therapy (nebulizer)
  An oxygen-powered nebulizer that aerosolizes the liquid bronchodilator to small particle size that can reach the alveoli
  Oxygen source
  Mask or mouthpiece with liquid reservoir
  Bronchodilator drugs
    Albuterol solution (1.25 mg/3mL, 2.5 mg/3 mL, 5 mg/mL solution for inhalation)
    Other inhaled bronchodilators include terbutaline, metaproterenol, and isoetharine

Inhalation therapy (MDI)
  MDI, mask and **spacer**
  Bronchodilator drugs
    Albuterol MDI (90 μg/puff)

Subcutaneous therapy
  Tuberculin (TB) or 3-mL syringe
  25- or 27-gauge needle
  Bronchodilator drugs
    Epinephrine (1:1,000)
    Another injectable bronchodilator is terbutaline

Rationale

Early bronchodilator therapy, on the scene and on the way to the ED, helps immediately open airways, relieve respiratory distress, and improve oxygen delivery. Inflammation and edema of small airways develop quickly if wheezing and bronchospasm are untreated. Early bronchodilator therapy may reduce the need for more aggressive hospital therapy, shorten ED and hospital times, and decrease chances of complications or death. *Continuous inhalation treatment with a nebulized beta agonist is the best initial approach with severe wheezing and respiratory distress.*

Preparation

Inhalation Therapy

1. Have the caregiver hold the child on his lap. An older child can sit alone.
2. Have the child in an upright position of comfort.

3. Explain what is happening. Most children need only inhalation bronchodilator therapy by oxygen-powered nebulizer or with an MDI.

Subcutaneous Therapy

1. Position the child on the caregiver's lap or straddling the caregiver's leg.
2. Expose the thigh or **deltoid** area for injection (see Procedure 14, Intramuscular and Subcutaneous Injections).

Possible Complications

Anxiety	Palpitations
Dizziness	Restlessness
Dysrhythmias	Tachycardia
Headache	Tremors
Hypertension	Vomiting
Nausea	

Procedure

7-1 Inhalation Therapy

1 If the child can cooperate, deliver nebulized bronchodilator through a mouthpiece. Alternatively, nebulize the bronchodilator and have the caregiver hold the mask to the child's face. Tape two tongue blades together to make a nose clip to help breathing through the mouthpiece.

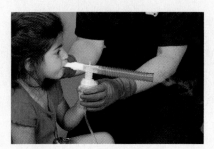

2 If an MDI is used, attach spacer and mask when the child is too young or unable to trigger aerosol effectively. Monitor respiratory rate, heart rate, and pulse oximetry during therapy.

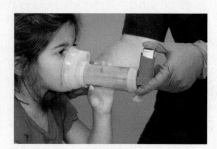

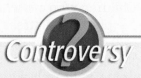

Controversy

The role of the MDI in out-of-hospital bronchodilator therapy is not known. While ED studies have shown that the MDI is as effective as inhaled drugs for most children, and it has not been studied in the out-of-hospital setting. MDI with mask and spacer, however, can probably deliver an adequate bronchodilator dose to most children older than 6 months of age.

Tip

Use bronchodilators for all infants and children who are wheezing from any cause.

Procedure

7-2 Subcutaneous Therapy

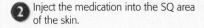

1 If the child cannot cooperate with inhalation therapy, give epinephrine by SQ injection. Use one of two anatomic locations: lateral aspect of deltoid in upper arms (older child) and anterior thigh.

2 Inject the medication into the SQ area of the skin.

Tip

Give an uncooperative child subcutaneous epinephrine.

Blip

Avoid injectable drugs in cooperative, wheezing patients. The procedure is painful and is no more effective than inhaled bronchodilators.

Procedure 8: Bag-Mask Ventilation

Introduction

Bag-mask ventilation is a highly effective way to deliver assisted ventilation to a child in respiratory failure. Oxygen at 60–95% concentration can be given safely by choosing a well-fitted mask, connecting the oxygen reservoir to a supplemental oxygen source at 15 L/min, disabling the pop-off valve, and ventilating at an age-appropriate rate.

Indications
Apnea or respiratory arrest
Respiratory failure
Cyanosis
Oxygen saturation (SaO_2) less than 90% despite administration of 100% oxygen by nonrebreathing mask

Contraindication
Complete airway obstruction

Equipment
Transparent masks with inflatable rim, sizes neonate through adult
Self-inflating resuscitator (bag), at least 450 mL volume

Rationale

Assisted ventilation is a way to oxygenate and ventilate a child who is unable to breathe adequately on his own. While the technique does not provide the definitive airway control that endotracheal intubation does, in many cases bag-mask ventilation will be the best technique for assisting ventilation during resuscitation and transport. Effective bag-mask ventilation is one of the prehospital professional's most useful skills in pediatric out-of-hospital care.

Preparation

1. Measure the mask on the patient. The mask should extend from the bridge of nose to the cleft of the chin, avoiding compression of the eyes. The right sized mask will have a small volume to minimize dead space and to prevent rebreathing of expired carbon dioxide. Transparency allows the rescuer to observe the child for cyanosis of the lips and for emesis.

2. Select an appropriate resuscitator bag. While a small child can be safely and effectively ventilated using a big bag, a small bag will not work for a large child. Pediatric tidal volume is approximately 8 mL/kg. The bag should have a volume of 450 to 750 mL. An adult bag (1200 mL) is acceptable for larger children or adolescents.

3. If a pop-off valve is present, it may need to be disabled to permit higher inspiratory pressures and achieve chest rise.

4. Connect one end of oxygen tubing to the oxygen device and the other end to the flow meter, set to 15 L/min.

Possible Complications

Hypoxia
Barotrauma
Gastric distention
Emesis and aspiration

Procedure

8-1 Bag-Mask Ventilation

1 Open airway. *Medical patient:* Use head-tilt/chin-lift maneuver. *Trauma patient:* Use jaw thrust with in-line manual stabilization.

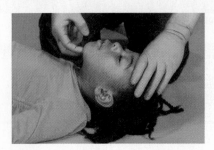

2 Ensure neutral positioning (sniffing position). Because infants and toddlers have large heads, place a small roll under the shoulders to achieve the sniffing position. Avoid hyperextension of the neck because this may cause airway obstruction or spinal injury.

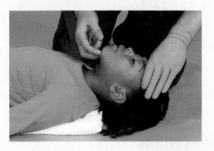

3 Insert appropriate airway adjunct if airway patency cannot be maintained with the head-tilt/chin-lift or jaw thrust maneuvers (see Procedure 4, Airway Adjuncts). Use an oropharyngeal (OP) airway if the patient does not have a gag reflex, or use a nasopharyngeal (NP) airway if the patient is older than 1 year of age and has an active gag reflex.

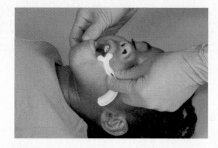

4 Begin ventilation.

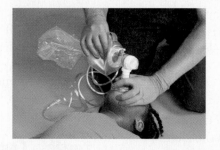

Blip

Avoid hyperextension of the neck, which may cause airway obstruction or spinal injury.

Tip

Use an OP or NP airway with the bag-mask device.

Procedure

8-2 Bag-Mask Ventilation Using One-rescuer Technique

1 Apply the mask to the face and get an airtight seal using the E-C clamp technique.

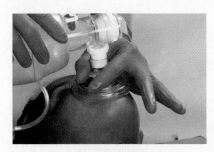

> **Tip**
>
> Pull the jaw into the mask, instead of pushing the mask into the face.

> **Tip**
>
> Seeing the chest rise is the best indicator of adequate tidal volume.

2 Pull the child's jaw into the mask, instead of pushing the mask into the face, to establish a seal. Failure to provide a tight seal may result in delivery of lower oxygen concentrations or an inadequate volume of air. Avoid placing pressure on soft tissues under the chin because this may compress the airway. Squeeze bag with the dominant hand, watching for chest rise. Squeeze the bag only until the chest rise is visible, then release. Say, "Squeeze, release, release" during ventilation to achieve the correct inspiratory volume and to allow for expiration. Child: 20 squeezes/minute. Infant: 30 squeezes/minute.

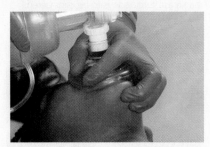

3 Assess effectiveness of ventilation. Look for adequate bilateral rise and fall of chest. Auscultate for lung sounds at the midaxillary line bilaterally. Monitor oxygen saturation.

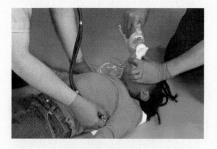

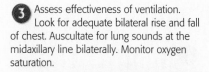

> **Controversy?**
>
> The relative value of bag-mask ventilation versus endotracheal intubation in respiratory failure is not known. Bag-mask ventilation may be as good as endotracheal tube ventilation in the out-of-hospital setting in children with acute illness or injury.

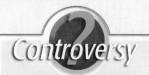

Procedure

8-3 Bag-Mask Ventilation Using Two-rescuer Technique

The two-rescuer technique is preferable in trauma patients or if the one-rescuer technique does not create an effective seal.

1 Rescuer applies the mask to the face and maintains a seal. *Medical patient:* Hold the mask to the face with the thumb and index fingers of both hands; use the other fingers to perform a chin lift (bilateral E-C clamp technique). *Trauma patient:* Perform a jaw thrust maneuver, lifting the jaw into the mask with both hands, while maintaining in-line manual stabilization.

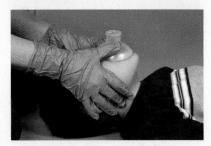

2 Pull the child's jaw into the mask, instead of pushing the mask into the face, to establish a seal. Avoid placing pressure on soft tissues under the chin because this may compress the airway.

3 Second rescuer ventilates. Avoid gastric distention. Watch the abdomen for signs of enlargement during ventilation. If this happens, reposition the airway and observe the chest rise carefully, squeezing the bag only until the chest starts to rise. If bag-mask ventilation is to be considered during transport, consider placement of an orogastric or nasogastric tube for gastric decompression.

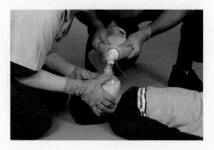

Tip

The two-rescuer technique is preferable in a trauma patient or if the one-rescuer technique does not get a good seal.

Blip

A bag less than 450 mL will not generate enough inspiratory pressure to ventilate a large child.

Procedure 9: Pulse Oximetry

Introduction

Pulse oximetry, which measures oxygenation and the pulse rate, can be a useful adjunct in the management of the ill or injured child. Use of the pulse oximeter does not replace clinical assessment of the child. Monitoring changes in pulse oximetry readings may help the prehospital professional to determine the patient's response to interventions and guide additional interventions.

There are caveats, however. Where there is suspected carbon monoxide (CO) poisoning, do not use pulse oximetry. The probe detects gaseous saturation of the hemoglobin molecule and does not discriminate between oxygen and carbon monoxide. A child with CO poisoning may have a pulse oximetry reading of 100% and be hypoxic. If the child is in shock, inadequate circulating red blood cells may have such low flow states that the pulse oximeter probe will be unable to sense flow, resulting in an inability to obtain a reading or waveform.

Indication
Need for oxygen therapy
Respiratory distress
Hypoxia
Major trauma
Other clinical conditions

Contraindication
Suspected carbon monoxide poisoning

Equipment
Pulse oximeter probes in sizes for newborns, infants, and children
Monitoring cable and pulse oximetry monitoring device

Relative Contraindications
Poor perfusion and/or anemia
Shock

Preparation

1. Prepare the child for application of the pulse oximeter probe. This may be explained as being similar to putting on a band-aid.

Possible Complications

Using incorrect probe placement
Poor perfusion with poor tracing or wave form
Inability to obtain a SpO_2 reading

Procedure

9-1 Pulse Oximetry

1 Obtain equipment in the appropriate size. Place probe on a fingertip, toe, earlobe, or forehead as indicated on the manufacturer's instructions.

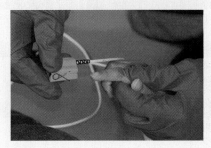

2 Connect the probe to the monitoring cable. Some portable monitoring devices have a reusable probe that has a spring-loaded clip for use only on a fingertip or toe. Note oxygen saturation (SpO_2) and document. If the monitoring device being used shows a waveform, observe for correlation with heart rate.

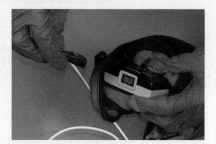

Tip

Use pulse oximetry in the primary assessment of every acutely ill or injured child.

Blip

Be careful not to overestimate oxygenation if the pulse oximetry is normal. If there is increased work of breathing or significantly increased respiratory rate, the child may be hypoxic but compensating.

Procedure 10: Orogastric and Nasogastric Tube Insertion

Introduction

Gastric tube insertion has many purposes, such as cleaning out the stomach and giving activated charcoal after a toxic ingestion, evaluation and treatment of gastrointestinal hemorrhage, and gastric **decompression** in cases of **bowel** obstruction or distention from assisted ventilation. In the out-of-hospital setting, gastric tube insertion has only one indication: decompression of the stomach during assisted ventilation. The tube may be placed into the stomach through the nose (nasogastric [NG] insertion) or through the mouth (orogastric [OG] insertion).

Indication

Abdominal distention associated with assisted ventilation

Contraindications

NG and OG insertion

Unconscious child with poor or no gag reflex and unsecured airway: In this case, do endotracheal intubation first to decrease risk of vomiting and aspiration.

Caustic ingestions: In a child who has ingested a caustic substance, there is a risk of esophageal damage with passage of the tube.

NG insertion

Perform OG insertion to avoid intracranial passage of the NG tube when the child has any of the following findings: severe head or facial trauma, as indicated by **midfacial** injuries, nasal bleeding, or clear nasal secretions.

Infants with nostrils too small to accommodate the tube: OG insertion is preferred for infants younger than 6 months of age.

Equipment

Gastric tube: A double-lumen sump tube is the best device for removing stomach contents.

30- to 60-mL syringe with funnel-tipped adaptor for manual removal of stomach contents through tube

Mechanical suction

Adhesive tape

Non-petroleum lubricant

Rationale

During assisted ventilation, it is common to inflate the stomach as well as the lungs with air. Gastric inflation with air slows downward movement of the diaphragm and decreases tidal volume, making ventilation more difficult and necessitating higher inspiratory pressures. In addition, inflation of the stomach with air increases the risk that the patient will vomit and aspirate. Gastric tube insertion with a NG or OG tube decompresses the stomach and makes assisted ventilation easier.

Preparation

1. Select the proper size tube. Sizing techniques are outlined in **Table P10-1**.
2. Measure the tube on the patient. The length of the tube should be the same as the distance from the lips or tip of the nose (depending on if the route OG or NG is used) to the left ear PLUS the distance from the left ear to the left upper quadrant of the abdomen, just below the **costal margin**.

3. Mark this length on the tube with a piece of tape. When the tip of the tube is in the stomach, the tape should be at the lips or nostrils.
4. Place the patient in a supine position.
5. Assess the gag reflex. If the patient is unconscious and has a poor or no gag reflex, perform endotracheal intubation before gastric tube insertion.

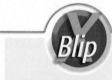

Do not perform gastric intubation on an unconscious patient because she is at risk for aspiration.

6. In a trauma patient:
   - Maintain in-line stabilization of the cervical spine if a neck injury is possible.
   - Choose the orotracheal route if the patient has severe head or facial trauma or has serious midfacial injuries.
7. Lubricate the end of the tube.

Table P10-1	Methods for Determining NG/OG Tube Size

1. Refer to a length-based resuscitation tape or resuscitation software (see Procedure 2).

2. Select a tube size that is the same as the size of the patient's nostril, through which it should pass with minimal resistance.

3. Use a tube size twice the endotracheal (ETT) tube size (a child who needs a 5.0-mm ETT tube needs a 10.0 French NG or OG tube).

Possible Complications

Placement of the tube into the trachea with hypoxia
Vomiting and aspiration of stomach contents
Airway bleeding/obstruction
Passage of tube into brain

Controversy

The value of NG and OG insertion is unproven. Although these procedures are routine in EDs, no studies have tested the benefit of easier ventilation against the potential complications of hypoxia from endotracheal intubation or aspiration of stomach contents.

Procedure

10-1 NG Insertion

1 Pass the tube gently through the nostril, directing the tube straight back. Do not angle the tube superiorly.

2 If the tube does not pass easily, try the opposite nostril, or a smaller tube. Never force the tube. If NG passage is unsuccessful, use the OG approach.

Never use force to pass an NG tube.

Procedure

10-2 OG Insertion

1 Insert the tube over the tongue, using a tongue blade if necessary to help insertion.

2 Advance the tube into the hypopharynx, then insert rapidly into the stomach. If coughing, choking, or change in voice occurs, immediately remove the tube. It may be in the trachea.

Perform OG insertion in infants younger than 6 months of age.

Procedure

10-3 Check Placement of NG or OG Tube

1 Check tube placement by aspirating stomach contents. Use a syringe with appropriate adaptor to quickly instill 10 to 20 mL of air through the tube while auscultating over the left upper quadrant. If there is a rush of air over the stomach region, the placement is correct. If correct placement cannot be verified, remove the tube.

2 Secure the tube to the bridge of the nose or to the cheek, using adhesive tape. Aspirate air from stomach, using a 30- to 60-cc catheter-tipped syringe, or connect to mechanical suction at low, continuous, or intermittent setting.

Talking or crying during the procedure is a good indication that the gastric tube is not in the trachea.

Procedure 11: Endotracheal Intubation

Introduction

Endotracheal intubation is the definitive advanced airway maneuver that is often a life-saving procedure for some critical patients. However, this procedure has important modifications and pitfalls in children. There are several anatomic considerations that make the pediatric airway different from the adult airway:

- The child's vocal cords are more anterior and superior.
- The tongue is larger.
- The mandible and oral cavity are smaller.
- The diameter and length of the trachea are less.
- The soft tissues are more fragile.

Performing the procedure quickly and safely in the field can be tricky. Inappropriate or unsuccessful intubation attempts may result in hypoxia or injury to the child's airway.

Indications

Respiratory or cardiopulmonary arrest
Respiratory failure
Inability to maintain patent airway
Loss of protective airway reflex
Need for prolonged hyperventilation
Need for endotracheal administration of resuscitative medications

Contraindications

Permanent tracheostomy (relative)
Good response to bag-mask ventilation and short transport time (relative)
Anatomic abnormalities that would probably prevent successful intubation (large tongue hematoma, massive facial injuries) (relative)

Rationale

Successful endotracheal tube (ETT) placement allows optimal oxygenation and ventilation, provides a tube for medication delivery, and decreases the risk of aspiration and loss of airway control. A properly placed and secured endotracheal tube is a good tool for managing critical patients, but the procedure can take a long time, and there are frequent and serious complications.

Preparation

1. Make sure oxygen delivery equipment is connected to an oxygen source.
2. Select an appropriately sized ETT (**Tables P11-1 and P11-2**) for oral endotracheal intubation.
3. For a properly selected uncuffed ETT:
   - Allow a minimal air leak. The absence of an air leak may indicate excessive pressure at the cricoid cartilage.
4. For a properly selected cuffed endotracheal tube:
   - For a cuffed ETT tube under size 6 mm, do not test or inflate cuff.
   - For cuffed ETT tube size 6 mm and over, check cuff for leaks, maintaining aseptic technique, as follows:
     ○ Inflate cuff with appropriate volume of air.
     ○ Remove syringe.
     ○ Feel cuff for integrity.
     ○ Deflate cuff.
     ○ Leave syringe with appropriate volume of air attached to the tube.
5. Attach blade to laryngoscope handle, and make sure the light works.
6. Test the large-bore rigid suction catheter.
7. Insert stylet into the ETT, stopping the stylet at least 1 cm from the end of the endotracheal tube.
8. Bend the ETT tube into gentle upward curve. In some cases, bend the tube into the shape of a hockey stick.
9. Lubricate tube with a water-soluble lubricant.
10. Prepare device for confirmation of ETT placement.
11. To predict correct ETT tube position at gum line, either:
    - Check resuscitation tape, refer to computer software, OR
    - Calculate ETT position with formula: gum line position (in cm) = ~3 × tube size
12. Have partner prepare for:
    - ongoing patient assessment
    - providing time counts for ventilation rates
    - watching monitors (heart rate, pulse oximetry)
    - handling suction devices
    - handling ETT

- applying gentle cricoid pressure
- stabilizing neck, if child has possible spinal trauma
13. Position patient (avoid hyperextension or hyperflexion of neck).

- Medical patient: Place the child in the "sniffing" position.
- If spinal trauma is possible: Place the child in neutral position with in-line manual stabilization.

Procedure

11-1 Insert Endotracheal Tube

1 Have partner oxygenate and ventilate patient 5 to 6 times with bag-mask device and 100% oxygen, at a rate of one ventilation every 2 seconds. Say "squeeze, release, release" to reinforce proper rate.

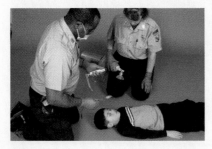

2 Grasp laryngoscope in left hand. Ask partner to stop ventilating and begin timing, giving 20 to 30 second counts.

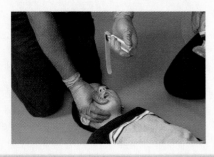

3 Open mouth by applying thumb pressure on chin; remove OP airway if present.

4 Have partner apply gentle cricoid pressure (Sellick maneuver) to prevent gastric reflux.

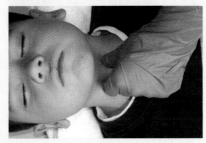

5 Hold laryngoscope in trigger finger position.

6 Insert pediatric straight laryngoscope blade into mouth.

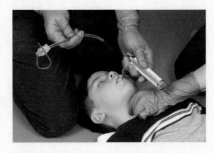

7 Lift tongue with blade.

8 Exert gentle traction upward along the axis of laryngoscope handle at a 45-degree angle. Do not use teeth or gums to gain leverage.

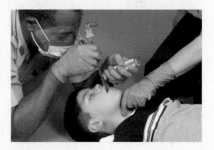

9 Advance blade straight along tongue. Continue looking at blade tip, until tip is just beyond epiglottis.

10 If there is difficulty seeing the vocal cords, you have three options. Advance or retract laryngoscope blade. Modify amount of cricoid pressure (Sellick maneuver). Remove vomitus, blood, other fluids, or particulate matter with rigid, large-bore suction device.

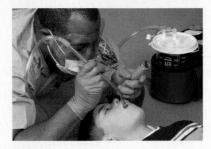

11 If gastric reflux appears near, increase cricoid pressure or stop laryngoscopy attempt.

12 Continue to look at vocal cords and suction.

Procedure

11-1 Insert Endotracheal Tube *(continued)*

13 Remove large solid matter with pediatric Magill forceps.

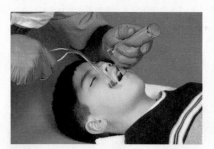

14 Insert ETT. Hold tube in dart-like fashion with right hand and insert tip of tube from right corner of mouth down between vocal cords. Do not insert tube in channel of laryngoscope blade because this blocks the view of the vocal cords. Watch the endotracheal tube go through the vocal cords. Advance tube until vocal cord marker on ETT is situated beyond the vocal cords. Look for centimeter marking on ETT in relation to the gum line.

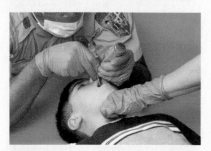

15 Remove laryngoscope blade, holding ETT in place.

16 Remove stylet from ETT.

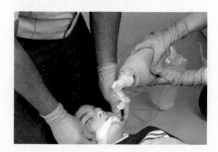

17 Inflate cuff with pilot balloon. (If cuffed ETT tube is under size 6 mm, do not inflate balloon.) If cuff was inflated, remove syringe and check "pilot" balloon for inflation. Maintain tube position by holding ETT against upper lip. If large amount of fluid is evident in ETT, use a suction catheter to clear the airway. Have partner maintain ETT position and ventilate patient with bag-mask device.

18 Record tube position on permanent record. Use centimeter mark at teeth or gum line or mark on ETT with indelible pen.

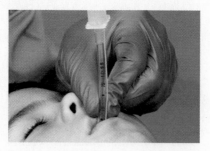

19 Assess correct position in trachea. Do general patient evaluation (appearance, heart rate, pulse oximetry). Look for bilateral chest rise. Make sure there are no bubbling, gurgling sounds in epigastric area indicating air-water interface (check for 2 breaths). Auscultate for bilateral lung sounds at the midaxillary line, third intercostal space (check for 2 breaths on right and then 2 breaths on left). Use device to confirm endotracheal positioning.

20 Secure tube with tape or commercially available endotracheal tube securing device. Reassess proper location of tube and make sure the patient is stable.

Indications for Tube Removal

Immediate Tube Removal

- No chest rise with ventilation.
- Presence of epigastric gurgling sounds.
- Failure to confirm endotracheal placement with detection device.
- Vomitus in ETT.

Blip

Beware of inadequate spinal stabilization during intubation attempts in trauma patients.

Blip

Never assume the endotracheal tube is in the trachea unless you see the tube passing through the vocal cords.

Procedure

11-2 Secure Endotracheal Tube

1 Insert correctly-sized oral airway (see Procedure 5, Airway Adjuncts) and make sure ETT is not compressed. Do not use a bite block in pediatric patients. Carefully hold the ETT in place while the second rescuer secures.

2 In medical patients, one method of securing the ETT is by wrapping the tape around the patient's neck.

3 Bring tape up to opposite side of face and wrap around the tube twice, crimping end of tape so it can be easily removed.

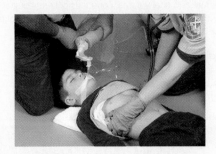

Procedure

11-3 Reconfirm Endotracheal Tube Placement

1 Recheck to make sure there is no bubbling, gurgling noise in epigastric area (air-water interface) for two breaths.

2 Reassess breath sounds bilaterally at the midaxillary line, third intercostal space (two breaths on right and then two breaths on left). Take extra care handling an ETT in a pediatric patient because it can be easily dislodged. Reassess after patient is in ambulance (and after change of position or change in patient status). Report and record findings.

Equipment

Uncuffed endotracheal tubes in pediatric sizes (2.0–5.0, in addition to cuffed adult sizes (6.0–8.0)
Pediatric laryngoscope with fresh batteries
Pediatric laryngoscope blades, curved (sizes 2–4) and straight (sizes 0–4)
Light bulb
Large-bore rigid suction catheter
Suction catheters, sizes 5–12 French
Pediatric stylets
Water-soluble lubricant
Oropharyngeal airways
Pediatric bag-mask device, at least 450 mL volume
Pediatric face masks
Adhesive tape

Commercial endotracheal tube securing devices
Skin adhesive
Pulse oximeter
Oxygen source
Device for confirmation of ETT placement

Possible Complications

Aspiration of stomach contents
Dislodgment of ETT from trachea
Esophageal intubation
Hypoxia
Increased intracranial pressure
Laryngeal, tracheal, pharyngeal, or esophageal injury
Teeth and mouth injury
Vocal cord injury

Procedure

11-4 Extubation

1 Postresuscitation extubation is rarely indicated in the field. All three situations must be present: spontaneous breathing with adequate rate and tidal volume; conscious patient; coughing and gagging with inability to maintain oxygenation and ventilation. Ensure rigid large-bore suction device is functioning.

2 Suction oropharynx.

3 Turn patient on left side.

4 Deflate cuff completely (if cuff is inflated).

5 Remove ETT quickly at end-inspiratory phase, while suctioning.

Table P11-1	Suggested Endotracheal Tube (ETT) and Suction Catheter Sizes	
Age	**ETT Size (mm)**	**Suction Catheter Size (French)**
Premature newborn	2.0–2.5	5
Newborn	3.0–3.5	6–8
6 months	3.5	8
12–18 months	4.0	8
3 years	4.5	8
5 years	5.0	10
6 years	5.5	10
8 years	6.0	10
12 years	6.5	10
16 years	7.0–8.0	12

Tip

Make sure proper equipment is available and functioning prior to intubation attempt.

Maintain gentle cricoid pressure until appropriate tube location is confirmed.

Chest rise is the best indication of correct endotracheal placement of the endotracheal tube.

Always reassess tube location after patient movement or when there is a change in patient status.

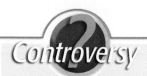

Controversy

The value of performing endotracheal intubation in children in the out-of-hospital setting is controversial. More studies are necessary to define which groups of children will benefit from this procedure, especially in light of the well-known risks of hypoxia, esophageal intubation, tube dislodgment, and airway injury as well as transport delay.

Table P11-2	Selecting Endotracheal Tube Size

Remembering numbers

    Newborns and infants:
        Preterm infants: 2.0- or 2.5-mm tube
        Term newborns or small infants: 3.0- or 3.5-mm tube

    Infants 6–12 months: 3.5-mm tube

    Infants 12–18 months: 4.0-mm tube

    Children >1 year:

OR
Use the resuscitation tape or resuscitation software (see Procedure 2).

OR
The diameter of the tracheal tube is approximately the same size as the child's fingernail on the fifth finger.

$$\text{Size} = \frac{(\text{age in years})}{4} + 4 \text{ (formula for child over 2 years of age)}$$

Procedure 12: Confirmation of Endotracheal Tube Placement

Introduction

Performing pediatric endotracheal intubation in the out-of-hospital setting may be difficult or impossible even for experienced prehospital professionals. Confirming position of the endotracheal tube (ETT) in the trachea is a major challenge because esophageal intubation is a common and dangerous complication of endotracheal intubation. Currently there are four methods to confirm placement of the ETT:

1. Clinical assessment
2. Use of exhaled carbon dioxide detection device
3. Use of digital capnometry
4. Use of esophageal aspiration bulb or syringe

Indication
Endotracheal intubation

Contraindication
An adult carbon dioxide detector device cannot be left in place in a child weighing less than 15 kg

Equipment
Stethoscope
Esophageal detector bulb or syringe OR
Colorimetric end-tidal carbon dioxide detector device

Rationale

A properly positioned ETT makes it possible to effectively oxygenate and ventilate children with critical illnesses or injuries. Esophageal placement of a ETT, on the other hand, is usually harmful or fatal. Moreover, if the child is moved, a correctly placed ETT may easily dislodge from the trachea to the esophagus. Delayed detection may result in hypoxia. Clinical assessment of placement of the ETT is inaccurate, especially in infants and small children. Often, there is a lot of noise in the surrounding area (family members, loud music next door, traffic) that may make it hard to hear breath sounds. Also, breath sounds may be transmitted from the esophagus or stomach throughout the chest of a child and mislead the listener. Fortunately, several mechanical adjuncts are available to supplement clinical assessment and help confirm correct ETT placement in the trachea.

Preparation

1. Intubate the infant or child with a correctly sized ETT (see Procedure 11, Endotracheal Intubation).
2. Determine weight of the patient.
3. Suction any fluid from the ETT.

Esophageal Detector (Aspiration) Bulb or Syringe

1. Remove esophageal detector bulb or syringe from packaging.

Colorimetric Exhaled Carbon Dioxide Detector

1. Determine correct size of the carbon dioxide detector.
   - Use a pediatric device if the child weighs less than 15 kg.
   - Use an adult device if the child weighs 15 kg or more.
   - If an adult device is used on a small child, remove after 6 breaths (initial confirmation of placement).
2. Check the expiration date on the carbon dioxide detector package.
3. Remove the carbon dioxide detector from its packaging.
4. Inspect the carbon dioxide detector prior to use for:
   - bright purple color
   - dryness

Digital Capnometry

1. Place sensor as indicated by manufacturer.
2. Attach sensor probe to monitoring cable.
3. Observe for square waveform that indicates correct ETT placement.
4. Absence of square waveform indicates improperly placed ETT or low exhaled CO_2

Procedure

12-1 Clinical Assessment

1 Look for bilateral rise and fall of the chest. Remove ETT if there is no chest rise with assisted ventilation. Listen for breath sounds over the stomach. If gurgling is present (like a straw in milk), the ETT is in the esophagus. If breath sounds only are present in the stomach, continue your assessment and do not remove the tube unless there is noticeable gastric distention with ventilation.

2 Listen for breath sounds in the right midaxillary line, then in the left midaxillary line. If breath sounds are equal, secure the tube. If breath sounds are greater on the right side than on the left side, then the tube may be in the right mainstem bronchus. Slowly pull back the ETT until breath sounds are equal.

Blip

Do not remove the endotracheal tube just because breath sounds are heard in the stomach. They may be transmitted sounds from the lungs.

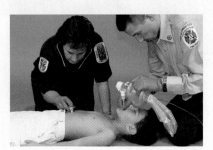
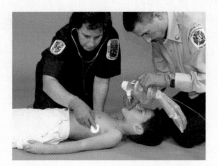

Procedure

12-2 Esophageal Detector Bulb or Syringe

1 Attach the device to the end of the ETT.

2 Aspirate slowly over 3 to 5 seconds. If resistance is felt, then the ETT is in the esophagus. Remove it. If air is aspirated, the ETT is in the trachea. Secure it.

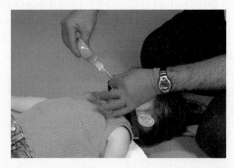
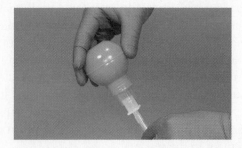

Possible Complications

A faulty device or misinterpretation of results of carbon-dioxide detector or esophageal detector device may result in incorrect endotracheal tube placement or incorrectly removing a ETT that was correctly placed.

Rebreathing carbon dioxide may cause hypercarbia in an infant weighing less than 15 kg if an adult-sized detector is left inline.

Blip

Do not use an esophageal detector bulb or syringe if the child weighs less than 20 kg.

Tip

If the child weighs less than 15 kg, use a pediatric device. If the child weighs 15 kg or more, use an adult device.

Procedure

12-3 Carbon Dioxide Detector Device

1 Attach the device to the end of the ETT and attach the other end to the bag-mask device.

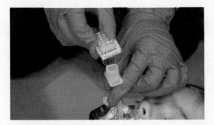

2 Begin ventilation.

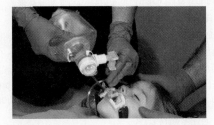

3 Observe the carbon dioxide detector for color change during exhalation. Read only after a total of six breaths. Check the color and act accordingly (**Table P12-1**). Regardless of whether the ETT is in the trachea the carbon dioxide detector will change to a purple color when 100% oxygen is squeezed through the bag device and ETT into the lungs.

The color on exhalation is the one to pay attention to because the color in the expiratory phase of breathing reflects carbon dioxide production. However, do not leave an adult carbon dioxide detector in place after initial confirmation of tube position on a patient weighing less than 15 kg because the adult device has too much dead space and an infant can rebreathe carbon dioxide if it is left in line. Leave the carbon dioxide detector in line for transport unless the transport time exceeds 60 minutes. Document observations and interventions.

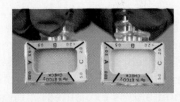

Table P12-1	Use of Colorimetric Exhaled Carbon Dioxide Detector in Endotracheal Tube Placement	
Color	**Patient with Pulse**	**Patient without Pulse**
Yellow	Yes—tube correctly placed Leave tube in place and secure it	Yes—tube correctly placed Leave tube in place and secure it
Tan	Think about it Ventilate six more times (while reassessing tube placement) Reassess detector for color change. If still tan, leave tube in place and secure Attempt to correct any possible cause of low perfusion or low carbon dioxide	Think about it Ventilate six more times (while reassessing tube placement) Reassess detector for color change. If still tan, leave tube in place and secure Attempt to correct cause of low perfusion or low carbon dioxide

Purple	Problem—tube incorrectly placed
	Extubate
	Ventilate with bag-mask device
	Reintubate
		Problem—tube may be incorrectly placed, or the child is dead and not producing measurable amounts of carbon dioxide
		Look at vocal cords with laryngoscope
		If tube is incorrectly placed:
		    Extubate
		    Ventilate with bag-mask device
		    Reintubate
		If tube is between vocal cords, and vocal cord marker is below vocal cords:
		    Leave tube in place
		    Check adequacy of CPR
		    Proceed with ALS protocol

 Tip

Remove the carbon dioxide detector from the endotracheal tube if endotracheal drugs are given, because a wet detector may not show a correct color change from purple to yellow.

 Tip

If the child is dead, no color change will occur, even if placement is correct, because there is no carbon dioxide being produced.

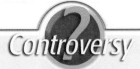 **Controversy**

An important controversy is whether a carbon dioxide detector or esophageal detector (aspiration) bulb or syringe is better. There is not enough data on efficacy, safety, and feasibility to clearly support one technique alone.

Procedure 13: Advanced Airway Techniques

Introduction

Rarely, standard bag-mask ventilation fails and endotracheal intubation is difficult or impossible. Examples of such patients are children with massive head trauma and airway edema or hematomas of the mouth or upper airway, children with multisytem injuries and long transport times, or infants with significant congenital or acquired airway abnormalities that cannot be ventilated. In such dire circumstances, some EMS systems allow prehospital professionals to perform advanced airway techniques. These include use of the **laryngeal mask airway (LMA),** the **gum elastic bougie,** the **lighted stylet** and **rapid sequence intubation (RSI).** **Needle cricothyrotomy** is another option and is explained in detail in this procedure. None of these techniques have been well evaluated in children in the out-of-hospital setting, and each procedure has important benefits, limitations, and contraindications.

Indications
A child who requires ventilation
Failed bag-mask ventilation
Failed ETI attempt

Contraindications
Upper airway obstruction
An awake patient with intact airway reflexes
Patients requiring high pressures to ventilate (asthma, bronchiolitis)
A relative contraindication is a full stomach. The LMA does not fully protect against aspiration.

Equipment
LMA have three disposable sizes, 3, 4 and 5
There are four reusable sizes, 1, 1.5, 2 and 2.5
Water soluble lubricant
Syringe
Oxygen source
Suction
Ventilation bag
Monitors (pulse oximeter)

Characteristics of children that are red flags for possible problems managing the airway include the following history or physical findings:

History:

1. Past history of difficult intubation or problems with ventilation.
2. Children with congenital anomalies affecting facial bones, and oropharyngeal structures including the tongue.
3. History of recurrent stridor or upper airway obstruction.

Physical Findings:

1. Unable to open the mouth widely.
2. Difficulty in fully extending the neck.
3. Presence of a large tongue or dysmorphic facial features.
4. Inability to visualize the entire uvula when depressing the tongue with a tongue blade.
5. Trauma to the face, mouth, tongue, or neck

Laryngeal Mask Airway (LMA)

The LMA is a device used frequently in EDs and hospitals to ventilate children. It consists of a tube with a distal inflatable mask that is inserted into the mouth. When the mask is inflated, air goes into the trachea. A bag-mask device can then be connected to the tube to provide rescue breathing. There is little out-of-hospital experience with LMAs, and the few reported trials are in adults. Hence, the safety and efficacy of this procedure in children in the out-of-hospital setting are unknown. However, the procedure is simple and fast, the success rates in hospitals are excellent, and the risks are small. EMS systems may soon be introducing the LMA for pediatric rescue breathing, and it may be an easier rescue technique than ETI in children who cannot be effectively ventilated by a bag-mask device. This technique requires special equipment and special training. Also, the epiglottis may flip over and interfere with good positioning of the LMA device.

Preparation

1. Measure the mask on the patient (see **Table 13-1** for sizing). The mask should extend from the bridge of the nose to the cleft of the chin, avoiding compression of the eyes. The right size mask will have a small volume, to minimize dead space and to prevent rebreathing of expired carbon dioxide. Transparency allows the rescuer to observe the child for cyanosis of the lips and for emesis.

2. Select an appropriate resuscitator bag: While a small child can be safely and effectively ventilated using a big bag, a small bag will not work for a large child. Pediatric tidal volume is approximately 8 mL/kg. The bag should have a volume of 450 to 750 mL. An adult bag (1200 mL) is okay for larger children or adolescents.

3. Connect the bag device to the end of the LMA.

4. Connect the oxygen tubing.

5. Open airway. Medical patient: Use head-tilt/chin-lift maneuver. Trauma patient: Use jaw thrust with in-line manual stabilization. Ensure neutral positioning (sniffing position). Because infants and toddlers have large heads, place a small roll under the shoulders to achieve the sniffing position. Avoid hyperextension of the neck because this may cause airway obstruction or spinal injury. Insert appropriate airway adjunct if airway patency cannot be maintained with chin-lift/jaw thrust maneuver (see Procedure 4). Use an oropharyngeal (OP) airway if the patient does not have a gag reflex or use a nasopharyngeal (NP) airway if the patient is less than 1 year of age and has an active gag reflex.

TABLE P13-1	LMA Size/Cuff Volume by Weight	
LMA Size	**Cuff Volume**	**Weight of Patient**
1	4 mL	<5kg
1.5	7 mL	5–10 kg
2	10 mL	10–20 kg
2.5	14 mL	20–30 kg
3	20 mL	30–50 kg
4	30 mL	50–70 kg
5	40 mL	>70 kg

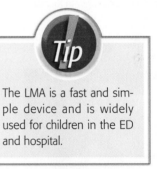

Tip

The LMA is a fast and simple device and is widely used for children in the ED and hospital.

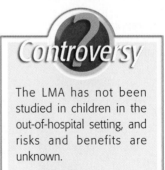

Controversy

The LMA has not been studied in children in the out-of-hospital setting, and risks and benefits are unknown.

Procedure

13-1 LMA-Fastrach Insertion

1 Deflate the cuff of the mask and apply a water-soluble lubricant to the posterior surface. Rub the lubricant over the anterior hard palate.

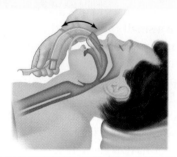

2 Ensure the curved metal tube is in contact with the chin and the mask tip is flat against the palate prior to rotation.

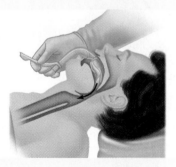

3 Swing the mask into place with a circular motion, maintaining pressure against the palate and the posterior pharynx.

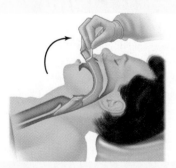

4 Visually inspect and inflate ETT to verify cuff integrity and symmetry. Deflate cuff, lubricate ETT, and pass through LMA-Fastrach tube (rotate with up/down movement) to distribute lubricant. Pass the ETT to the 15-cm depth marker or the transverse line on the LMA-Fastrach ETT, which corresponds to passage of tube tip through the epiglottic elevating bar.

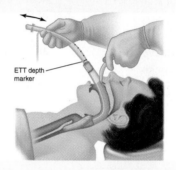

ETT depth marker

5 Use the handle to gently lift the device 2 to 5 cm as the ETT is advanced. Carefully advance until intubation is complete. Do not force. Inflate ETT cuff and confirm intubation.

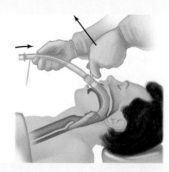

6 Remove ETT connector and gently ease the LMA-Fastrach out over the ETT into the oral cavity. Use a stabilizer rod to hold the ETT in position as LMA-Fastrach is withdrawn over the tube.

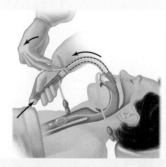

7 Remove the stabilizer rod and hold onto the ETT at the level of the incisors.

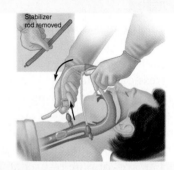

Stabilizer rod removed

8 Remove the LMA-Fastrach completely, gently unthreading the inflation line and the pilot balloon of the ETT.

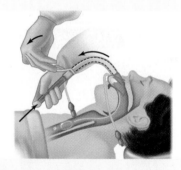

9 Replace the ETT connector.

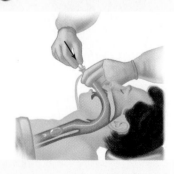

Gum Elastic Bougie

Sometimes it is difficult to visualize the vocal cords for ETI. There are many reasons for failure to see the anatomy, especially if the child has muscle tone. The gum elastic bougie or endotracheal tube introducer is a long flexible stylet that facilitates insertion of an endotracheal tube. There are several versions of this device that are available and may prove useful in facilitating intubation. The cartilaginous rings structure of the trachea allows the operator to feel the gum elastic bougie in the correct location. The semi-rigid tube or rod can be angled to pass into the trachea and as the device brushes against the tracheal rings, the rod can be palpated to be in position. Once in place, the device serves as a guide for placement of the endotracheal tube (ETT). The available equipment restricts use to patients over 14 years. Airway injury is a risk as well.

Indications
A child who requires endotracheal intubation and visualization of the cords or insertion of the ETT is difficult or impossible.

Contraindications
A child who is breathing effectively or has good bag-mask or LMA ventilation

Equipment
Gum elastic bougie device Endotracheal intubation (ETI) equipment

Preparation

1. Prepare the child for ETI (Procedure 11).
2. Ensure the gum elastic bougie points upward in a "J" shape configuration.

Procedure

13-2 Gum Elastic Bougie Device

1. Place the lubricated ETT over the straight end of the gum elastic bougie.

2. Visualize the cords with laryngoscopy.

3. Insert the "J" shaped end of the gum elastic bougie through the cords, advancing the device until clicks are palpated indicating the presence of tracheal rings.

4. Slide the ETT over the gum elastic bougie into the trachea.

5. Remove the laryngoscope then the gum elastic bougie.

6. Ensure the ETT is in the trachea by end-tidal CO_2 detection or an esophageal aspirator device, and that the tube has a correct position at the lips.

7. Secure the ETT.

Tip

A gum elastic bougie is particularly helpful when a very anterior placed larynx makes visualization of the vocal cords difficult.

Blip

The available equipment restricts use to patients over 14 years.

Lighted Stylet

The lighted stylet utilizes a stylet with a fiber-optic tip that is brightly illuminated as the tube is passed into the trachea. It is a blind intubation technique and uses the light's position visualized on the external area of the neck over the trachea to determine positioning. The technique does not require airway visualization. The lighted stylet is particularly useful when copious blood or secretions obstruct direct laryngoscopy.

Preparation

1. Follow ETI procedure (Procedure 11).

Indications

An adjunct for the difficult airway when direct visualization of the vocal cords is impossible due to secretions or blood obstructing the view.

Contraindications

Major facial trauma
Laryngeal fracture
Upper airway obstruction

Equipment

Lighted stylet of appropriate diameter to fit through an endotracheal tube
All equipment described under endotracheal intubation.

Procedure

13-3 Lighted Stylet

1 Select an appropriate size endotracheal tube that allows a lighted stylet to fit within the lumen. (Smallest possible size for use is 5.5 mm inner diameter)

2 Apply a water soluble lubricant to the opening of the endotracheal tube to allow easy advancement of the stylet without sticking. Test the light source on the stylet.

3 Insert the lighted stylet so that the light source is at the tip of the endotracheal tube.

4 Bend the endotracheal tube/stylet assembly to a sharp angle of greater than 90 degrees. Place the bend at the same distance as the distance from the patient's thyroid cartilage to the angle of their mandible.

5 Apply gentle cricoid pressure. Darken the ambulance or treatment room. Place the patient's head in a neutral position, lift the jaw forward to elevate the tongue and epiglottis while inserting the ETT/stylet assembly into the mouth.

6 If the mouth is easily opened, the stylet can be introduced in the midline and advanced over the base of the tongue. If this is difficult, the ETT/stylet assembly can be turned 90 degrees, advanced into the oropharynx and turned for insertion when the angle of the assembly reaches the base of the tongue.

7 As the assembly is passed into the trachea, observe for a circular "tracheal glow" that can be observed on the skin over the larynx and trachea.

Tip

The brightness of the glow that confirms appropriate endotracheal tube placement can be assessed by shining the light through the patient's cheek prior to insertion of the tube.

Blip

A lighted stylet positioned in the periform fossa or *velecula* will not provide appropriate tracheal glow. A very obese patient may also make it difficult to see the characteristic tracheal glow.

Rapid Sequence Intubation (RSI)

RSI is a technique for relaxing a child's muscles for facilitation of ETI. There are several options in medications (**Table P13-2**). A common drug combination is etomidate and succinylcholine. The medications have important benefits and risks. The induced muscular paralysis allows the prehospital professional to insert an ETT with no resistance, and hence will improve success and decrease complications. There is wide experience with RSI in adult, but limited experience in children. RSI will render the patient apneic. *Therefore, if RSI fails, bag-mask ventilation is essential for the child to* *survive. Medication doses vary with the changing weight of the child. Medication complications are important causes of error.*

Preparation

1. Prepare the child for ETI (Procedure 11).
2. Double check suction, oxygen source, oxygen tubing, endotracheal confirmation device, and monitor.
3. Ensure stable IV or IO line.
4. Double check doses per kg based upon length/weight calculation (Procedure 2).

Indications
Failed ETI
Severe head trauma required hyperventilation

Contraindications
Abnormal airway anatomy
Upper airway obstruction
Laryngeal fracture

Equipment
ETI equipment
RSI medications

TABLE P13-2	Common Drugs for Rapid Sequence Intubation	
Drug	**Type**	**Dose**
Succinylcholine	Paralytic	1–2 mg/kg/dose IV
Rocuronium	Paralytic	1 mg/kg IV
Midazolam	Sedative	0.05–0.1 mg/kg IV, IO, or IM
Diazepam	Sedative	0.1 mg/kg IV or IO
Atropine	Anticholinergic	0.01–0.02 mg/kg IV or IO 0.1 mg minimum 0.5 mg maximum (child) 1 mg maximum (adolescent)

Procedure

13-4 Rapid Sequence Intubation (RSI)

1 Administer atropine and sedative drug.

2 Administer paralyzing agent.

3 Do ETI when muscles are paralyzed.

Tip

The induced muscular paralysis from RSI allows the pre-hospital professional to insert an ETT with no resistance, and hence will improve success and decrease complications from forced insertion attempts.

Blip

If RSI fails, bag-mask ventilation is essential for the child to survive.

Procedure 14: Intramuscular and Subcutaneous Injections

Introduction

The intramuscular (IM) or subcutaneous (SQ) route is acceptable for giving several important medications to children. These medications include epinephrine, diphenhydramine, and morphine sulfate. The IM or SQ routes have limitations, but when inhalation, IV, or IO delivery of medication is not possible, IM or SQ administration may be life-saving.

Indication

Administration of medications when vascular access is not possible or practical

Contraindications

Poor perfusion
Availability of alternative effective routes: oral, inhalation, IV, or IO

Equipment

Tuberculin or 3-mL syringe
22- or 25-gauge needle
• 1 to 1-½ inch for IM injection
25- or 30-gauge needle
• ⅝-inch for SQ injection

Rationale

IM or SQ administration allows the medication to absorb slowly but steadily. IM medications are absorbed more quickly than are SQ medications. The advantages of IM and SQ techniques are easy delivery and high safety. The disadvantages are poor patient acceptance and delayed effect. Avoid IM or SQ medications in patients with low perfusion because absorption is unpredictable. Sometimes, in situations involving a child with low venous pressures, such as in anaphylaxis, IM or SQ is an excellent first choice for delivery while vascular access is attempted.

The SQ route (for example, for epinephrine in bronchospasm) has few complications because it avoids contact with tendons, nerves, and blood vessels. The IM route may result in nerve damage, particularly if the injection is in the buttocks of an infant or small child.

Preparation

1. Explain the procedure using developmentally appropriate terminology. Avoid using the word "shot" because the child may associate this with being shot by a gun. Be honest and tell the child it will hurt but be over as quickly as possible. Describe the needle stick as a pinch or a bee sting.
2. Select the medication, reaffirm if the child is allergic to any medications.

3. Select the appropriate syringe and needle. Keep needles out of the child's sight.
   Needle Length for IM Injection
   • For the **ventrogluteal** or **dorsogluteal** sites, use a needle slightly longer than one half of the distance between the thumb and finger when the skin at the injection site is grasped.
   • For the **deltoid** and **vastus lateralis** sites, use a 1-inch needle if the skin is grasped. If the muscle is stretched, use a ⅝-inch needle.
   Needle Length for SQ Injection
   • Use the smallest needle size (25- or 30-gauge) with a ⅝-inch length.
4. Cleanse the top of the medication vial with an alcohol wipe or open the **ampule**.
5. Withdraw the appropriate volume of medication, based on the child's mg/kg dose. Calculate the dose or obtain from a length-based resuscitation tape or resuscitation software (see Procedure 2). Expel all but 0.1 mL of air from the syringe.
   • The maximum volume SQ is 0.5 to 1.0 mL.
   • The maximum volume IM is:
     ◦ 2.0 mL in older children
     ◦ 1.0 mL in small children and older infants
     ◦ 0.5 mL in small infants

6. Select the appropriate injection site (**Table P14-1**). Consider the following factors:
- The volume of medication
- The condition of the muscle
- The type of medication
- The child's ability to be properly positioned

7. Position and secure the child. Consider letting the caregiver hold the child in one of the following ways:

- Have the child sit on the caregiver's lap, facing to the side. Put one of the child's arms around the caregiver's waist and have the caregiver hold the child close to her chest. The caregiver can hold the child's arm or legs.
- Position the child straddling the caregiver's lap, sitting chest to chest. Tell the caregiver to hug the child. The caregiver can help to hold an arm or leg.

Procedure

14-1 IM Injection

1 The vastus lateralis site is preferable. Use the ventrogluteal or dorsogluteal sites if the thigh muscle is not accessible in children over 3 years.

2 Stretch the skin and insert the needle at a 90-degree angle.

3 Release the skin and pull back on the plunger to aspirate for blood.

4 If no blood appears, inject the medication. If blood appears, remove the syringe and start the procedure again.

5 Gently massage the area after the needle is removed.

Tip

Select the injection site based on age, anatomic considerations, and volume of medication to be given.

Tip

Put pressure on the site after the needle is removed, and massage the area to increase absorption.

Procedure

14-2 SQ Injection

1 Use the area over the deltoid or anterior thigh.

Blip

Avoid injecting close to a major nerve because it may cause nerve damage.

2 Gently grasp the skin and insert the needle.

3 Insert the needle into the SQ area of the skin.

4 Release the skin and pull back on the plunger to aspirate for blood.

5 If no blood appears, inject the medication. If blood appears, remove the syringe and start the procedure over.

Possible Complications

Abscess (rare)
Cellulitis
Damage to blood vessel, nerve, or tendon

Redness or swelling at the site
Adverse reaction to the medication
Pain at site

Procedure

14-3 After the Injection

1 Praise the child. Apply an adhesive bandage to the site.

2 Dispose of the syringe.

3 Write down the name of the medication, dosage, route, time, and any effects.

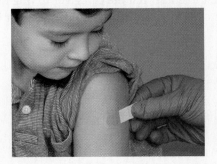

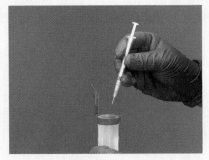

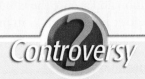

Controversy

Some experts believe that the dorsogluteal site should not be used until the child has been walking for at least one year.

Table P14-1	Appropriate Sites for IM and SQ Injections			
Site	**Indications**	**Landmarks**	**Considerations**	**Disadvantages**
Vastus lateralis muscle: Largest muscle group in children under 3 years of age	Use in infants and small children Preferred site for all ages	Palpate the greater trochanter and the knee joint; divide the distance into thirds Use middle third for injection site	Can be use for SQ or IM injections	Thrombosis of the femoral artery More painful than deltoid or gluteal sites.
Ventrogluteal muscle: Large muscle with few nerves and blood vessels	Use in children over 3 years of age	Have the child lie on his side and bend the upper leg forward in front of the lower leg Palpate greater trochanter and anterior and posterior iliac crests Place palm over greater trochanter with fingers open in a V shape pointing toward iliac crests Inject into center of the V shape	Well-defined landmarks to identify the site	None
Dorsogluteal site	Use in children over 3 years of age	Have the child lie on his stomach and rotate his legs and toes inward Palpate greater trochanter and posterior iliac spine; draw an imaginary line between these two points Inject lateral and above the imaginary line	In an older child, larger volumes of medication (2 mL) can be injected because the muscle mass is larger.	Contraindicated in children under 3 years of age and those who have not been walking for at least 1 year Medication may inadvertently be given SQ in older child with a large muscle mass Do not damage the sciatic nerve, which tracks out from the lower lumbar spine and goes underneath the gluteal muscles
Deltoid	Use for small volumes of medication. Used in children 18 months of age and older	Palpate the shoulder and go two fingerbreadths below Give the injection in the upper third of the muscle	Usually used for SQ injections Faster absorption rate than gluteal site Fewer side effects from the injection and less painful site	May damage the radial nerve in young children Because of the limited muscle mass, only small volumes of medication can be injected

Procedure 15: Intravenous Access

Introduction

Establishing intravenous (IV) access is a time-honored method of fluid and drug administration. However, unlike the situation with an adult, securing IV access in a pediatric patient is often difficult or impossible in the out-of-hospital setting. Fortunately, the majority of pediatric patients do not require IV access before ED arrival and many out-of-hospital medications do not require an IV route for administration.

Indications
Cardiopulmonary arrest
Shock
Cardiac dysrhythmia
Illness or injury possibly requiring immediate IV drug or fluid administration

Contraindications
Availability of another reliable administration route
Brief transport time
Consider vascular access on the way to the ED in the following situations:
    Multisystem injury
    Compensated shock
    Cardiogenic shock
    Newly born with circulatory depression from hypovolemia

Equipment
IV catheters, 14- to 24-gauge
IV tubing (**macrodrip** or **microdrip**)
IV solution
Rubber band or elastic band **tourniquet**
Adhesive tape or occlusive dressing
Gauze pad
Pediatric arm board

Rationale

IV access makes it easier to give medications and provides a route for fluid therapy in illness or injuries where there is possible blood or fluid loss. IV delivery is the gold standard for giving medications because it permits rapid and predictable onset of action for most important drugs. The indications for IV access must be carefully weighed against common complications and risks associated with the procedure. These include diversion from airway and breathing management, possible delays to ED care, and pain to the child. Also, there is a risk to the prehospital professional from exposure to blood-borne pathogens. However, in certain children, such as the critically ill child with shock, IV therapy in the field can be life-saving.

Preparation

1. Assemble the equipment. Select the appropriate IV solution and tubing.
   - Inspect the solution for cloudiness, expiration date, leakage, or contamination.
   - Use microdrip IV tubing for giving medication.
   - For fluid administration, use a macrodrip.
   - For medication administration consider a saline lock: male luer lock device with injection port and normal saline flush.
   - Spike the fluid bag with the tubing, clamp the tubing, squeeze the drip chamber until it is half full, open the clamp, and flush the tubing.
   - Select the appropriate catheter, depending on need for fluid volume. Use a smaller catheter when only medications are indicated.

Tip

If IV access is for giving medication only, use microdrip tubing. For giving fluid, use macrodrip tubing

2. Prepare the child and family for the procedure. Use developmentally appropriate language to explain the procedure.

3. Select the site.
   - The scalp is an excellent site in newly borns.
   - The best sites in the infant are the hands, antecubital fossa, and saphenous vein at the ankle or feet. The **dorsum** (back) of the hand is

a good site in chubby infants. To access that site, grasp the child's hand with the fingers closed and flex the wrist downward.

- In toddlers and older children, potential sites are the hands and antecubital areas. Use the child's nondominant extremity if possible. The external **jugular** veins are good sites.
- Avoid inserting the catheter over a joint.
- Consider the antecubital fossa when fluid boluses are required because veins that are more distal in the forearm or hand are usually smaller.
- Hand veins are often mobile under the skin and may move with contact with the catheter.

4. Position the patient supine, or in the caregiver's lap if the child is under school age. Secure the child's legs to avoid kicking. For external jugular cannulation, place the child in a slight head-down position. The caregiver can help hold the child and immobilize the insertion site.

5. Apply the rubber band or tourniquet proximal to the entry site. Do not make it too tight. The tourniquet should not block arterial flow. If it is necessary to make the vein more visible, do the following:
   - Place the extremity in a dependent position.
   - Tap or massage the site.
   - Ask the older child to clench and unclench his fist.

6. Cleanse the site with antiseptic solution.

Procedure

15-1 Intravenous Access

1 Insert the needle. Stabilize the vein by pulling the skin taut distally from the insertion site. Insert the catheter through the skin with the bevel up, at a 30-degree angle. Insert the catheter slowly; blood return may be delayed for a few seconds. When there is a flashback of blood, advance the needle and catheter into the vein and then remove the needle. Never pull the catheter back over the needle because this may cause shearing of the catheter tip. Release the tourniquet. Compress the vein proximal to the site to prevent blood loss through the catheter while connecting the tubing. It is also helpful to position a gauze pad under the catheter at this time. Connect the tubing or male luer lock to the catheter. If a saline lock (male luer lock with injection port) is used, a 2–5 mL saline flush should be used to maintain patency.

2 Stabilize the catheter with tape or occlusive dressing. Avoid placing an excess amount of tape or gauze over the site because it obstructs the view of the site. Use a clear medicine cup or other device to protect the site while allowing access and visualization.

3 Immobilize the extremity. Be careful not to apply the tape too tightly, as this will block the flow of blood through the vein.

4 Monitor the solution drip rate to avoid giving too much or too little fluid.

5 Dispose of the needle.

Troubleshooting

1. If the fluid is not infusing properly, assess the following:
   - Make sure the tourniquet has been released.
   - Make sure the child's arm is not bent.
   - Make sure the tape is not too tight.
   - Make sure the tubing is not kinked.
   - Make sure the clamp is open.
   - Lower the fluid bag below the extremity and assess for a backflow of blood into the tubing.
   - Raise the fluid bag higher if possible.

2. If none of the above measures are effective, discontinue the IV and restart in another site.

Blip

Never delay transport in any critically injured infant or child; consider IV attempts on the way to the hospital.

Tip

Reward and comfort the child after the procedure.

Possible Complications

Pain

Infiltration: Look for pain or edema at the site, inability to infuse fluids, or lack of blood return. Discontinue IV and insert at another site.

Hypothermia from giving too much room-temperature fluid to an infant

Skin infection

Thrombophlebitis

Inadvertent fluid overload

Catheter shear

Inadvertent arterial puncture

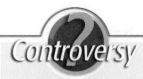

Controversy

Few children require IV access in the field or on the way to the ED. Injured children must always be transported before attempting IV access. For ill children, especially if there is a short transport time, it is controversial which ones need IV access, and whether IV access should be attempted on scene or on the way to the hospital.

Blip

Do not use words like "stick" or "needle" when describing the procedure to the child. Instead, consider an explanation such as, "I will be putting a soft tube into your arm to give your veins a drink."

Blip

Be careful not to secure the tape too tightly to immobilize the extremity, as this will block blood flow in the vein.

Tip

Position the child and secure the site before beginning the procedure.

Procedure 16: Intraosseous Needle Insertion

Introduction

Establishing vascular access is often difficult or impossible during life-threatening emergencies in infants and young children. The intraosseous (IO), intramedullary, or marrow route for the delivery of resuscitation fluids and medications has been used for over 50 years in children and adults. Many studies have confirmed that the intraosseous space is an excellent route for medications and fluids. The primary technical problem is successfully piercing the bony cortex (outer layer of the bone) in older children. The bones of neonates and infants are usually soft and the intraosseous space is relatively large, so needle insertion is easy in children of these younger age groups. Good equipment, preparation, and effective technique are especially important for success.

Indication
Severe illness or injury requiring immediate drugs or fluids, when IV access is impossible or unlikely to be successful

Contraindications
Available secure IV line
Extremity deformity in same bone as insertion site

Equipment
14- to 16-gauge IO needles
Alcohol swab for cleaning the skin
Normal saline and IV tubing
10-cc syringe
Stopcock (optional)

Rationale

Using an IO needle to give drugs or fluids is an excellent alternative to cannulating peripheral veins in critically ill or injured children. The IO space is highly vascular and functions as a noncollapsible vein. Needle insertion into this space is quick, simple, effective, and usually quite safe. There are several possible sites, but the easiest location is the proximal tibial. The IO space is suitable for infusion of almost all parenteral medications, crystalloid fluids, or blood products—which are quickly absorbed from small veins of the bone into the central circulation. Complications are usually minor and infrequent.

Preparation

Tibia and Femur Sites
1. Place the patient in the supine position.
2. Put a small towel roll under the knee.
3. Prepare the skin over the insertion site.

Possible Complications

Compartment syndrome
Failed infusion
Growth plate injury
Bone infection
Skin infection
Bony fracture

Procedure

16-1 Proximal Tibia Site

1 Use the flat surface of the proximal medial tibia, medial to the tibial tuberosity on the flat side of the bone.

2 Introduce the IO needle in the skin, directed away from the growth plate or pointing toward the foot.

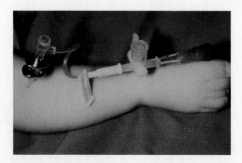

Procedure

16-2 Distal Tibia Site

1 Use the flat surface of the medial distal tibia above the medial malleous.

2 Introduce the IO needle in the skin directed away from the growth plate or towards the knee.

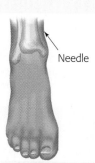

Needle

Procedure

16-3 Distal Femur Site

1 Use the distal third of the femur, estimate distance through soft tissue to reach bony surface of femur, and ensure that IO needle has been adjusted to a length that will allow bony penetration.

2 Introduce the IO needle in the skin, directed away from the growth plate or pointing towards the trunk.

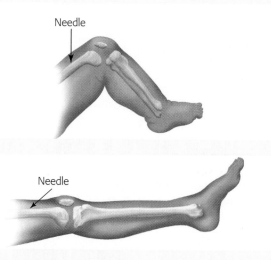

Needle

Needle

Controversy

There are no data that compare intraosseous infusions of fluids and medications to IV administration. While intraosseous access is easy, quick, and safe, it is painful in a conscious child and therefore is only practical in a critically ill or injured child.

Procedure

16-4 Method to Access All Sites

1 Pierce the bony cortex with a firm, twisting motion. Use a back-and-forth twisting motion to enter the marrow space. Do not push hard on the needle. A "pop" may be felt as the needle passes through the bony cortex and into the marrow cavity.

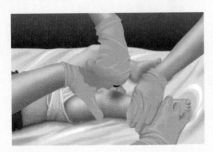

2 Remove the stylet and aspirate marrow contents. Keep any bone marrow aspirate for glucose check or for other tests in the ED. Sometimes marrow cannot be aspirated. Confirm correct placement by infusing 10 mL of normal saline without resistance.

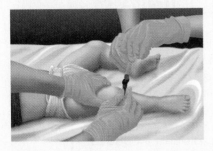

3 Attach IV line to the hub, or to a stopcock, and infuse fluids or drugs directly into intraosseous space.

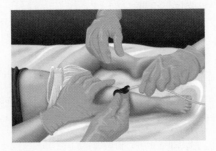

4 Secure the needle to the overlying skin with tape. Monitor the calf to ensure that there is no swelling to indicate leakage of fluid.

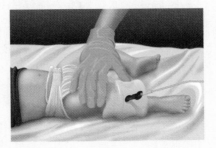

Tip

When placing the IO needle, use firm pressure and a twisting motion.

Blip

Insert the IO needle gently. Too much force may push the needle all the way through the bone and into the soft tissues.

Procedure 17: Cardiopulmonary Resuscitation

Introduction

Cardiopulmonary arrest (CPA) occurs when a patient's heart and lungs stop functioning. In children, CPA usually begins as a primary respiratory arrest. This is in contrast to adults, in whom CPA or "sudden death" is almost always a primary cardiac event that occurs with onset of ventricular fibrillation and an abrupt change in the heart's electrical activity. Because cessation of effective breathing is the precipitating factor in pediatric CPA, airway management and ventilation are to children in CPA what defibrillation is to adults. Cardiopulmonary resuscitation (CPR) refers to basic airway management, artificial ventilation, and chest compressions to provide oxygen and circulation to core organs: the heart, brain, and lungs. In children, CPR has been shown to improve survival from drowning, and it may also benefit patients in CPA from other causes.

Indications
Newly born, neonate, infant, or child of any age who is apneic and pulseless
Newly born with a heart rate less than 60 beats/min and not improving after standard newborn care
Neonate, infants and children with a heart rate less than 60 beats/min and shock

Contraindication
Newly born, infant, or child with effective perfusion (palpable central or peripheral pulse)

Equipment
Mouth-to-mask device
Bag-mask device, infant or child
Airway adjuncts
Appropriate mask sizes

Rationale

CPR encompasses the basic procedures for sustaining critical oxygenation, ventilation, and perfusion recommended by the American Heart Association. The pediatric techniques are slightly modified from the adult techniques to reflect the known differences in CPA between age groups. Furthermore, there are specific differences between infants and children, including number of rescuers, placement of hands and fingers, rates of ventilation, and rates and depth of chest compressions.

Preparation

1. Position a child on a hard surface. Position a neonate or infant on a hard surface or on the forearm of the rescuer with the hand supporting the head.

Procedure

17-1 Assess Responsiveness

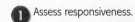 Assess responsiveness.

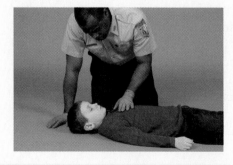

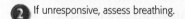 If unresponsive, assess breathing.

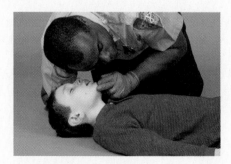

Procedure

17-2 Assess Breathing

① Open airway using either the head-tilt/chin-lift maneuver (medical patient) or modified jaw thrust maneuver (trauma patient) to achieve a neutral position.

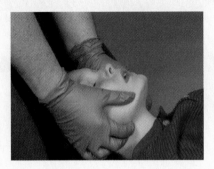

② If spinal injury is possible, have a second rescuer maintain manual spinal stabilization.

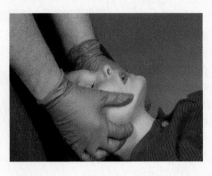

③ Look, listen, and feel for signs of breathing.

④ Remove any obvious obstructions, such as loose teeth or vomitus.

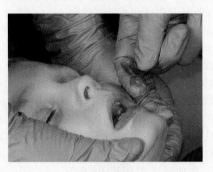

Tip

Manipulation of the head to keep the airway in a neutral position is essential for effective ventilation. A towel roll under the shoulders of the infant or small child may help maintain neutral head position.

Compression Rates

These are the timing rates for single rescuers, not the actual number of compressions delivered each minute because of pauses for ventilations and reassessments.

- Newly born: At least 120 compressions/min
- Neonate and infant: 100 compressions/min
- Child 1–8 years: 100 compressions/min
- Child over 8 years: 80 to 100 compressions/min

Possible Complications

Coronary vessel injury
Diaphragm injury
Hemopericardium
Hemothorax
Interference with ventilation
Liver injury
Myocardial injury
Pneumothorax
Rib fractures
Spleen injury
Sternal fracture

Procedure

17-3 Ventilation Rate

1 If not breathing, begin mouth-to-mask ventilation, or perform bag-mask ventilation with 100% oxygen. Give two initial breaths.

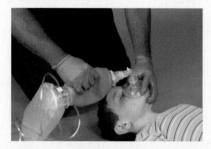

2 If breaths do not expand the chest, reposition the head and attempt again. If breaths are still ineffective, suction the mouth with a bulb syringe or flexible suction catheter (newly born) or a large-bore rigid suction catheter (neonates, infants, and children) and attempt breaths again.

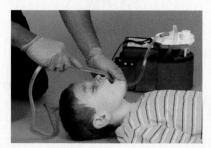

3 If breaths now expand the chest, assess pulse.

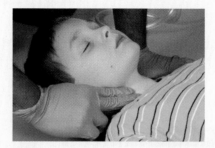

4 If pulse is present, but the victim is still not breathing, continue ventilations. Give one every 2 seconds in newly born; one every 3 seconds for neonates, infants, and children age 8 years and younger; one every 5 seconds for children older than 8 years.

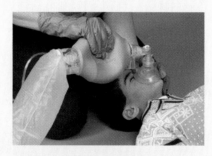

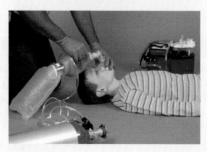

5 Slowly repeat "squeeze-release-release" to time bag-mask ventilation rate.

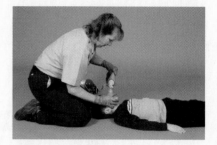

6 Use the E-C clamp technique to achieve a good mask seal and watch for adequate chest rise to ensure effective ventilation.

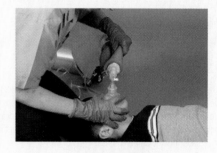

Tip

Continuously assess effectiveness of CPR by ensuring chest rise and feeling for a palpable pulse.

Procedure

17-4 Compression Rate

1 Check central pulse. Newly born: umbilical cord stump or listen to **precordium.** Neonate and infant: brachial pulse or femoral pulse. Child: carotid pulse.

2 If pulse is absent or if heart rate is less than 60 beats/min, with shock or poor peripheral perfusion, begin chest compressions. Newly born: 3 compressions:1 ventilation. Neonate, infant, and child: 5 compressions:1 ventilation. Use proper compression technique, compression-ventilation ratio, depth of compression, and compression-release ratio (**Tables P17-1 and P17-2**).

Table P17-1	Delivered Compression-Ventilation Ratios per Minute*		
Age	Rate of Compressions (min)	Rate of Ventilations (min)	Compression-Ventilation Ratio
Newly born (<1 month)	120	30	3:1
Neonate and infant (1–12 months)	100	20	5:1
Child 1–8 years	100	20	5:1
Child over 8 years			
One rescuer	80–100	10–12	15:2
Two rescuers	80–100	12	5:1

*The rate of compressions and the actual number of compressions delivered per minute are different. The rate of compressions refers to the timing of compressions when they are being performed, and the rate does not account for pauses for breathing. Delivered compressions are the actual number of compressions delivered per minute after accounting for breathing. The ratios are calculated from the timing rates, not the delivered rates.

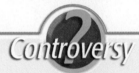

The value of CPR in children is unproven for any condition except drowning. There are no available studies to compare the effectiveness of different types of ventilation or compression techniques.

A potential problem when using the thumbs for chest compression with the fingers encircling the back is restriction of ventilation if more than the thumbs and fingertips are touching the chest and back.

Table P17-2	Parameters for BLS Resuscitation in Children			
Age	Compressions (min)	Ventilations (min)	Depth (in)	Hand Placement for Compression
Newly born (< 1 month)	120	30	0.50–0.75	2 fingers at midsternum, 1 finger below nipple line, or 2 thumbs at midsternum with hands encircling chest
Neonate (1–28 days)	100	20	0.5–1.0	2 fingers at midsternum, 1 finger below nipple line, or 2 thumbs at midsternum with hands encircling chest
Infant (1–12 months)	100	20	0.5–1.0	2 fingers at midsternum, 1 finger below nipple line, or 2 thumbs at midsternum with hands encircling chest
Child 1–8 years	100	20	1.0–1.5	3 fingers or heel of 1 hand at midsternum, 2 fingers above xiphoid process
Child over 8 years			1.5–2.0	Heel of both hands at midsternum, 2 fingers above xiphoid process
One rescuer	80–100	10–12		
Two rescuers	80–100	12		

Procedure

17-5 Finger or Hand Placement

1 Newly born: Use the two thumb method for the newborn. The two finger method is acceptable, but should be used when the two thumb method is not easily accomplished. Compression depth should be one third of chest depth. Two thumb technique: encircle the chest and use thumbs just below the **intermammary** line with the fingers supporting the spine. Two finger technique: Use two or three fingers on the **sternum** just below the intermammary line, with the other hand supporting the spine.

2 Neonate and infant: Use the two finger technique described above. Compression depth should be one third to one half the depth of the chest.

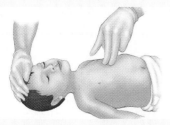

3 Child (1 to 8 years old): Use the heel of one hand on the sternum above the xiphoid process. Compression depth should be one third to one half the depth of the chest.

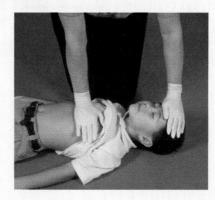

4 Child (> 8 years): Use the heel of both hands on the sternum above the xiphoid process.

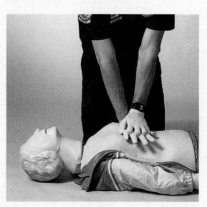

Procedure

17-6 Compressions

1 The depth of chest compressions should be approximately one third to one half the depth of the chest. Compressions should be deep enough to produce a palpable brachial, femoral, or carotid pulse. Newly born: 0.5 to 0.75 inch. Neonate and infant: 0.5 to 1.0 inch. 1–8 years: 1.0 to 1.5 inches. Over 8 years: 1.5 to 2.0 inches. The compression-release ratio is 1:1, which means that the time when there is no pressure on the chest should be as long as a compression. Coordinate ventilations with compressions: Allow 1.0 to 1.5 seconds for one ventilation after every five compressions.

2 Use the two-rescuer technique when possible.

3 Reassessment: Check pulse after approximately 1 minute or after every 20 compression-ventilation cycles.

A common problem in the transition from one-rescuer to two-rescuer child CPR is the lack of coordination between ventilations and compressions.

Procedure 18: AED and Defibrillation

Introduction

Synchronized **cardioversion for tachydysrhythmias** has long been part of adult emergency care and is one of the most effective treatments for sudden cardiac arrest from ventricular dysrhythmias. However, ventricular dysrhythmias are rare in children, especially in infants, and pediatric supraventricular tachycardia (SVT) is usually treatable with medical therapy. For these reasons, pediatric synchronized cardioversion is not often indicated. However, when a child develops ventricular fibrillation or pulseless ventricular tachycardia, defibrillation (unsynchronized cardioversion) may be lifesaving. Also, synchronized cardioversion may resuscitate a child in shock with SVT. Use the **synchronized** mode when there is SVT or ventricular tachycardia with a pulse, and the **asynchronized** (defibrillation) mode for ventricular fibrillation or ventricular tachycardia without a pulse.

Indications
Ventricular fibrillation
Pulseless ventricular tachycardia
SVT with shock and no vascular access rapidly available
Ventricular tachycardia with shock and unresponsiveness with pulse and no vascular access rapidly available
Atrial fibrillation or atrial flutter with shock

Contraindication
Conscious patient with good perfusion

Equipment
Automatic external defibrillator
Standard defibrillator
Newer models feature lower power outputs to deliver lower energy countershocks

Rationale

When a child's heart deteriorates into ventricular tachycardia or fibrillation, there is usually a severe systemic insult such as profound hypoxia, ischemia, electrocution, or myocarditis. Death may result if treatment is delayed. SVT, in contrast, is usually a more stable cardiac rhythm. When the child is pulseless and has ventricular fibrillation or ventricular tachycardia, perform defibrillation as quickly as possible with the appropriate technique. If a child has SVT or ventricular tachycardia and shock, use synchronized cardioversion. Do not attempt to perform synchronized cardioversion on a child with SVT who is well perfused.

Preparation

1. Open airway and ventilate with bag-mask device with 100% oxygen while assembling equipment for cardioversion or defibrillation.
2. If child is pulseless, begin closed-chest compressions, until automatic external defibrillator (AED) or conventional defibrillator is available.

Do not deliver synchronized cardioversion to a conscious child with SVT or ventricular tachycardia unless the child is in shock and has no IV or IO access rapidly available for medical treatment.

For a child with ventricular fibrillation or pulseless ventricular tachycardia, use the asynchronized (defibrillation) mode.

Procedure

18-1 Conventional Defibrillator Use

1 Apply the paddles directly to the skin. Place one paddle on the anterior chest wall on the right side of the sternum inferior to the clavicle and the other paddle on the left midclavicular line at the level of the **xiphoid process**. As another option, use the anterior-posterior position.

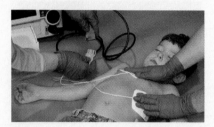

2 Clear the nearby area to avoid shocking someone. Announce, "I am going to shock on three. One, I am clear. Two, you are clear. Three, everybody is clear."

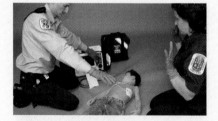

3 Begin recording rhythm. Deliver the electrical countershock with firm pressure.

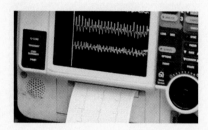

4 Assess the patient for evidence of **reperfusion** and check the monitor for the rhythm.

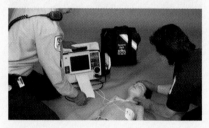

5 If the first electrical shock is unsuccessful, deliver additional electrical countershocks as per EMS protocol. Give specific dysrhythmia treatment with epinephrine or other drugs, as per EMS protocol. Treat bradycardia or other dysrhythmias.

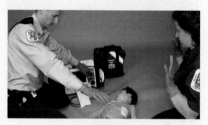

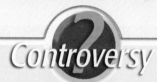

Controversy?

The preferred paddle location in children is controversial and no study in humans has compared the two techniques. Anterior chest wall placement has the advantage of a supine child and easier airway management. Anterior-posterior placement may allow larger paddles and more effective delivery of the charge.

Preparation

Conventional Defibrillator Use

1. Select the proper paddle size. Use the 8-cm adult paddles if these will fit on the chest wall; otherwise, use the 4.5-cm pediatric paddles (**Table P18-1**).
2. Prep paddles or skin electrodes with electrode jelly, paste, or saline-soaked gauze pads, or use self-adhesive defibrillator pads. Do not let jelly or paste from one site touch the other and form an "electrical bridge" between sites, which could result in ineffective defibrillation or skin burns.
3. Establish appropriate electrical charge (**Table P18-2**).
4. Select synchronized or asynchronized mode.
5. Properly charge pack and stop chest compressions.

Table P18-1	Paddle Size
8-cm adult paddles (Use in children over 12 months of age or weighing more than 10 kg) On anterior chest wall, OR Anterior-posterior	
4.5-cm pediatric paddles (Use in infants up to 12 months of age or weighing less than 10 kg) on the anterior chest wall	

Blip

Failure to firmly apply paddles to the chest wall will decrease effective delivery of charge.

Procedure

18-2 One Rescuer with an AED

For children under 8 years of age use a child-pad cable system if available. There are inadequate data to recommend AED use for the child less than 1 year of age.

1 Verify unresponsiveness.

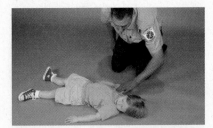

2 Open the airway, and check for breathing.

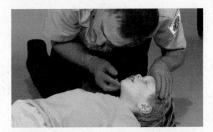

3 If the victim is not breathing effectively, give two ventilations.

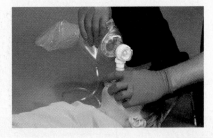

4 Check for signs of circulation. If there are no signs of circulation, attach the AED and proceed with the AED treatment algorithm. The AED operator should take the following actions.

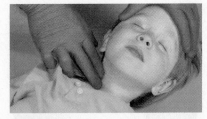

5 **POWER ON** the AED and follow voice prompts. Some devices will turn on when the AED lid or carrying case is opened.

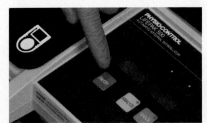

6 **ATTACH** the AED. Select the correct pads for victim's size and age (adult vs. child). Peel the backing from the pads. Attach the adhesive pads to the victim as shown on the pads. (If only adult pads are available, and they overlap when placed on the chest, use an anterior [chest] and posterior [back] placement.) Attach the electrode cable to the AED (if not preconnected).

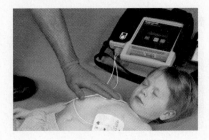

7 Allow the AED to **ANALYZE** the victim's rhythm ("clear" victim during analysis). **Deliver a SHOCK if needed** ("clear" victim before shock).

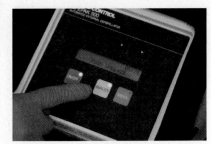

Reasonable variations in this sequence are acceptable.

Table P18-2	Appropriate Electrical Charge for Countershock	
Dysrhythmia	**Mode**	**Charge**
Ventricular fibrillation Ventricular tachycardia without a pulse	Defibrillation (asynchronized)	2 J/kg, then 4 J/kg, then 4 J/kg, as needed. Then 4 J/kg 30–60 seconds after each dose of epinephrine.
Ventricular tachycardia with pulse SVT Atrial fibrillation and atrial flutter with shock	Synchronized	0.5–1.0 J/kg. Repeat as needed.

Possible Complications

Ineffective delivery of countershock because of failure to charge, improper positioning on the chest, incorrect paddle size, or improper **conduction** medium

Burns on the chest wall

Failure to "clear" before voltage discharge, leading to electrical shock of a team member or bystander

Tachydysrhythmia

Bradycardia

Myocardial damage or necrosis

Cardiogenic shock

Embolic phenomena

Procedure

18-3 Two Rescuer AED Sequence of Action

Reprinted with permission from *AHA BLS for HCP text*, 2001 (updated version with AED for children); 99–105.

1 **Verify unresponsiveness.** If victim is unresponsive, have partner call 9-1-1. Get AED.

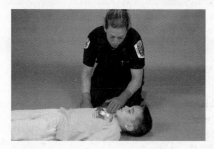

2 **Open airway:** head-tilt/chin-lift (or jaw thrust if trauma is suspected).

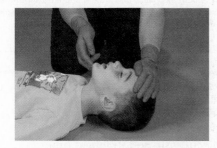

3 **Check for effective breathing:** provide breathing if needed. Check for breathing (look, listen, and feel). If not breathing, give two slow breaths. A mouth-to-mask device should be available in the AED carrying case.

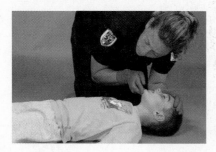

4 **Check for signs of circulation:** if no signs of circulation are present, perform these steps. Perform chest compressions and prepare to attach the AED. If there is any doubt that the signs of circulation are present, the first rescuer initiates chest compressions while the second rescuer prepares to use the AED. Remove clothing covering the victim's chest to provide chest compressions and apply the AED electrode pads.

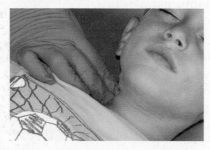

5 **Attempt defibrillation with the AED** if no signs of circulation are present. Place the AED near the rescuer who will be operating it. The AED is usually placed on the side of the victim opposite the rescuer who is performing CPR. The rescuer begins performing CPR while the rescuer who was performing CPR prepares to operate the AED. (It is acceptable to reverse these roles.)

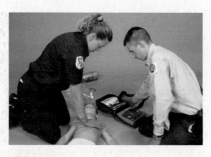

6 **The AED operator takes the following actions. POWER ON** the AED first (some devices will turn on automatically when the AED lid or carrying case is opened).

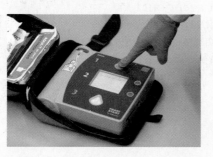

7 **ATTACH** the AED to the victim. Select correct pads for the victim's size and age. Peel the backing from the pads. Ask the rescuer performing CPR to stop chest compressions. Attach the adhesive pads to the victim as shown on the pads. (If only adult pads are available, and they overlap when placed on the chest, use an anterior [chest] and posterior [back] placement.) Attach the AED connecting cables to the AED (if not preconnected). **ANALYZE** rhythm. Clear the victim before and during analysis. Check that no one is touching the victim. Press the ANALYZE button to start rhythm analysis (some brands of AEDs do not require this step). *"Shock Indicated" message.* Clear the victim once more before pushing the SHOCK button (I'm clear, you're clear, everybody's clear"). Check that no one is touching the victim. Press the SHOCK button (victim may display muscle contractions). Press the ANALYZE and SHOCK buttons up to two more times if the AED signals "shock advised" or "shock indicated." (Clear the victim before each analysis and shock.) *"No Shock Indicated" message.* Check for signs of circulation (including a pulse). If signs of circulation are present, check breathing. If breathing is inadequate, assist breathing. If breathing is adequate, place the victim in the recovery position, with the AED attached.

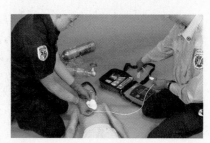

8 If no signs of circulation are present, resume CPR for 1 minute, then recheck for signs of circulation. If there are still no signs of circulation, analyze rhythm, then follow the *"shock indicated"* or *"no shock indicated"* steps as appropriate.

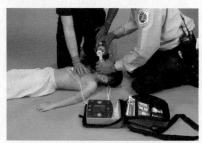

Procedure 19: Endotracheal Tube Drug Instillation

Introduction

The ability of the airways of the lungs to absorb medicines has been recognized for over a century. Giving medication through an endotracheal tube is a simple alternative to IV or IO drug delivery in a cardiopulmonary resuscitation. The airways are well vascularized and can absorb certain emergency medications. Drug dosages and dilutions in endotracheal (ET) delivery are different from IV or IO administration. ET drug delivery has been deemphasized, while this route of administration is better than no drug delivery, it is less effective than IV or IO. Once vascular access has been achieved, consideration should be given to repeating drugs if there has been no response to the ET drug delivery.

Indications
Cardiopulmonary resuscitation
Lack of IV or IO access

Contraindication
Functioning IV or IO access

Equipment
Endotracheal tube
Long catheter (feeding tube, suction catheter, nasogastric [NG] tube, or umbilical catheter)
Catheter size (in French units): approximately 2 times ET tube size (in mm) **(Table P19-1)**
Desired drug/**diluent** mixture
Normal saline or sterile water
Self-inflating ventilation device
Use 1 to 3 mL of diluent in infants, and 5 to 10 mL in older children. Use a minimum of 1 to 3 mL of diluent to ensure distribution and a maximum of 1.0 mL/kg (to approximately 30 mL total dose) to prevent problems with gas exchange in lungs.

Table P19-1	Suggested Catheter Size per Tracheal Tube
Endotracheal Tube Size (mm)	Catheter Size (Fr)
2.5	5
3.0	6
3.5–4.5	8
5.0–6.5	10
7.0	12

Rationale

If neither IV nor IO access is available for giving drugs during cardiopulmonary resuscitation, the ET route is a good alternative for pediatric drugs: atropine, naloxone, and epinephrine. The absorption, blood levels, onset, and duration of action are different with each drug. ET doses are unique for each agent, and are higher than IV or IO doses because absorption is not as good. While ET drugs are probably not as effective as IV or IO drugs, they can help improve the chances of successful resuscitation while IV or IO access is established.

Preparation

1. Intubate the patient.
2. Stabilize and secure the endotracheal tube.
3. Preoxygenate and ventilate.

Possible Complications

Hypoxia
Hypercarbia
Pneumonitis
Tracheal injury
Adverse side effects of drug itself

Endotracheal drug administration is a potential route for medications during early phases of resuscitation.

IV and IO are better routes of drug administration than the ET route.

Procedure

19-1 Endotracheal Drug Delivery

1 Draw the calculated drug dose into a syringe.

2 Dilute the medication with the proper diluent (diluting agent, either normal saline or sterile water).

3 Insert tip of small feeding tube or catheter past distal tip of ETT.

4 Instill solution directly into the trachea.

5 Follow with positive-pressure breaths.

6 Ventilate three times with self-inflating ventilation device to disperse the solution into the entire lung. Repeat medications if indicated.

Blip

Never give sodium bicarbonate by the endotracheal tube.

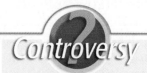

Controversy

The absorption and extent of central delivery of drugs given via endotracheal tube is not known and dose recommendations have not been validated by scientific studies on children.

Procedure 20: Rectal Administration of Benzodiazepines

Introduction

Rectal drug administration is a well-known delivery technique in children and is useful for many medications, including antipyretics and **anticonvulsants.** The only rectal medication approved in most EMS systems is diazepam for pediatric status epilepticus. Studies have compared the use of rectal lorazepam to rectal diazepam, and preliminary evidence showed that lorazepam may be safer and more effective than diazepam rectally for status epilepticus. Status epilepticus is a major pediatric medical emergency that may benefit from quick treatment. Although the first priority is airway and breathing, additional therapy may include medication to terminate the seizure. There remains significant controversy over the administration of rectal drugs from both a safety and effectiveness stance. Rectal diazepam is an effective route with few added complications when other routes of administration are not immediately available.

Indication
Status epilepticus

Contraindications
Newborn age (a month or less) (relative)
Recent rectal surgery (e.g., for **Hirschsprung disease, imperforate anus**) (relative)

Equipment
Lubricant
Tuberculin syringe, or 14- to 20-gauge over-the-needle catheter with 3- to 5-mL syringe
IV solution of diazepam
Tape (optional)

Rationale

Establishing IV or IO access is often time consuming and may delay delivery of essential advanced life support (ALS) drugs, especially in infants and toddlers. The rectum is an effective alternative route for emergency drug administration. The **rectum** is highly **vascularized**, and certain drugs are quickly absorbed through the lining or mucosa. Diazepam is a lipid-soluble benzodiazepine that is reliably absorbed through the rectum and will terminate most seizures without further treatment. It will take a few minutes longer to stop the seizure after rectal administration of diazepam as compared to IV diazepam. Occasionally, as with the IV diazepam preparation, more than one dose of rectal diazepam is necessary because of the drug's short duration of action.

Controversy

The relative effectiveness and safety of rectal diazepam or lorazepam versus intramuscular midazolam are not known.

Rectal lorazepam also has been used in the treatment of status epilepticus. This is less frequently encountered in the out-of-hospital setting due to the manufacturer's recommendations to keep this drug refrigerated. Lorazepam may be stored for up to thirty days unrefrigerated.

Tip

The most serious potential complication of rectal diazepam is respiratory depression, which is usually from the drug, but may be from the prolonged seizure, or the underlying cause of the seizure.

Preparation

1. Use the pediatric resuscitation tape or resuscitation software to determine the weight of the child (see Procedure 2), or establish the patient's weight from information provided by the caregiver.
2. Draw up the calculated dose of IV medication into a disposable tuberculin syringe or 3- to 5-mL syringe.

3. Lubricate the syringe or catheter:
   - If using the tuberculin syringe as the administration device, remove needle and apply lubricant to the tip of the syringe.
   - If using a 3- to 5-mL syringe (or tuberculin syringe, to draw up medication only), remove needle, attach over-the-needle catheter (plastic portion only), and lubricate catheter.

Possible Complications

Respiratory depression
Administration that is too high with inadequate serum level
Rectal tearing

Procedure

20-1 Rectal Administration of Benzodiazepines

1 Position the patient in the decubitus position, knee-chest position, or supine position with a second prehospital professional or the caregiver holding the legs apart.

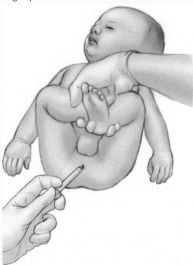

2 Carefully introduce the syringe or over-the-needle catheter approximately 5 cm (2 in) into the rectum. Inject the solution into the rectum. Remove the syringe. Hold buttocks closed for 10 seconds. Tape buttocks closed (optional).

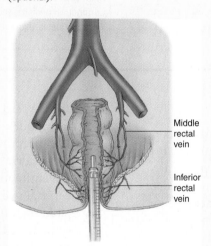

Middle rectal vein

Inferior rectal vein

Tip

The rectal dose of diazepam is 0.5 mg/kg, to a maximum dose of 20 mg. Onset of action for rectal diazepam is slower.

Blip

Administration of diazepam too high into the rectum may decrease its anticonvulsant effect, because the drug may be absorbed differently and broken down more quickly in the liver.

Procedure 21: Spinal Stabilization

Introduction

Spinal injury may be subtle or difficult to recognize because of altered level of consciousness, distracting injuries, or lack of obvious signs. Failure to recognize potential spinal injury can lead to death or permanent disability. Spinal stabilization is therefore essential for every child who sustains a suspicious mechanism of injury (where the head, neck, or spine may be involved), who has pain or tenderness of the spine, or who has signs or symptoms of weakness or loss of sensation.

Indications

Any significant mechanism of injury above the clavicles, including the head, neck, face, or axial spine
Acute weakness or loss of sensation after an injury
Pain or tenderness to the neck or spine
Deformity to the neck or spine
Altered level of consciousness after an injury

Contraindications

The combative child is a relative contraindication because forceful restraint of a combative child with spinal or head injury can worsen the injury.
If the risks of agitation and increased spinal movement from full spinal stabilization are greater than the benefits, consider more acceptable but less definitive stabilization options, and document the circumstances clearly.

Equipment

Long spine board
Padding materials (blankets, towels)
Rigid cervical collars in pediatric sizes
Straps with fastening device
Wide tape (2-in or 3-in)
Optional equipment
Head cushions from a cervical spine stabilization device (CID)
Commercial pediatric spinal stabilization device
Vest-type stabilization device

Rationale

The spinal column is made of 33 articulating bones, and its structure changes significantly during childhood growth. The age of the child and the physical state of spinal growth are important factors in the incidence and types of pediatric spinal injuries. Whenever the mechanism of injury, signs, or symptoms suggests possible spinal injury, the entire spine must be stabilized. This is best performed with the patient supine on a rigid spine board and in a neutral, in-line position. In field situations where this stabilization technique is not possible, maintain the anatomic stability of the entire spinal column as carefully as possible, and use age-specific considerations in approaching the child to minimize spinal movement.

Preparation

1. If the child is unstable or the environment is unsafe, quickly remove the patient onto the long spine board using manual spinal stabilization techniques.

2. If the depth of the patient's head is greater than that of the torso, arrange padding on the board to keep the entire lower spine and pelvis in line with the cervical spine and parallel to the board. This padding must cover the entire surface of the long spine board from the patient's shoulders to the hips.

3. Prepare the child and caregiver for the procedure by explaining actions. Make a game of it for an alert, cooperative child.

Possible Complications

Airway obstruction
Impairment of ventilation
Obscuring hemorrhage or other injuries
Spinal injury from improper technique
Back pain

Procedure

21-1 Initial Manual Spinal Stabilization

1 Gently align the head and neck into a neutral position similar to the "sniffing position." Do not force neutral position if there is resistance to movement, crepitus, or increased spinal pain.

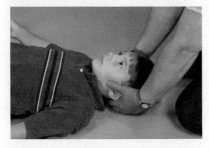

2 Have an additional rescuer(s) restrain other body parts as needed to reduce motion.

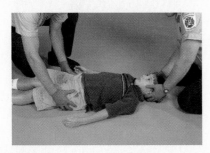

3 Have a second rescuer apply a size-appropriate rigid cervical collar. Evaluate the neck area that will be covered by the cervical collar. Determine the appropriate size with the manufacturer's recommendations. If a correctly sized cervical collar is unavailable, move on to the next step.

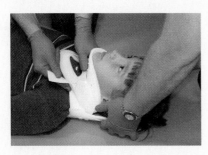

4 Transfer the patient as a unit onto a spine board or alternate stabilization device that is long enough to support the patient's full length. Perform the clinical assessment of the patient's back, buttocks, and breath sounds during the logroll process. Be prepared to treat injuries. After placing the child on the board, pad all open spaces under the patient before securing the patient to the board.

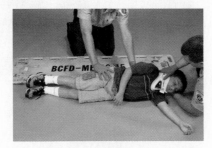

Tip

Reassure nervous children that the spinal stabilization is only temporary, but it is necessary. Try distraction.

Tip

Assign one rescuer to in-line neck stabilization of a combative child.

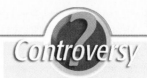
Controversy

The indications for long-board spinal stabilization of infants and toddlers are unknown. Infants and young children cannot verbally communicate symptoms such as weakness, numbness, or pain, so the threshold for spinal stabilization must be lower than for the older child. However, restraining a conscious child on a long board will cause pain and agitation in a short time.

Blip

Do not accept the labeled sizes for cervical collars ("pediatric" or "infant"). Measure each patient individually.

Procedure

21-2 Securing a Patient to a Spinal Stabilization Device

1 Secure the patient's body to the board while manually maintaining the neutral alignment of the head and neck. To secure against lateral movement, pad along the patient's sides to the edge of the board, especially along the pelvis and legs.

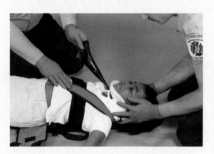

2 Stabilize the cervical spine by using blanket rolls, or blocks from the CID, to restrict lateral head motion and rotation and to prevent upward motion of the shoulders. Do not pad the young child's head because the large **occiput** will flex the neck and bend the airway out of neutral position. Secure against axial shifts if the board needs to be tilted (going down stairs, fitting into a small elevator, or for elevating the head in cases of head injury).

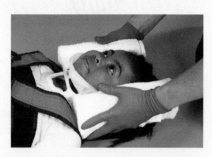

3 Place straps across the patient at the level of the **axilla**, pelvis, and legs. Do not place straps over the abdomen or use straps to impair movement of the diaphragm.

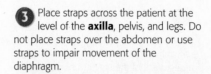
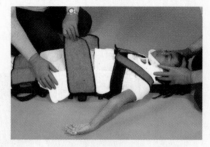

Blip

Do not use sandbags or weighted material because of the risk of injury in the event of movement.

Blip

Never place tape across the child's neck, as this may obstruct the airway.

4 Further secure the head with tape directly above the patient's eyebrows. Avoid chin straps that may complicate airway maintenance in case of emesis.

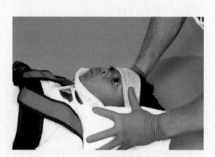

Tip

When using tape, use the longest strips possible to maximize adhesive surface and security.

Procedure

21-3 Pediatric Spinal Stabilization Using a Vest-type Stabilization Device

1 Perform the steps for initial spinal stabilization. Remove the vest device from its case. Open the head and body flaps. If the child's legs are longer than the device, place the device on a long spine board.

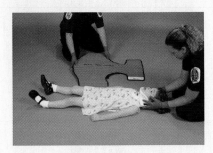

2 If padding is required to keep the child in neutral position, place it on the device.

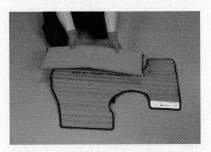

3 Using standard techniques (logroll, pivot onto board), move the patient as a unit onto the device.

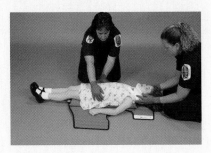

4 Lift the body flaps up and fold them inward on themselves along the lateral sides of the patient. This will ensure that the abdomen and chest are not restricted.

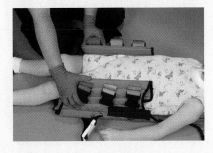

5 Secure the body flaps across the patient's trunk with tape or the attached straps. Make sure not to restrict the child's diaphragm or breathing.

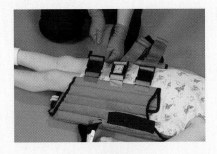

6 Lift the head flaps up along the child's head, and then fold the flaps down to the side so that the top edges are even with the child's forehead.

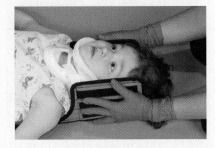

7 Place a strap across the child's forehead, connecting it across both sides of the head flaps. Secure the stabilized child to a long spine board.

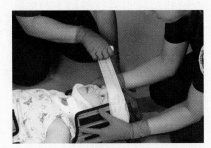

Controversy

The effectiveness and safety of the vest-type spinal stabilization device is controversial. The device is supposed to provide added restraint to a long spine board, but risks and benefits are not established.

Tip

Pad the patient to make the child as wide as the board.

Procedure

21-4 Releasing and Monitoring Spinal Stabilization

1 Do not release manual head and neck stabilization until the entire spine is properly stabilized.

2 Reassess airway, breathing, and circulation for possible compromise due to spinal stabilization technique.

3 Assess the patient's distal neurologic status before and after spinal stabilization.

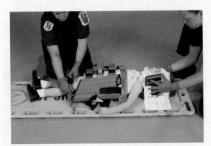

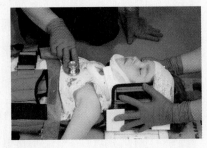

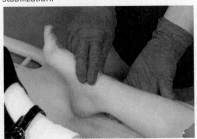

Blip

Never release manual neck stabilization until the entire spine is properly stabilized.

Procedure 22: Needle Thoracostomy

Introduction

A pneumothorax occurs when air gets between the two pleural membranes of the lung, a potential space that is empty under normal breathing conditions. Tension pneumothorax develops when the air in the pleural space has enough pressure to shift the internal contents of the chest and impair the function of the lungs, heart, and great vessels. Reduction in blood return to the heart and diminished cardiopulmonary function will result in shock and cardiopulmonary arrest if the tension pneumothorax is untreated. The child with tension pneumothorax has usually had positive-pressure ventilation in the field and will have physiologic abnormalities on assessment, with evidence of increased work of breathing and hypoxia. Classical adult physical findings, such as a shifted trachea or diminished breath sounds on the affected side, may not be detectable in an infant or child. If cardiac output is severely impaired by the tension pneumothorax, the child will also exhibit shock.

Indications

Penetrating chest-wall injury in a child with poor perfusion accompanied by respiratory distress and hypoxia

Blunt chest-wall injury in a child with respiratory distress and hypoxia that worsens with assisted ventilation

Contraindication

History of a severe bleeding disorder such as hemophilia (relative)

Equipment

14- or 16-gauge over-the-needle catheter
30-mL syringe
Povidone-iodine solution

Rationale

When the mechanism of injury, signs, and symptoms suggest tension pneumothorax in a child, create an opening between the pleural space and the atmosphere to immediately reduce elevated air pressure. This will help re-expand the lung, improve venous return, and restore cardiopulmonary function. The easiest method for creating a communication between the pleural space and the outside atmosphere is by producing an open pneumothorax. The technique requires inserting a large-bore needle into the pleural space and leaving it open to the air. This procedure is more frequently indicated after a penetrating injury than a blunt injury.

Preparation

1. Position the child supine.
2. Raise the arm above the head on the affected side, and have the caregiver or second rescuer hold it.
3. Select the site:
   - second intercostal space at the midclavicular line OR
   - fourth intercostal space at the anterior axillary line

4. Before preparing the site, count the ribs twice to ensure proper site location. The nipple is usually at the fourth intercostal space.
5. Prepare the site with povidone-iodine solution.

Possible Complications

Open pneumothorax
Hemothorax
Diaphragm penetration
Bowel penetration
Hemopericardium
Coronary vessel injury

Do not insert the needle *under* the rib margin because the vessels and nerves there are easily injured. Insert *above* the rib.

Procedure

22-1 Needle Thoracostomy

1 Attach the needle, with stylet in place, to the syringe.

2 Insert the needle through the skin at 90 degrees and advance until the tip hits a rib.

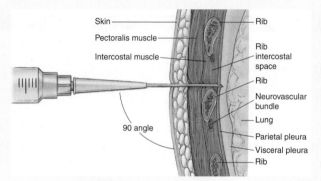

Skin — Rib
Pectoralis muscle — Rib intercostal space
Intercostal muscle — Rib
Neurovascular bundle
90 angle — Lung
Parietal pleura
Visceral pleura
Rib

3 Advance the needle over the top of the rib margin.

4 Push the needle tip into the pleural space. A slight "pop" is usually felt when the needle pierces the outside pleural membrane, or parietal pleura.

5 Pull back the plunger of the needle to aspirate air.

6 Remove the syringe and stylet and leave the catheter in the pleural space, anchored in the chest wall.

7 Monitor work of breathing, circulation to skin, heart rate, respiratory rate, and blood pressure. Consider doing contralateral needle thoracostomy if the child does not improve.

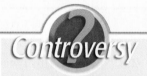

Controversy

The frequency of tension pneumothorax after blunt chest-wall injury is not known, and the indications for needle thoracostomy in this out-of-hospital situation are controversial.

Blip

Feeling for a midline trachea and listening for breath sounds are inaccurate ways to assess for pneumothorax in an infant or young child.

Tip

Suspect a tension pneumothorax when a child with chest injury worsens with assisted ventilation.

Procedure 23: Removing and Replacing a Tracheostomy Tube

Introduction

Children with tracheostomy tubes are increasingly common in the out-of-hospital setting. Most of these children live at home and have trained caregivers. Rarely, a tracheostomy tube problem occurs with a technology-assisted child (TAC) and 9-1-1 is activated.

Indications

Decannulation
Obstruction

Contraindications

Inadequately sized tract or stoma for insertion of a new tracheostomy tube; in this case, insert an endotracheal tube
Lack of a replacement tracheostomy tube or appropriately sized endotracheal tube

Equipment

Suction device
Sterile suction catheters
Oxygen
Bag-mask device, standard pediatric and adult mask sizes
Tracheostomy cannulas, appropriately sized for patient
Endotracheal tubes, standard pediatric and adult sizes
Laryngoscope handle with blades
Tape or tracheostomy ties
Gauze pads
5- or 10-mL syringe
Water-soluble lubricant
Scissors
Sterile saline
Stethoscope

Procedure

23-1 Removing an Old Tracheostomy Tube

1 Position the child with the head and neck hyperextended to expose the **tracheostomy** site.

2 Apply oxygen over the mouth and nose, and occlude (close off) the stoma or tracheostomy tube.

3 If the existing tube has a cuff, deflate it. Connect a 5- to 10-mL syringe to the valve on the pilot balloon. Draw air out until the balloon collapses. Cutting the balloon will not deflate the cuff.

4 Cut or untie the cloth ties that hold the tracheostomy tube in place.

5 Withdraw the tracheostomy tube using a slow, steady, outward and downward motion.

6 Assess airway for patency and adequate ventilation.

7 Provide oxygen and ventilation through the stoma as needed.

Rationale

Treatment of a tracheostomy tube problem usually requires simple techniques, such as suctioning or removal of the old tube and replacement with a new tube. Partial airway obstruction from clogging of the old tube may not be relieved by suctioning alone, or it may be impossible to ventilate a child through an existing tracheostomy tube because of **decannulation** or complete obstruction. Under these conditions, the prehospital professional must place a new tracheostomy tube to save the child's life.

Preparation

1. Ask the caregiver if there are any special problems with the child's trachea or special requirements involving the child's tracheostomy.
2. Ask the caregiver if a replacement tracheostomy tube is available.
3. Speak directly to the child about what to expect and attempt to enlist her cooperation.

Procedure

23-2 Replacing the Tracheostomy Tube

Insert a tracheostomy tube of the same size and model whenever possible. If this is not available, use a smaller tube or an endotracheal tube of the same outer diameter as the tracheostomy tube.

1 If the tube uses an insertion obturator, place this in the tube. If the tube has an inner and outer cannula, use the outer cannula and obturator for insertion.

2 Moisten or lubricate the tip of the tube (and obturator) with water, sterile saline, or a water-soluble lubricant.

3 Hold the device by the flange (wings) or hold the actual tube like a pencil.

4 Gently insert the tube with an arching motion (follow the curvature of the tube) posteriorly and then downward. Slight traction on the skin above or below the stoma may help.

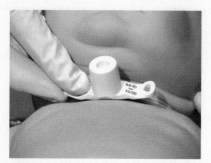

5 Once the tube is in place, remove the obturator, attach the bag-mask device, and attempt to ventilate. If the tube uses an inner cannula, insert to allow mechanical ventilation with a bag-mask device.

6 Check for proper placement by watching for bilateral chest rise, listening for equal breath sounds, and observing the patient. Signs of improper placement include lack of chest rise, unusual resistance to assisted ventilation, air in the surrounding tissues, and lack of patient improvement.

7 If the tube cannot be inserted, withdraw the tube, administer oxygen, and ventilate as needed.

8 Use a smaller-size tracheostomy tube for the second attempt. If still unsuccessful with a smaller tracheostomy tube, insert an endotracheal tube through the stoma. Check the length of the original tracheostomy tube, note the markings on the endotracheal tube, and advance it to the same depth as the original tube. The inserted portion of the endotracheal tube will be approximately half the distance needed for oral insertion. Do not advance the tube too far, or it may go into the right mainstem bronchus.

Tip

Talk to the caregiver about the size and type of tracheostomy tube and about known problems with the stoma or tube.

If unable to reinsert a tracheostomy tube, use a similarly sized endotracheal tube.

Keep the suction catheter close at hand.

9 If still unsuccessful, use a suction catheter as a guide. Insert a small, sterile suction catheter through the tracheostomy tube. Without applying suction, insert the suction catheter into the stoma. Slide the tracheostomy tube along the suction catheter and into the stoma, until it is in the proper position. Remove the suction catheter. Assess ventilation through the tracheostomy tube.

10 If still unsuccessful, consider orotracheal intubation or transport the patient with ventilation through the stoma using a stoma mask or newborn mask, or through bag-mask device over the nose and mouth while covering the stoma with a sterile gauze.

11 After proper placement, cut the ends of the tracheostomy ties or tape diagonally (allows for easy insertion), pass through eyelets (openings) on the flanges, and tie around the patient's neck, so that only a little finger can pass between the ties and the neck.

Blip

Do not use an esophageal detector bulb or syringe if the child weighs less than 20 kg.

Do not force a large tracheostomy tube through a new stoma site.

Do not advance an endotracheal tube too far through the stoma.

Possible Complications

Creation of a false **lumen**
Subcutaneous air
Pneumomediastinum

Pneumothorax
Bleeding at insertion site
Bleeding through tube
Right mainstem intubation with endotracheal tube

Note: The following drugs may be used for pediatric prehospital care. Certain drugs may not be available in some EMS systems per local policy. The drugs in tables designated by a green bar are core drugs commonly used in EMS systems. The drugs designated by a yellow bar are optional drugs that are sometimes used for children in EMS systems.

Acetaminophen, APAP, Paracetamol

Use: Analgesic, Antipyretic

Recommended Dose
10–15 mg/kg
Maximum Dose
1 g

Precaution: Ensure proper concentration.
Adverse Reactions: Nausea, vomiting

Activated Charcoal

Use: Gastric decontamination

Recommended Dose
Initial dose:
< 12 years: 1–2 g/kg
Maximum Dose
100 g

Precaution: Based on local EMS policy, the prehospital professional should consult either medical oversight or poison control (1-800-222-1222). Iron, lithium, alcohols, ethylene glycol, alkalis, flouride, mineral acids, and potassium do not bind to activated charcoal. Avoid aspiration. If airway reflexes are impaired, the risk of administering activated charcoal may outweigh the benefits. Commercially available preparations of activated charcoal often contain sorbitol as a cathartic. Fatal hypernatremic dehydration has been reported after repeated doses of charcoal with sorbitol.

Adverse Reactions: Constipation, obstruction, intestinal bezoar, diarrhea, dehydration, pulmonary aspiration

Adenosine

Use: Paroxysmal supraventricular tachycardia (PSVT)

Recommended Dose
0.1 mg/kg rapid IV or IO bolus over 1–2 seconds. Repeat at 0.2 mg/kg.
Maximum Dose
First Dose: 6 mg
Second Dose: 12 mg

Precaution: Use continous cardiac monitoring.
Avoid use in second or third degree AV block, sick sinus syndrome.
Adverse Reactions: Nausea, hypotension, dyspnea, bronchospasm, chest pain/pressure, tingling, heart block, dysrhythmias, facial flushing, metallic taste.
Bronchoconstriction may occur in asthmatics.

Albuterol (Salbutamol)

Use: Prevention and acute relief of bronchospasm, Prophylaxis for exercise-induced bronchospasm.

Recommended Dose
Nebulizer solution (1.25 mg/3 mL, 2.5 mg/3 mL, 5 mg/mL)
Minimum Dose: 2.5 mg every 20 minutes for 3 doses, repeat at dose of 0.15–0.3 mg/kg up to 10 mg every 1–4 hours as needed. Dilute in minimum of 2–3 mL of saline for adequate nebulization. May use continuously for status asthmaticus.
MDI: 4–8 puffs (90 µg/puff) every 15–20 minutes for 3 doses. Repeat every 1–4 hours as needed.
Maximum Dose
Not established for status asthmaticus

Precaution: Tremors common
Adverse Reactions: Nausea, palpitations, headache, dizziness, tremor, tachycardia

Amiodarone

Use: Life-threatening ventricular arrhythmias: ventricular fibrillation or tachycardia

Recommended Dose
5 mg/kg IV or IO push for cardiac arrest. 5 mg/kg IV or IO infusion over 20–60 minutes for wide complex tachycardia
Maximum Dose
15 mg/kg/day

Precaution: Must dilute with 20 mL of 5% dextrose prior to administration to avoid thrombophlebitis. May cause hypotension and prolonged Q-T interval. Should not use in combination with procainamide. Contraindicated in severe sinus node, dysfunction, marked sinus bradycardia, second and third degree AV block.
Adverse Reactions: Hypotension, bradycardia, dysrhythmias, vomiting

Aspirin

Use: Analgesic, Antipyretic

Recommended Dose
10–15 mg/kg
Maximum Dose
1 g

Precaution: Avoid use in children < 16 years with chickenpox or viral illness due to association with Reye's Syndrome.
Adverse Reactions: Nausea, vomiting, abdominal pain, ulcers, rash, urticaria, bronchospasm

Atropine

Use: Sinus bradycardia, Chemical nerve gas and organophosphate pesticide poisoning

Recommended Dose
0.01–0.02 mg/kg/IV or IO.
Minimum single dose of 0.1 mg.
May repeat dose every 5 minutes to maximum total dose of 1 mg for a child and 2 mg for an adolescent or adult.

Maximum Dose
Single Dose: 0.5 mg for a child,
1 mg for an adolescent.

Precaution: Atropine sulfate comes in different concentrations, calculate dosage accordingly. Avoid in tachydysrhythmias. Caution in children with brain damage or spastic paralysis. Anticholinesterase poisonings may require large doses of atropine (maximum dose above does not apply) and the addition of pralidoxime.

Adverse Reactions: Dry mouth, blurred vision, tachycardia, constipation, urinary retention

Calcium Chloride

Use: Ionized hypocalcemia, Hyperkalemia, Hypermagnesemia, Calcium channel blocker toxicity.
Recommended for cardiac resuscitation only in cases of documented hyperkalemia, hypocalcemia, or calcium channel blocker toxicity.

Recommended Dose
20 mg/kg IV or IO slowly (if using10% CaCl, dose is 0.2 mL/kg). Inject slowly while monitoring heart rate, Repeat dose as necessary for desired clinical effects.

Maximum Dose
1000 mg is usual maximum

Precaution: Stop injection if symptomatic bradycardia occurs. Calcium chloride administration results in a more rapid increase in ionized calcium concentrations than calcium gluconate and is preferred for the critically ill child.
Extravascular administration can result in severe skin injury. Highly irritating to tissues. Avoid scalp vein, small hand or foot veins for IV administration.

Adverse Reactions: Tissue extravasation and necrosis; May exacerbate metabolic acidosis. Hypotension, bradycardia, arrhythmias, ventricular fibrillation

Calcium Gluconate (preferred in neonates)

Use: Ionized hypocalcemia, Hyperkalemia, Hypermagnesemia, Calcium channel blocker toxicity.
Recommended for cardiac resuscitation only in cases of documented hyperkalemia, hypocalcemia, or calcium channel blocker toxicity.

Recommended Dose
60 mg/kg IV or IO slowly (if using 10% calcium gluconate, dose is 0.6 mL/kg). Inject slowly while monitoring heart rate.
Repeat dose as necessary for desired clinical effects.

Maximum Dose
1000 mg is usual maximum

Precaution: Stop injection if symptomatic bradycardia occurs. Calcium chloride administration results in a more rapid increase in ionized calcium concentrations than calcium gluconate and is preferred for the critically ill child. Extravascular administration can result in severe skin injury. Highly irritating to tissues. Avoid scalp vein, small hand or foot veins for IV administration.

Adverse Reactions: Tissue extravasation and necrosis, hypotension, bradycardia, arrhythmias, ventricular fibrillation

Dexamethasone

Use: Croup, Asthma

Recommended Dose
Croup:
0.15–0.6 mg/kg IV, IM, or PO
Asthma:
0.6–1.0 mg/kg IV or IM

Maximum Dose
16 mg/day

Precaution: Long acting glucocorticoid

Adverse Reactions: Sodium and fluid retention, hyperglycemia

Diazepam

Use: Seizures, Agitation

Recommended Dose
IV: 0.1 mg/kg every 5–10 minutes. Administer over approximately 2 minutes to avoid pain at intravenous site.
PR: 0.5 mg/kg up to 20 mg

Maximum Dose
IV: 5 mg/dose
PR: 20 mg

Precaution: There is an increased incidence of apnea when combined with other sedative agents or when given rapidly. Be prepared to provide respiratory support. Monitor oxygen saturation. Avoid extravasation to prevent venous thrombosis or phlebitis. Avoid rapid administration to prevent hypotension or respiratory arrest. Avoid prolonged use of parenteral diazepam because it contains 40% propylene glycol as a diluent.

Adverse Reactions: Respiratory depression, drowsiness, bradycardia, hypotension, apnea, pain at injection site

Diphenhydramine

Use: Anaphylaxis, Antihistamine

Recommended Dose
1–2 mg/kg IV or IO slow push

Maximum Dose
IV: 50 mg

Precaution: May case sedation and respiratory suppression especially if using other sedative agents. May cause hypotension. Overdosage may cause hallucinations and seizures. Rapid IV administration may precipitate seizures. All doses may cause paradoxical excitement or agitation.

Adverse Reactions: Drowsiness, dry mouth, constipation, urinary retention

Dopamine

Use: Hypotension, Shock

Recommended Dose
Neonate: 2–10 µg/kg/min IV or IO infusion
Children: 2–20 µg/kg/min IV or IO infusion
Titrate up to desired effect:
  5 µg/kg/min = low dose
  10 µg/kg/min = moderate dose
  20 µg/kg/min = high dose

Maximum Dose
20 µg/kg/min

Precaution: Infusion rates greater than 20 µg/kg/minute may produce extreme peripheral vasoconstriction and ischemia. Mix with great caution. Extravascular administration can result in severe skin injury. Avoid small veins. Dopamine is inactivated in an alkaline solution. Correct hypovolemia prior to use.

Adverse Reactions: Ectopic beats, tachycardia, palpitations, vasoconstriction, dyspnea, vomiting

Epinephrine

Use: Croup, Anaphylaxis, Acute asthma, Cardiac arrest

Recommended Dose
Anaphylaxis:
  IM, SQ: 0.01 mg/kg/dose = 0.01 mL/kg/dose of 1:1000 (max 0.3 mg = 0.3 mL). Repeat dose every 5–20 minutes.
Croup:
  0.25–0.5 mg/kg of 1:1000 in 3 mL of NS by inhalation (max 5 mL/dose)
Cardiac arrest:
  0.01 mg/kg = 0.1 mL/kg of 1:10,000 IV or IO OR 0.1 mg/kg = 0.1 mL/kg of 1:1000 ET. Except in newly born use 0.01–0.03 mg/kg = 0.1–0.3 mL/kg of 1:10,000.
Racemic epinephrine (2.25%) for croup:
  0.5 mg/kg = 0.5 mL/kg by inhalation (maximum 5 mL) in 2 mL of NS by inhalation.

Precaution: Use length-based resuscitation tape or computerized software to verify correct dose. Read concentration on label carefully. Incompatible with alkaline solutions. Extravascular administration can result in severe skin injury.
Anaphylaxis: Some anaphylactic reactions require large doses of epinephrine that may be administered IV.
Cardiac Arrest: If administered through an endotracheal tube, follow the dose with saline flush or dilute in isotonic saline flush (1 to 5 mL) based on patient length/weight.

Adverse Reactions: Tachycardia, palpitations, cardiac dysrhythmias, diaphoresis, vomiting, headache, dizziness

Fentanyl

Use: Analgesic, Anesthetic for intubation and maintenance

Recommended Dose
IV: 1–5 µg/kg/dose every 30–60 minutes

Maximum Dose
Titrate to effect

Precaution: There is an increased incidence of apnea when combined with other sedative agents, particularly benzodiazepines. Avoid rapid IV infusion; inject slowly over several minutes. If given rapidly, may cause chest wall or glottic rigidity, which may be reversed with a muscle relaxant.

Adverse Reactions: Apnea, bradycardia, nausea, vomiting

Flumazenil

Use: Reverse sedative effects of benzodiazepines

Recommended Dose
IV: 0.01–0.02 mg/mL over 15 seconds; repeat every 1 min prn. When IV access is unavailable, may be given IM.

Maximum Dose
0.2 mg/dose and to cumulative total dose of 0.05 mg/kg or 1 mg

Precaution: May precipitate acute withdrawal in dependent patients. May precipitate seizures in high risk patients on chronic benzodiazepine, sedative/hypnotics or other coingestants in an overdose. Observe for resedation. Avoid single bolus injection.

Adverse Reactions: Rebound sedation or respiratory depression due to its short duration of action.

Fosphenytoin

Use: Seizures, Status epilepticus

Recommended Dose

Status epilepticus:
20 phenytoin equivalents (PE) mg/kg IV or IO over 7 minutes (3 mg/kg/min); not to exceed 150 mg/min. May be given IM.

Maximum Dose

1000 mg

Precaution: Rate of infusion should not exceed 3/mg/kg/min. Reduce rate of infusion if heart rate decreases by 10 bpm. Dosages and concentrations are expressed as phenytoin sodium equivalents. Rapid IV administration may produce hypotension.

Adverse Reactions: Hypotension, bradycardia, central nervous system depression, ataxia, dizziness, headache, paresthesia, pruritus. Itching is common and is controlled by reducing flow rate.

Furosemide

Use: Fluid overload, Congestive heart failure, Diuresis, Edema, Pulmonary Edema, Hypertension

Recommended Dose

Children: 1–2 mg/kg IV, IO, or IM

Maximum Dose

10 mg

Precaution: Do not give to child with hypovolemia. Contraindicated in anuria.

Adverse Reactions: Hypotension, electrolyte depletion, alkalosis, tinnitus, ototoxic

Glucagon

Use: Beta-blocker or Calcium channel blocker overdose, Hypoglycemia

Recommended Dose

Hypoglycemia due to insulin excess:
Children: 0.03–0.1 mg/kg IV, IO, IM, or SQ; repeat every 15 minutes if needed for clinical effect. Total 3 doses.
Beta-blocker or calcium channel blocker overdose:
IV: 0.03–0.15 mg/kg followed by 0.07 mg/kg/h (maximum of 5 mg/h) infusion.

Maximum Dose

Pediatric: 1 mg

Precaution: Use immediately after reconstitution. Caution in patients with pheochromocytoma.

Adverse Reactions: Nausea, vomiting

Glucose (Dextrose)

Use: Hypoglycemia

Recommended Dose

Newly born: 2 mL/kg 10% dextrose IV or IO push
Neonate: 5 mL/kg 10% dextrose IV or IO push
< 2 years: 2 mL/kg 25% dextrose IV or IO push
> 2 years: 1 mL/kg 50% dextrose IV or IO push

Maximum Dose

Doses guided by repeated serum glucose level determinations

Precaution: Depending on situation hypoglycemia may re-occur.

Adverse Reactions: Hyperglycemia

Ibuprofen

Use: Analgesic, Antipyretic

Recommended Dose

5–10 mg/kg/dose PO

Maximum Dose

800 mg

Precaution: Cross reacts with aspirin allergy, gastrointestinal bleeding. Liquid products may contain alcohol.

Adverse Reactions: Vomiting, gastritis, ulcer formation, rash

Ipratropium

Use: Asthma

Recommended Dose

Nebulized solution (0.5 mg/2.5 mL)
Children < 12 years: 0.25 mg nebulized every 20 minutes for 3 doses
Children > 12 years: 0.5 mg nebulized every 20 minutes for 3 doses

Maximum Dose

0.5 mg

Precaution: Use with albuterol every 20 min x 3.

Adverse Reactions: Tachycardia, dry mouth, headache, cough, hoarseness, blurred vision

Ketamine

Use: Anesthesia for intubation

Recommended Dose
IV: 1–2 mg/kg for intubation
IM: 3–5 mg/kg

Maximum Dose
Highest dose in dose range is maximum dose to administer.

Precaution: Emergence reactions may occur up to 24 hours postoperatively: delirium, hallucinations, vivid dreams. Avoid use in patients with increased ICP, increased intraocular pressure, or bowel obstruction.

Adverse Reactions: Hallucinations, tonic-clonic movements, nausea, vomiting, decreased cough reflex, nystagmus, tachycardia, bronchospasm, hypertension, bradycardia, hypotension, apnea. May cause purposeless movements.

Lidocaine (Lignocaine)

Use: Ventricular tachycardia, Ventricular fibrillation, Wide-complex PSVT

Recommended Dose
Children: IV/IO/ET Loading Dose = 1 mg/kg; repeat in 10–15 minutes for 2 doses if needed; IV continuous infusion after loading dose: 20–50 μg/kg/min
ET: 2–2.5 times the IV dose

Maximum Dose
IV: 3 mg/kg/dose

Precaution: Contraindicated in complete heart block and wide complex tachycardia due to accessory conduction pathways. Excessive dosage may result in myocardial depression, hypotension, agitation, or seizures. Hypersensitivity to amide anesthetics. If administered through an endotracheal tube, follow the dose with saline flush or dilute in ostonic saline flush (1 to 5 mL) based on patient size.

Adverse Reactions: Arrhythmias, seizures, respiratory depression or arrest

Lorazepam

Use: Anticonvulsant, Anxiety, Sedation

Recommended Dose
Status epilepticus:
Neonates: 0.05 mg/kg IV or IO over 2–5 minutes
Infants and Children: 0.05–0.1 mg/kg IV or IO over 2–5 minutes; max: 4 mg/dose; repeat 0.05 mg/kg second dose in 10–15 minutes if needed

Maximum Dose
4 mg/dose

Precaution: Beware of respiratory depression. There is an increased incidence of apnea when combined with other sedative agents. Monitor oxygen saturation and be prepared to provide respiratory support. May be reversed with flumazenil.

Adverse Reactions: Bradycardia, hypotension, apnea, confusion, hallucinations, myoclonic jerking in preterm infants

Mannitol

Use: Diuresis, Reduces intracranial pressure

Recommended Dose
IV: 0.25–1 g/kg

Maximum Dose
1 g/kg body weight

Precaution: Inspect vials for crystals. Use 5 micron filter for 20% solutions or greater. Avoid excessive fluid loss with diuresis to prevent dehydration and electrolyte imbalance.

Adverse Reactions: Dehydration, fluid and electrolyte imbalance, headache, hypovolemia, seizures, water intoxication

Methylprednisolone

Use: Asthma, Croup

Recommended Dose
Status asthmaticus:
1–2 mg/kg/dose IV or IO

Maximum Dose
60 mg

Precaution: Rapid IV push of high doses in < 20 minutes may cause hypotension, arrhythmias, and sudden death.

Adverse Reactions: Edema, pituitary-adrenal suppression, hypokalemia, peptic ulcer, nausea, vomiting

Midazolam

Use: Anxiety, Seizures

Recommended Dose

Status epilepticus:
    IV, IO, or IM: 0.05–0.15 mg/kg
Sedation:
    IV, IO, or IM: 0.05–0.1 mg/kg

Maximum Dose

6 months–5 years: 6 mg
> 6 years: 10 mg

Precaution: Avoid rapid IV administration which may produce respiratory arrest and seizures. There is an increased incidence of apnea when combined with other sedative agents, particularly benzodiapines. Be prepared to provide respiratory support, regardless of route of administration. Monitor oxygen saturation. May be reversed with flumazenil. Myoclonus may occur in premature infants. Paradoxical excitation may occur in children. May be reversed with flumazenil.

Adverse Reactions: Bradycardia, hypotension, cardiac arrest, apnea, respiratory depression

Morphine

Use: Severe acute and chronic pain, Pulmonary edema

Recommended Dose

Neonates: 0.05 mg/kg IM, IV, IO, SQ
Infants and Children: 0.1–0.2 mg/kg IM, IV, IO, SQ
Adolescents: 3–4 mg IV or IO, repeat in 5 minutes as needed

Maximum Dose

Neonates: 0.1 mg/kg
Infants, children, and adolescents: 10 mg

Precaution: Pediatric patients are more sensitive to the effects of opiates. Hypersensitivity to similar opiates. Some products may contain sulfites. There is an increased incidence of apnea when combined with other sedative agents, particularly benzodiapines. Be prepared to provide respiratory support, regardless of route of administration. Monitor oxygen saturation. May be reversed with naloxone.

Adverse Reactions: Respiratory depression, hypotension, rash

Naloxone

Use: Opiate intoxication

Recommended Dose

Pediatric: 0.1 mg/kg/dose IV, IO, IM, ET, SQ

Maximum Dose

2 mg

Precaution: Dilute to 1–2 mL with normal saline for ET use. May induce acute withdrawal in opioid dependency. Patients who receive naloxone should be continuously observed for renarcotization for at least 2 hours after last dose of naloxone. Doses may be repeated as needed to maintain opiate reversal. IM absorption may be erratic. Do not administer naloxone to a newly born whose mother is suspected of recently abusing drugs due to risk of acute withdrawal in the infant.

Nitrous oxide, Dinitrogen oxide, Nitrogen oxide, N_2O, Laughing gas

Use: Analgesia, Sedation

Recommended Dose

25–50% with oxygen 50:50

Maximum Dose

70–80%

Precaution: Asphyxiation may occur

Adverse Reactions: Malignant hyperthermia, cardiac dysrhythmias, nausea, vomiting, delirium

Norepinephrine

Use: Distributive shock

Recommended Dose

0.05–0.1 µg/kg/min IV, titrate to desired response

Maximum Dose

1–2 µg/kg/min

Precaution: Double check concentration and infusion rate. Avoid scalp veins.

Adverse Reactions: Bradycardia, hypertension, arrhythmias, palpitations, pallor, ischemic necrosis, organ ischemia

Phenobarbital, Phenobarbitone

Use: Status epilepticus, Sedation

Recommended Dose

20 mg/kg IV or IO over 20 min (1 mg/kg/min); not to exceed 50 mg/min

Maximum Dose

1000 mg

Precaution: There is an increased incidence of apnea when combined with other sedative agents. Be prepared to provide respiratory support. Monitor oxygen saturation. Avoid extravasation because parenteral solutions are very alkaline. Be prepared to support respirations.

Adverse Reactions: Drowsiness, hypotension, apnea, paradoxical excitation

Phenytoin, Sodium Diphenylhydantoin (DPH)

Use: Status epilepticus

Recommended Dose
Neonate: 10 mg/kg
Children: 20 mg/kg IV or IO over 20 min
(1 mg/kg/min); not to exceed 50 mg/min
Maximum Dose
1000 mg

Precaution: Incompatible with glucose solutions. Monitor heart rate and reduce infusion if rate decreases by 10 beats/min. Rapid IV administration may trigger ventricular fibrillation and cardiac arrest. Avoid extravasation. Injections may contain propylene glycol and benzyl alcohol.

Adverse Reactions: Bradycardia, hypotension, arrhythmias, cardiovascular collapse, nystagmus, drowsiness

Pralidoxime Chloride, 2-PAM, 2-Pyridine Aldoxime Methochloride

Use: Organophosphate poisoning, Carbamate insecticide poisoning with nicotinic symptoms, Cholinesterase

Recommended Dose
25–50 mg/kg, up to 1 g, IV over
  5–30 minutes, then 10 mg/kg/hr or repeat load
  every 1–2 hours.
Maximum Dose
1 g/dose
Large total amounts may be required in a severe
  poisoning.

Precaution: Rapid IV administration may cause tachycardia, laryngospasm, muscle rigidity and transient neuromuscular blockade. IV route preferred, but may be given IM or SC when IV route is not immediately accessible.

Adverse Reactions: Nausea, headache, dizziness, diplopia, hyperventilation

Rocuronium Bromide

Use: Adjunct to general anesthesia to facilitate tracheal intubation and provide skeletal muscle relaxation during mechanical ventilation.

Recommended Dose
IV: 1 mg/kg
Maximum Dose
1.2 mg/kg

Precaution: Ventilatory support is necessary. Prepare to respond with airway management. Do not mix with alkaline solutions. May interact with certain antibiotics that have neuromuscular blocking actions (e.g., aminoglycosides) and enhance neuromuscular blockade. Toxicity may be increased in patients with pulmonary disease.

Adverse Reactions: Muscle weakness, hypotension or hypertension, arrhythmias, tachycardia, bronchospasm, hiccoughs

Sodium Bicarbonate

Use: Cyclic antidepressant overdose, Hyperkalemia

Recommended Dose
Pediatric: 1–2 mEq/kg IV or IO slowly
Maximum Dose
50 mEq/dose

Precaution: Do not mix with calcium, dopamine, epinephrine. May cause tissue necrosis from IV extravasation. Caution with renal impairment. No more than 0.5 mEq/mL for neonatal use.

Adverse Reactions: Cerebral hemorrhage, edema, hypernatremia, hypokalemia, hypocalcemia, metabolic alkalosis

Succinylcholine, Suxamethonium

Use: Adjunct to general anesthesia, Endotracheal intubation, Mechanical ventilation

Recommended Dose
IV: 1–2 mg/kg/dose

Precaution: Contraindications in conditions associated with increased ICP, severe burns, spinal cord injury, neuromuscular disease, myopathy, or malignant hyperthemia. When these contraindications exist, use a nondepolarizing muscle relaxant such as rocuronium. Ventilatory support is necessary. If cardiac arrest occurs immediately after administration of succinylcholine, hyperkalemia must be suspected (particularly in males under 9 years of age). Toxicity is increased in patients with muscle injury, muscle myopathies, rhabdomyolysis, or low pseudocholinesterase levels. Children are more susceptible to developing bradycardia, cardiac arrest, and myoglobinemia. Atropine is recommended prior to the administration of succinylcholine in children.

Adverse Reactions: Bradycardia, hypotension, arrhythmias, apnea, cardiac arrest, hyperkalemia, malignant hyperthermia

Glossary

abdomen the anatomic portion of the anterior trunk below the ribs and above the pelvis; it contains the stomach, lower part of the esophagus, small and large intestines, liver, gall bladder, spleen, pancreas, and bladder.

abdominal excursions the work of abdominal muscles in infants during the breathing cycle.

abrasion a portion of skin or of a mucous membrane scraped away as a result of injury.

absorb to take in or suck up.

acceleration-deceleration injury a type of injury caused when a moving body part, such as the head, stops its forward motion suddenly.

acetaminophen a synthetic drug with antipyretic and analgesic actions similar to aspirin, used in patients with sensitivity to aspirin.

acid a corrosive substance with low ph.

acidosis excessive acidity of body fluids due to an accumulation of acids (as in diabetic acidosis or renal disease) or an excessive loss of bicarbonate (as in renal disease).

acrocyanosis cyanosis of the extremities; acrocyanosis of the hands and feet may be normal in the infant within the first hour after birth.

activation phase first of three phases in disaster response. This is the notification and initial response phase which includes establishment of the Incident Command System organization and scene assessment.

additional assessment includes a focused history and physical exam, a detailed physical exam (if the child is injured), and the ongoing assessment.

adenoidal lymphoid tissue in the back of the mouth and oropharynx.

adrenaline synonym for epinephrine. A hormone produced by the body that increases pulse rate and blood pressure; mediates the "fight-or-flight" response of the sympathetic nervous system when the body is under stress.

adrenergic agents drugs that mimic the effects of epinephrine (adrenaline) and norepinephrine.

afebrile seizures a seizure not accompanied by a fever.

agent something that causes an effect; thus, bacteria that cause a disease are said to be agents of the specific disease. An injury agent is the energy causing the damage, such as thermal energy from a burn. A drug is a pharmacologic agent.

agonist a substance that stimulates or activates a specialized receptor on a cell.

airway adjunct an artificial device to maintain an open airway.

alkali a strong base with a high ph, usually corrosive to tissues.

alveoli the air sacs of the lungs in which the exchange of oxygen and carbon dioxide takes place.

amniotic fluid the liquid contained in the amnion, inside the uterus. This fluid is sterile, transparent, and almost colorless. The liquid surrounds and protects the fetus from injury and helps maintain an even temperature.

analgesia, analgesic a drug that relieves pain.

anaphylactic reaction an extreme, life-threatening systemic allergic reaction that may include shock and respiratory failure.

anaphylaxis a severe form of hypersensitivity reaction that produces dangerous physiologic changes, such as bronchospasm, shock, and airway edema.

anatomic relating to the anatomy or structure of an organism.

ancillary something that assists another action or effect but is not essential to the accomplishment of the action.

antecubital fossa the triangular area lying anterior to and below the elbow, bounded medially by the pronator teres muscle and laterally by the brachioradialis muscles.

anteroposterior (AP) from front-to-back. For example, an AP x-ray of the chest is taken from front-to-back.

antibiotic any of a variety of natural or synthetic substances that inhibit growth of, or destroy, bacteria that are responsible for infectious diseases.

anticonvulsant agent that prevents or stops convulsions.

antigen protein recognized by the immune system which causes an allergic reaction.

antipyretic an agent that reduces fever.

antivenin a serum that counteracts the effect of venom from an animal or insect.

anxiolysis reduction of anxiety, agitation, or tension.

Apgar score a system of scoring a newly born's physiologic condition at 1 minute and 5 minutes after birth. The heart rate, respiration, muscle tone, response to stimuli, and color are each rated 0, 1, or 2. The maximum total score is 10.

apnea a temporary cessation of breathing.

apneic characterized by absence of breathing.

apparent life-threatening event (ALTE) an unexplained sudden episode of color change (cyanosis or pallor), tone change (limpness, stiffness), or apnea that required mouth-to-mouth resuscitation or vigorous stimulation.

asphyxia a condition caused by insufficient oxygen.

aspiration the process of sucking in. Foreign bodies may be aspirated into the nose, throat, or lungs on inspiration.

assessment evaluation.

asthma a disease caused by increased responsiveness of the tracheobronchial tree to various stimuli. The result is paroxysmal constriction of the bronchial airways. Clinically, there is severe dyspnea accompanied by wheezing.

asymmetric without symmetry.

asystole cardiac standstill; absence of contractions of the heart.

asystolic arrest cardiac standstill; absence of a heartbeat.

ataxia an abnormal gait.

atrioventricular heart block blockage of the electrical impulse from the atrium of the heart to the ventricle.

atrium one of two (right and left) upper chambers of the heart. The right atrium receives blood from the vena cava and delivers it to the right ventricle, which, in turn, pumps blood into the blood vessels of the lungs. The left atrium receives blood from pulmonary veins and delivers it to the left ventricle, which, in turn, pumps blood into the body.

auscultate to listen, as with a stethoscope.

auscultation the process of listening for sounds within the body with a stethoscope.

AVPU scale the components of the AVPU scale are used to assess the level of consciousness: Alert, Voice, Painful, Unresponsive.

avulsion a tearing away of a part or structure.

axial loading vertical pressure on the spine.

axillary temperature the temperature taken in the armpit.

axonal shearing a tearing of axons or nerve sheaths, caused by sudden movement, to produce severe brain injury.

baseline a known or initial value with which subsequent observations can be compared.

basilar skull fracture a fracture into the base of the skull, sometimes associated with brain hemorrhage or brain injury.

Battle sign bruising behind the ear; an indication of basilar skull fracture.

belly breathing a type of breathing using abdominal muscles that is normal in infants.

benzodiazepines a family of sedative-hypnotic drugs useful for treatment of seizures and agitation.

bezoar a hard mass of entangled material sometimes found in the stomach and intestines.

bilateral pertaining to, affecting, or relating to two sides.

biological agents organisms that cause disease, including viruses, bacteria, and toxins.

biological pathogens a microorganism that can cause disease in a host.

blood pressure the perfusing pressure of blood.

brachial pertaining to a main artery and vein of the arm.

bradycardia a slow heartbeat.

brain death cessation of brain function.

brain perfusion blood circulation in the brain.

brain stem the stemlike part of the brain that connects the cerebral hemispheres with the spinal cord.

brain stem functions bodily functions controlled by the brain stem that are necessary for life, such as breathing.

brain stem herniation bulging and compression of brain tissue; causes breathing to stop and death of the patient.

breech a newborn presentation that is not the head, usually the buttocks.

bronchiolitis inflammation of the bronchioles by a virus.

bronchoconstriction narrowing of the bronchial tubes.

bronchodilator a drug that helps open the airways to improve air movement and reduce wheezing.

bronchopulmonary dysplasia (BPD) iatrogenic chronic lung disease that develops in premature infants following a period of oxygen therapy.

bronchovesicular pertaining to the tree of pulmonary passages.

buckle fracture a minor fracture only partially through the bone, in which the top layer of bone on one side is compressed, forming a slight angle or "buckle" in the surface.

bulging fontanelle a protuberance of brain contents through the immature opening of bone in the front of the skull; this sign suggests increased intracranial pressure.

button a type of gastrostomy tube.

calcium channel blockers a family of drugs that helps reduce the speed of conduction through the heart and the overall work of the heart.

cannulating to introduce a catheter through a vein or passageway.

capillary refill time (CRT) a test that evaluates distal circulatory system function performed by pushing on an area such as a nail bed and watching the speed of its return of pinkness after releasing the pressure.

cardiac arrest the cessation of cardiac mechanical activity, determined by the inability to palpate a central pulse, unresponsiveness, and apnea.

cardiac dysrhythmia an abnormal cardiac rhythm.

cardiogenic shock a reduced cardiac output secondary to abnormal cardiac function.

cardiomyopathy disease of the myocardium, especially due to primary disease of the heart muscle.

cardiotonic affecting the heart.

cartilage a specialized type of dense connective tissue, softer than bone, that is common in the skeletons of children.

cartilaginous growth plates the horizontal part of the bone which grows as the human body matures.

cathartic a purgative agent for the bowel.

caustic corrosive and burning; destructive to living tissue.

central cyanosis slightly bluish, grayish, or dark purple discoloration of the skin (on the trunk and face) due to presence of hypoxia.

central nervous system (CNS) CNS consists of the brain and spinal cord; it controls vital body functions.

central venous catheter catheter inserted into the vena cava to permit intermittent or continuous monitoring of central venous pressure and to facilitate obtaining blood samples for chemical analysis.

cerebral cortex the higher brain; the source of the senses, thinking, feeling, and voluntary movement.

cerebral spinal fluid (CSF) shunt tube that suctions fluid manufactured in the ventricles of the brain from the subarachnoid space to drain in another part of the anatomy outside of the brain, such as the peritoneum. This lowers pressure in the brain.

cerebrospinal fluid a water cushion protecting the brain and spinal cord from physical impact.

cervical of, pertaining to, or in the region of the high spine.

chest wall the musculoskeletal framework of the chest.

child maltreatment a general term applying to all forms of child abuse and neglect.

child neglect failure by those responsible for caring for a child to provide for the child's nutritional, emotional, and physical needs.

child protective services (CPS) this agency is the community legal organization responsible for protection, rehabilitation, and prevention of child maltreatment and neglect. CPS has the legal authority temporarily to remove from home children at risk for injury or neglect and to secure foster placement.

children with special health care needs (CSHCN) those who have or are at increased risk for a chronic, physical, developmental, behavioral, or emotional condition and who also require health and related services of a type or amount beyond that required by children generally.

cholinergic crisis a crisis involving cholinergic drugs or "nerve gases" designed for chemical warfare. Cholinergic agents overstimulate normal body functions that are controlled by the parasympathetic nerves.

cholinergic impulses description of a neuron that secretes the neurotransmitter acetylcholine.

circadian rhythm the regular recurrence, in cycles of about 24 hours, of biological processes or activities, such as sensitivity to drugs and stimuli, hormone secretion, sleeping, feeding, etc. This rhythm seems to be set by a biological clock that seems to be set by recurring daylight and darkness.

clavicles the collarbone; a bone, curved like the letter f, that articulates with the sternum and scapula.

coin rubbing cultural ritual intended to treat an illness by rubbing hot coins, often on the back, which produces rounded and oblong red, patch, flat skin lesions.

commotio cordis sudden cardiac arrest from a blunt, nonpenetrating blow to the chest. The basis of the cardiac arrest is ventricular fibrillation (a chaotically abnormal heart rhythm) triggered by chest wall impact immediately over the anatomic position of the heart.

compensated shock a clinical state in which there are clinical signs of inadequate tissue perfusion, but the patient's blood pressure is in the normal range.

compensatory mechanisms physiologic responses, initiated to help return the body's vital functions to normal after a severe insult to breathing, perfusion, or metabolic function.

complex febrile seizure unusual form of convulsion that occurs in association with a rapid increase in body temperature.

complex partial seizure characterized by alteration of consciousness with or without complex focal motor activity.

compression a squeezing together; state of being pressed together.

concussion a brain injury causing any type of altered state of consciousness.

congenital present at birth.

congential anomalies an anatomic structure that is unusual or different at birth.

congenital heart disease heart disease that is present from birth.

congestive heart failure a disorder in which the heart loses part of its ability to effectively pump blood, usually as a result of damage to the heart muscle and usually resulting in a backup of fluid into the lungs.

consent for care permission to render care.

constipation infrequent defecation with passage of unduly hard and dry fecal material.

contact burn a thermal burn from direct contact with a hot object, fluid, or gas.

contraindications a condition indicating that a treatment is inappropriate.

core perfusion blood circulation in the core of the human body.

corrosive producing corrosion or destruction of tissue.

cortical pertaining to or of the outer layer of the brain.

crackles rales. Lung sounds that suggest fluid in alveoli.

cranium (physeal plates) the area of the head above the ears and eyes; the skull. The cranium contains the brain.

crepitus the noise or feel of gas in soft tissues.

critical incident stress management (CISM) a process that confronts the responses to critical incidents and defuses them, directing the emergency service personnel toward physical and emotional equilibrium.

croup a childhood viral disease characterized by edema of the upper airways with barking cough, difficult breathing, and stridor.

crowning stage in delivery when the fetal head presents at the vaginal opening.

CSF otorrhea leakage of CSF from the ear; a sign of basilar skull fracture.

cyanosis slightly bluish, grayish, slatelike, or dark purple discoloration of the skin due to presence of hypoxia.

cyanotic heart disease a type of congenital heart disease with a right to left shunt resulting in partially oxygenated blood in the systemic circulation.

cyclic antidepressants a type of antidepressant drug that may cause coma, seizures, and conduction disturbances if taken in an overdose.

decerebrate a posture characterized by extension of the arms and legs; indicates pressure on the brain stem and may appear in patients with severe brain swelling.

decompensated shock a severe shock state that will rapidly progress to cardiac arrest if not rapidly corrected.

decompensation failure of the heart to maintain adequate bodily functions after a physiologic insult.

decontamination the process of removing a poison.

decorticate a posture characterized by flexion of the arms and extension of the legs; indicates pressure on the brain stem and may appear in patients with severe brain trauma.

defibrillator an electrical device that produces defibrillation of the heart; it may be used externally or in the form of an automatic implanted defibrillator.

demarcated a defined area in a boundary

dendrite a projection from a neuron that makes connections with an adjacent cell.

dependent lower region of the body; the part closest to the ground.

diabetes mellitus a metabolic disorder in which the ability to metabolize sugar is impaired, usually because of a lack of insulin.

diabetic ketoacidosis a form of acidosis in uncontrolled diabetes in which certain acids accumulate when insulin is not available.

diagnostic testing tests used to determine the cause of an illness or disorder.

diaphoretic a state of excessive perspiration because of high physiologic stress.

diaphragm the muscle separating the chest from the abdominal cavity, which allows breathing.

diaphysis the shaft of a long bone.

diastolic pressure the pressure that remains in the arteries during the relaxing phase of the heart's cycle (diastole) when the left ventricle is at rest.

diffuse axonal injury a diffuse injury in discrete regions of the brain following high-speed, long-duration deceleration injuries.

dilated widened.

diptheria an acute infectious disease of childhood characterized by fever, upper airway obstruction, and respiratory distress.

direct medical oversight on-line, real-time supervision of the prehospital professional's practice by base hospital physicians or nurses.

dirty bomb name given to a bomb that is used as a radiological dispersal device (RDD).

disaster a widespread event that disrupts community resources and functions, in turn threatening public safety, citizens' lives, and property.

distal farthest from the center.

distal extremities structures that are farther from the trunk or nearer to the free end of the extremity.

distention inflation, enlargement.

distributive shock a clinical state characterized by maldistribution of blood volume and vascular tone.

diving reflex submersion of the face and nose in water to produce a vagal reaction; used to terminate an important dysrhythmia of childhood called supraventricular tachycardia.

Do Not Resuscitate written documentation giving permission to medical personnel not to attempt resuscitation in the event of cardiac arrest.

Down syndrome (DS) a congenital disorder in which a person is born with three copies of chromosome 21 (trisomy 21). Clinical features include moderate to severe mental retardation, slanting eyes, a broad short skull, broad hands and short fingers. Other congenital abnormalities include heart defects and oesophageal atresia.

dressings protective covering for diseased or injured parts.

dysphagia inability to swallow or difficulty in swallowing.

dysrhythmias abnormal, disordered rhythm.

edema a local or generalized collection of tissue fluid.

effortless tachypnea tachypnea, without the signs of increased work of breathing; this represents the child's attempt to blow off extra carbon dioxide to correct the acidosis generated by poor perfusion.

electrocardiogram (ECG) a 12-lead electo-cardiographic recording used to evaluate the heart and its rhythm.

emancipated minor person legally under age but recognized by the state as having the legal capacity to consent for self (usually over 14 years of age).

emergency exception rule *see* doctrine of implied consent.

emesis vomiting.

emotional abuse the intentional infliction of emotional harm to a child.

emotional neglect the intentional omission of emotional support to a child.

empathy the awareness of and insight into the feelings, emotions, and behavior of another person.

EMS-EMSC Continuum the linked community services set up to prevent and treat childhood emergencies. The continuum includes prevention, the primary physician, out-of-hospital care, ED care, hospital care, and rehabilitation.

encephalitis inflammation of the brain.

endotracheal intubation a method of intubation in which an endotracheal tube (ETT) is placed through a patient's mouth, directly through the larynx between the vocal cords, and into the trachea, to open and maintain an airway.

enterovirus species of virus that causes gastrointestinal or respiratory disease in children.

envenomation the act of injecting venom, such as by a snake or insect.

environment the surroundings, conditions, or influences that affect an organism or an injury.

environmental assessment evaluation of the scene to draw clues about what is wrong and the best route to take for treatment. Gathering information by observing things like damage to a vehicle or medication bottles in the patient's home.

epiglottis a thin, leaf-shaped structure located immediately posterior to the root of the tongue that prevents food and secretions from entering the trachea.

epiglottitis inflammation of the epiglottis.

epilepsy a condition of recurrent seizures.

epiphysis the ends of long bone.

esophagus a muscular canal that carries food from the pharynx to the stomach.

etiology cause and origin of disease.

evaporation change from liquid to vapor.

exhalation the process of breathing out.

extensor posturing a posture characterized by extension of the arms and legs; indicates pressure on the brain stem and may appear in patients with severe brain trauma.

extraocular movement of the eyes in various directions.

febrile seizure convulsions that result from sudden high fevers in children.

feeding tube a tube placed into the stomach through the mouth, nose, or skin.

fetal placental transfusion the transfusion of blood from the baby to the placenta, leading to a decrease in the infant's blood volume. This can occur if the baby is held higher than the uterus or womb prior to clamping the cord.

fetus a human or mammal in an early form of intrauterine development.

flaccidity weak, lax, and soft.

flail chest an unstable condition of the chest wall due to two or more fractures on each affected rib resulting in ineffective breathing.

flexion the act of bending.

flexor posturing a posture characterized by flexion of the arms and extension of the legs; indicates pressure on the brain stem and may appear in patients with severe brain trauma.

flexural creases the creases behind the knees or inside the elbows.

fontanelle a soft spot of undeveloped bone lying between the cranial bones of the skull of a fetus or infant.

fulminant pneumonia sudden and intense inflammation of the lungs with consolidation.

gag reflex the protective reflex that keeps food, fluid, or secretions from getting into the trachea.

gastric decompression the removal of air and other contents from the stomach.

gastric feeding tube an advanced airway adjunct that provides a channel directly into a patient's stomach, allowing removal of gas, blood, and toxins, or insertion medications and nutrition.

gastroenteritis inflammation of the stomach and intestinal tract.

gastroesophageal reflux a condition in which the liquid content of the stomach regurgitates (backs up, or refluxes) into the esophagus.

gastrointestinal (GI) decontamination the removal of poison from the stomach.

gastrostomy tube (G-tube) a feeding tube placed directly through the wall of the abdomen used in patients who cannot ingest liquids or solids.

general assessment consists of the Pediatric Assessment Triangle. The latter is an observational (visual and auditory) approach to the patient composed of noting the child's general appearance, work of breathing, and circulation. The outcome of this general assessment is the development of an initial impression of the patient's underlying cardiopulmonary and neurologic status. The PAT helps identify the general category of the patient's physiologic problem (e.g., respiratory or circulatory) and the urgency for treatment and/or transport.

generalized seizure characterized by manifestations that indicate involvement of both cerebral hemispheres.

gestation the length of time from conception to birth.

glial cells specialized cells that surround neurons, providing mechanical and physical support and electrical insulation between neurons.

glottis the sound-producing apparatus of the larynx, consisting of two vocal folds.

glucagon a hormone that has the property of increasing the concentration of sugar in the blood.

greenstick fracture a fracture involving only part of the outer layer or cortex of a bone.

grunting a short, low-pitched sound at the end of exhalation, present in children with moderate to severe hypoxia; it reflects poor gas exchange because of fluid in the lower airways and air sacs.

hazardous materials (HazMat) any substance that is toxic, poisonous, radioactive, flammable, or explosive and causes injury or death with exposure.

head bobbing the head lifts and tilts back during inspiration, then moves forward during expiration; a sign of increased work of breathing.

hematocrit a measure of red blood cell mass in the serum. An average figure for humans is 45 percent.

hematoma a swelling or mass of blood (usually clotted) confined to a organ, tissue, or space and caused by a break in a blood vessel.

hemodynamically stable not changing or fluctuating in relation to the mechanics of blood circulation.

hemopericardium accumulation of blood around the heart muscle in the pericardial sac.

hemophilia a congenital condition in which the patient lacks one or more of the blood's normal clotting factors.

hemostat instrument clamp; in its closed position it squeezes tissues or vessels and arrests the flow of blood.

hepatomegaly enlargement of the liver.

hives wheals; an itchy rash caused by contact with or ingestion of an allergic substance or food.

homeostasis the maintenance of a relatively stable internal physiologic environment.

host the organism acted upon in an injury or illness process.

hydrocarbon a basic organic compound made up only of hydrogen and carbon.

hydrocephalus the increased accumulation of cerebrospinal fluid within the ventricles of the brain.

hydrochloric acid a powerful and corrosive aqueous solution of hydrogen chloride (HCl).

hymenoptera insects such as bees, ants, and wasps.

hypercarbia increased amount of carbon dioxide in the blood.

hyperglycemia an increase of blood sugar levels, as in diabetes mellitus.

hyperoxia increased oxygen in the blood.

hypnotic pertaining to sleep or sedation.

hypocarbia decreased carbon dioxide in the blood, usually from an excess rate of ventilation.

hypoglycemia low blood sugar.

hypoperfusion inadequate circulation.

hypotension decrease of systolic and diastolic blood pressure below normal for age, representing decompensated shock.

hypothermia having a body temperature below normal range.

hypotonia reduced muscular tension.

hypovolemia diminished blood volume.

hypovolemic shock a clinical state of reduced intravascular volume.

hypoxemia a decreased oxygen saturation in blood detected by pulse oximetry or direct measurement of oxygen saturation in an arterial blood gas sample.

hypoxia a pathological condition in which the body as a whole (generalized hypoxia) or region of the body (tissue hypoxia) is deprived of an adequate oxygen supply.

hypoxic stress a subnormal concentration of oxygen.

idiopathic brain stem herniation bulging of tissue through the lowest part of the brain with no known cause.

impending herniation syndrome clinical state in which there is severely abnormal brain pressure, just before the moment of tissue herniation and compression of brain tissue

implementation phase second of the three phases in disaster response. Activities during this phase include: search and rescue, victim triage, initial stabilization and transport, and definitive management of scene hazards and victims.

implied consent a type of consent in which a patient who is unable to give consent is given treatment under the legal assumption that he or she would want treatment if thinking in a normal way.

Incident Commander (IC) the individual who has overall command of the scene in the field.

Incident Command System (ICS) an organizational system to help control, direct, and coordinate emergency responders and resources; known more generally as an incident management system (IMS).

indirect medical oversight off-line physician or nurse support for the prehospital professional's practice. This type of oversight can be in either a prospective (before) or retrospective (after) form.

indwelling central venous catheter small, flexible plastic tube inserted into the large vein above the heart, usually the subclavian vein, through which access to the blood stream can be made. This catheter is left in place and allows drugs and blood products to be given and blood samples withdrawn painlessly.

informed consent permission for treatment given by a competent patient after the potential risks, benefits, and alternatives to treatment have been explained.

infusion a liquid substance introduced into the body for therapeutic or diagnostic purposes.

initial assessment the part of the assessment process that helps to identify any immediately or potentially life-threatening conditions in order to initiate lifesaving care.

inspiratory the process of moving air into the lungs.

intracranial within the skull.

intranasal within the nasal cavity.

intercostal between the ribs.

intercurrent intervening.

intra-abdominal within the abdomen.

intracranial within the cranium or skull.

intracranial hypertension increased pressure of the cerebrospinal fluid that impairs brain function.

intramuscular medications injections into a muscle; a medication delivery route.

intraosseous within the marrow cavity of a bone; intramedullary.

intravascular volume the water portion of the circulatory system surrounding the blood cells.

in utero within the uterus.

ipecac an oral medicine to induce vomiting; this medicine is no longer recommended for use by prehospital professionals.

ischemia deficiency of blood supply.

jaundice a condition characterized by yellowness of skin, whites of eyes, mucous membranes, and body fluids due to deposition of excess bilirubin in the blood (hyperbilirubinemia).

jugular venous distension a prominence of the jugular veins as they fill with blood; if patient is not supine, indication that the blood may be having difficulty flowing back into the right side of the heart. This can be caused by pericardial tamponade, tension pneumothorax, or right-sided heart failure.

lactic acidosis the metabolic acidotic state resulting from the accumulation of lactic acid secondary to anaerobic cellular metabolism.

laryngoscope an instrument for examining the larynx.

laryngoscopy an examination of the interior of the larynx.

larynx the enlarged upper end of the trachea, below the root of the tongue, that contains the vocal cords.

lateral pertaining to the side.

lateral decubitus position the position with the patient on his or her side.

lateral diameters the width side-to-side.

legal authority the ability to make medical decisions under the law.

legal mandate mandatory order or requirement by statute, regulation, or public agency.

lethargy listlessness; weakness.

leukemia a cancerous condition in which certain cell lines begin to grow abnormally fast and invade other tissues.

lividity dark skin discoloration, as from venous pooling and lack of circulation.

localizes when a patient is able to respond to the site of a specific noxious or painful stimulus (e.g., when a patient reaches for and pushes away the hand that is pinching them during a neurologic exam).

lye corrosive, alkaline cleaning liquid.

malaise discomfort, uneasiness, or generalized ill feeling, often indicative of infection.

malposition when something is in an incorrect or abnormal position.

mandible the horseshoe-shaped bone forming the lower jaw.

mannitol a strong sugar solution used as an osmotic diuretic to draw out abnormal free water, such as for reduction of water in the brain to decrease cerebrospinal fluid pressure.

mature minor a person without the formal legal status of an emancipated minor, but having similar characteristics: married, pregnant, on active-duty status in the armed service, or 15 years or older and living separate and apart from his or her guardians. This person has the legal right to give consent for treatment as well as the legal right to refuse.

meconium the bowel contents of a fetus. The presence of meconium in amniotic fluid means the fetus may have suffered some type of stress, such as hypoxia, and may be depressed and need to be resuscitated.

mediastinum the space between the lungs, in the center of the chest, that contains the heart, trachea, mainstem bronchi, part of the esophagus, and large blood vessels.

medical home an approach to providing health care services in a high quality and cost-effective manner. Children and their families who have a medical home receive the care that they need from a pediatrician or physician that they know and trust. The pediatric health care professional and parents act as partners in a medical home to identify and access all the medical and nonmedical services needed to help children and their families achieve their maximum potential.

medical responsibility the moral and legal duty to provide medical care in an emergency.

medicolegal related to medical jurisprudence or forensic medicine.

meningitis inflammation of the membranes of the spinal cord or brain.

meningococcal sepsis blood-borne infection with the bacteria *Neisseria menigitidis* leading to sepsis (fever or hypothermia, shock, and hypotension).

meningococcemia infection of the blood stream by the bacteria *Neisseria menigitidis*. This is usually a severe infection characterized by fever, shock and a characteristic purpuric rash (bruising of the skin) with or without meningitis.

metabolic acidosis a metabolic state of acidosis resulting from retention of H+ or other positively charged ions not related to respiratory compromise.

midaxillary (line) imaginary vertical line drawn through the middle of the axilla (armpit), parallel to the midline.

military anti-shock trousers (MAST) a garment designed to put pressure on the lower extremities and abdomen in order to squeeze blood from the peripheral vessels so as to increase core organ circulation. This is no longer recommended in children.

minor a person not of legal age and thus requiring consent from a legal guardian for medical or surgical care.

minute ventilation the volume of air exchanged per minute. [minute ventilation = tidal volume × respiratory rate]

miosis abnormal contraction of pupils.

mongolian spots blue-gray areas of discoloration of the skin caused by abnormal pigment, not by trauma or bruising.

mortality death.

motor activity muscle use.

mottling a condition of abnormal skin circulation, caused by vasoconstriction or inadequate circulation.

multi-casualty incident (MCI) an emergency situation involving more than one patient, and which can place such great demand on equipment or personnel that the system is stretched to its limit or beyond.

multipara a woman who has had more than one live birth.

multisystem trauma injury involving more than one organ system, such as combined injury to the chest, abdomen, and brain.

myocardial depression when the heart muscle is not working adequately.

myocardial function a measure of how well the heart is working.

myocardial infarction the death of part of the heart muscle caused by partial or complete occlusion of one or more of the coronary arteries.

myocarditis inflammation of the myocardium.

narcotic an opiate drug that produces analgesia and sedation, as well as euphoria when used for recreational purposes.

nasal flaring flaring out of the nostrils, indicating increased work of breathing and hypoxia.

nasopharyngeal airway airway adjunct inserted into the nostril of a conscious patient who is not able to maintain a natural airway.

needle decompression the removal of air from a closed space, such as from the pleura.

neonatal seizures seizures that occur in neonates.

nerve agents a class of chemical called organophosphates; they function by blocking an essential enzyme in the nervous system, which causes the body's organs to become overstimulated and burn out.

neurovascular concerning both the nervous and vascular systems.

nonpulsatile fontanelle when the fontanelle or "soft spot" on an infant's head is full, usually tense and does not seem to beat or pulse with each beat of the heart.

nuclear bomb a bomb which is extremely powerful due to its use of atomic energy as a source of its explosive nature. In addition to the actual explosive force of the bomb, injury is caused in a wider area by the radiation released by the explosion.

obstetric having to do with pregnancy, delivery of a baby.

obstructive shock shock or inadequate tissue perfusion that is caused by a restriction to blood flow out from the heart (e.g., shock due to a critical coarctation or severe narrowing of the aorta which children may be born with).

obturator an inner stabilizing structure that gives stiffness to a hollow tube, to allow insertion or clearing of an obstruction.

occlusion the closure of a passage.

occlusive dressing a dressing that covers completely.

occult illness an illness that is not immediately obvious or is "hidden." An illness that does not have obvious symptoms.

operations administrative processes.

opiates *see* narcotics.

organophosphate insecticide a type of poison with cholinergic properties, used as an insecticide.

oropharynx the part of the pharynx lying between the soft palate and upper portion of the epiglottis.

ossification the formation of bone. An ossification center is an area where cartilage is transformed through calcification into a new area of bone.

osteogenesis imperfecta a genetic disorder in which the patient lacks sufficient collagen for proper strength of the bones.

pallor lack of color; paleness.

palpitation a rapid or throbbing pulsation, as an abnormally rapid throbbing or fluttering of the heart.

paradoxical irritability a marker for possible serious pediatric illness, consisting of a particular type of irritability where attempts to console further distress the child.

partially implanted device an indwelling line that is partially implanted under the skin and partially exposed above the skin.

pathophysiology the study of how disease or injury affects the body.

pedal related to the foot (e.g., pedal pulses are pulses found in the foot).

pediatric assessment triangle (PAT) assessment tool that allows an integrating rapid formation of a general impression of the type and level of illness or injury in an infant or child without touching him or her; consists of assessing appearance, work of breathing, and circulation to the skin.

pediatric critical care center a type of specialized center for children with advanced resources for care of critically ill children.

pediatric trauma center a type of specialized center for children with advanced resources for care of critically injured children.

pelvic fractures breaks through one or more bones of the pelvis (the hip bones and the sacrum and coccyx or lower parts of the spine).

perfusion blood circulation.

pericardial tamponade compression of the heart due to a buildup of blood or other fluid in the pericardial sac.

perinatal the period around birth; includes the time from 20 to 28 weeks of pregnancy through 1 to 4 weeks after birth.

perineum the structures occupying the pelvic floor.

periosteum the membrane, made up of a double layer of connective tissue, that covers all bones, except the articular surfaces.

peripheral cyanosis slightly bluish or dark purple discoloration of the skin (on the hands and feet only) due to presence of abnormal amounts of reduced hemoglobin in the blood.

peripheral vasoconstriction when the blood vessels in the outer extremities (hands and feet especially) constrict (get smaller in size through the contraction of the smooth muscle in the blood vessel walls) and therefore lead to a decrease in blood flow to those areas. This may produce acrocyanosis (bluish discoloration of the hands and feet) and prolonged capillary refill time.

peritoneum the membrane lining the abdominal cavity (parietal peritoneum) and covering the abdominal organs (visceral peritoneum).

petechiae small, purplish, nonblanching spots on the skin that appear in certain severe fevers and are indicative of possible sepsis.

petechial related to petechiae, small purplish, nonblanching spots on the skin. Petechiae represent small areas of hemorrhage into the skin and are usually seen with infections, especially sepsis.

petechial rash rash which contains petechiae, small areas of hemorrhage into the skin that do not blanch when they are pressed on.

pharynx passageway for air from nasal cavity to larynx and food from mouth to esophagus.

phencyclidine a hallucinogen, referred to as PCP or angel dust. Moderate doses cause elevated blood pressure, rapid pulse, increased skeletal muscle tone, and, sometimes, myoclonic jerks.

physical abuse *see* child abuse.

physical neglect *see* child neglect.

physiologic concerning body function.

plague an illness caused by infection with the bacteria *Yersinia pestis*. The disease is characterized by fever and chills followed by a severe illness with pneumonia, headache, and delirium. It is transmitted to humans by the bites of fleas from infected rodents and has a high fatality rate. It is an agent that could possibly be used as a weapon of bioterrorism.

pleura the serous membrane that enfolds both lungs and is reflected upon the walls of the thorax and diaphragm.

pleural space the space between the parietal and visceral layers of the pleura.

pneumomediastinum air or gas in the mediastinal tissues.

pneumonia an inflammation of the lungs caused primarily by bacteria, viruses, and chemical irritants.

pneumothorax a collection of air in the pleural cavity, which if under pressure may cause severe physiologic changes with poor venous return and inadequate cardiac output.

policies medicolegal operational standards to guide prehospital professionals intended to help with decision-making in difficult or legally sensitive field situations.

polypharmacy an ingestion involving more than one drug.

positive-pressure ventilation assisted ventilation.

posteriorly from the back, from behind, or from underneath.

postictal state the confused state of a patient after having a seizure.

postpartum after childbirth.

posttraumatic epilepsy a seizure disorder that occurs after a closed-head injury.

posturing abnormal body positioning after a brain injury; it may be in response to painful stimuli. Decorticate posturing is characterized by rigid flexion of the upper extremities and extension of the lower extremities. Decerebrate posturing is characterized by rigid extension of the arms and legs.

preterm pertaining to events occurring prior to the 37th week of gestation.

primary brain injury injury resulting from the direct biomechanical effects of the impact forces on the brain which result in direct impact or sudden movement causing shear stress of the brain.

primipara a woman who has had one live birth.

procedure a physical intervention.

prone lying horizontal with face downward.

propylene glycol a solvent in medicines.

protocol a step-by-step process for treatment.

proximal nearest the point of attachment, center of the body, or point of reference; opposite of distal.

pulmonary contusion a bruise of the lung.

pulmonary edema a build-up of fluid in the lungs.

pulmonary intoxicants toxins or poisons which may be absorbed through (e.g., by inhalation) or cause harm to the respiratory system.

pulseless electrical activity (PEA) an organized cardiac rhythm on the cardiac monitor in absence of a palpable pulse.

pulse oximeter a device to measure oxygen saturation in the blood.

pulse oximetry an assessment method that measures oxygen saturation of hemoglobin in the capillary beds.

purpura a rash that looks like bruising of the skin that is usually seen in overwhelming infections (sepsis) or when a patient has an inflammation of the blood vessels (vasculitis).

purpuric pertaining to bruising of the skin.

pus the liquid product of inflammation, generally yellow in color.

QRS complex the electrical shape of a major portion of the heart rhythm on the cardiac monitor, representing venticular electrical activity.

quadriplegia a condition that causes paralysis of all four extremities (both arms and both legs) usually due to an injury in the upper cervical portion of the spinal cord.

quality assurance (QA) a formalized process of reviewing patient care activities and patient outcomes in an attempt to promote high quality care and insure that the best possible outcomes are achieved while identifying and correcting actions that lead to poor patient care.

quality improvement (QI) a system of internal and external reviews and audits of all aspects of the system.

racemic including all isomers of a drug, such as epinephrine.

radial pertaining to the radius, the larger and more lateral of the two bones in the forearm.

reactivity the capacity for reacting to a stimulus.

recovery phase final of three phases in disaster response. Activities include: scene withdrawal, return to normal operations, and debriefing.

respiratory arrest the absence of respirations (i.e., apnea) with detectable cardiac activity.

respiratory depression a condition in which there is a slowing of the respiratory rate and decreased respiratory effort usually due to some effect on the respiratory center in the medulla of the brain. This may be caused by trauma, illness, or the effects of drugs (e.g., morphine or diazepam) or toxins (e.g., ethanol).

respiratory distress a clinical state characterized by increased respiratory rate, effort, and work of breathing.

respiratory failure a clinical state of inadequate oxygenation, ventilation, or both.

respiratory syncytial virus (RSV) a virus that commonly causes bronchiolitis; usually results in life-long immunity following exposure.

retractions physical drawing in of the chest wall between the ribs that occurs with increased work of breathing.

rhinorrhea thin watery discharge from the nose.

ricin neurotoxin derived from mash that is left from the castor bean. When introduced into the body, ricin causes pulmonary edema and respiratory and circulatory failure, leading to death.

salivation the act of secreting saliva.

saphenous veins two superficial veins, the great and small, passing up the leg.

scald a burn to skin or flesh caused by moist heat and hot vapors, as steam.

scopolamine an anticholinergic agent with action similar to atropine.

secondary brain injury injury to the brain resulting from factors occurring after the initial biomechanical effects of the primary brain injury.

secretion the process of producing liquid materials into the blood or body cavities.

sedative/hypnotic an agent that relaxes.

sepsis a pathological state, usually in a febrile patient, resulting from the presence of invading microorganisms or their poisonous products in the bloodstream.

septic shock shock from infection, involving hypotension and signs of inadequate organ perfusion.

serial examinations the act of repeatedly examining a patient to carefully watch and document the progression of signs or symptoms in an attempt to develop a diagnosis (e.g., serial examinations of the abdomen to decide if someone with abdominal trauma may have a perforation of the intestine) or to watch for a change in their condition (e.g., serial examinations of a child with a head injury to monitor their neurologic status and watch for signs of increasing intracranial pressure).

serum glucose the level of blood sugar.

sexual abuse rape, sexual assault, or sexual molestation. The abuser may be male, female, adult, or child, and the abused person may be of the same or opposite sex of the abuser.

shaken baby syndrome a syndrome seen in abused infants and children. The patient has been subjected to violent, whiplash-type shaking injuries inflicted by the abusing individual. This may cause coma, convulsions, and increased intracranial pressure due to tearing of the cerebral veins with consequent bleeding into the brain.

shock a clinical syndrome in which the blood flow and oxygen delivery are inadequate for normal organ function.

sickle cell disease a hereditary disease characterized by abnormal clumping together of deformed red blood cells. The patients have painful crises, anemia, infection-risks, and other serious complications.

simple febrile seizure a brief (less than 15 minutes), self-limited, generalized convulsion in a previously healthy child between the ages of 6 months and 6 years that is associated with the onset of or sudden increase in a fever. Children with simple febrile seizures have relatively short postictal periods after which they return to their baseline with a nonfocal neurologic examination.

simple partial seizures a focal (localized) seizure which involves a motor or sensory abnormality (e.g., twitching of one hand or a visual disturbance) in a patient who remains conscious. In children, partial seizures are usually motor seizures and frequently will progress to generalized seizures.

Sims position a semi-prone position with the patient on her side, with her opposite knee and thigh drawn well up to facilitate delivery of a baby.

sinus arrhythmia a variation in the resting heart rate often seen in children and adolescents. As the child breathes in the heart rate increases slightly and as they exhale the heart rate decreases. This is a normal variation in children and not truly an arrhythmia. On ECG each QRS complex is preceded by a P wave and there are no missed or skipped beats.

sinus tachycardia rapid heart rate in a child with normal conduction.

slurry a thin, watery mixture.

smallpox a rare, highly contagious viral disease; it is most contagious when blisters begin to form.

sniffing position an upright position in which the patient's head and chin are thrust slightly forward to keep the airway open; the child appears to be sniffing.

soft-tissue injuries injuries to the skin, fat, muscles, ligaments, and tendons.

somatic voluntary muscle groups that are under voluntary control and usually associated with the skeleton of the head and face, trunk, or extremities.

spasticity increased tone or contractions of muscles causing stiff and awkward movements.

spina bifida a congenital anomaly where the posterior elements of the vertebrae have failed to fuse together. The spinal cord and its associated coverings (meninges) may protrude through this defect in the vertebrae leading to a range of neurologic impairment in the lower extremities depending on the degree and level of the protrusion. When the defect is isolated to the bony structures without spinal cord or meningeal abnormality this is termed spina bifida occulta.

spinal shock a state of inadequate perfusion due to a spinal cord injury which is classically characterized by low blood pressure (hypotension) with a low heart rate (bradycardia) and loss of neurologic function below the point of spinal injury. Usually in patients with shock there is an increase in heart rate while in patients with spinal shock the expected tachycardia is absent.

spine the vertebral column.

spleen the major abdominal organ involved in the production and destruction of red blood cells and immune cells. It is filled with blood and can hemorrhage after injury.

splinting fixation with a splint.

status epilepticus a state of continuous seizures or multiple seizures without a return to consciousness for 30 minutes.

sterile free from living microorganisms.

stress forces that disrupt equilibrium or produce strain.

stridor a harsh sound during inspiration, high-pitched due to partial upper airway obstruction.

subcostal beneath the ribs.

subdural hemorrhage beneath the dura mater.

subglottic beneath the glottis.

sublingually under the tongue; a medication delivery route.

substernal situated beneath the sternum.

sucking chest wound an open or penetrating chest-wall wound through which air passes during inspiration and expiration.

suck reflex a primitive reflex of the newborn.

sudden infant death syndrome (SIDS) the abrupt and unexplained death of an apparently healthy infant under 1 year of age, remaining unexplained after a thorough case investigation, including performance of a complete autopsy, examination of the death scene, and review of the clinical history.

superior vena cava one of the two largest veins in the body that carries blood from the upper extremities, head, neck, and chest into the heart.

supine lying on the back with the face upward.

supraclavicular located above the clavical.

supraglottic the area above the glottis or true vocal cords.

suprasternal above the sternum.

suprasternal retractions when the muscles and skin above the sternum sink in above the manubrium as the patient attempts to breathe.

supraventricular tachycardia (SVT) an abnormal heart rhythm with a rapid, narrow QRS complex rate.

symmetry correspondence in shape, size, and relative position of parts on opposite sides of a body.

sympathomimetic agents adrenergic drugs; producing effects resembling those resulting from stimulation of the sympathetic nervous system, such as effects following the injection of epinephrine.

symphysis pubis the injunction of the pubic bones on midline in front; the bony eminence under the pubic hair.

symptomatic ventricular dysrhythmias abnormal ventricular electrical impulses (e.g., ventricular tachycardia) that are associated with symptoms on the part of the patient.

synaptic connections connections between two or more nerves (i.e., synapses).

tachycardia rapid heart rate.

tachypnea rapid respiration.

tamponade compression of tissues.

temporary protective custody when a legal guardian suffers from diminished judgement, law enforcement officers may place a minor in some form of temporary protective custody. While this may allow the prehospital professional to transport a minor to a medical facility for purposes of medical evaluation, it does not give the prehospital professional the right medically to treat a minor.

tension pneumothorax an accumulation of air or gas in the pleural cavity that progressively increases and causes serious hemodynamic changes.

thermoregulation heat regulation.

thoracic pertaining to the chest or thorax.

thoracic excursions the movements of the chest wall (rib cage and muscles) associated with respirations.

thoracostomy resection of the chest wall to allow drainage of the chest cavity.

thready weak.

tidal volume the amount of air that is exchanged with each breath.

titratable the ability to adjust the desired effect of an agent by giving more or less of that agent as needed over time (e.g., using an intravenous catheter to slowly give more analgesic or sedative agents until a patient is just quiet enough to effectively complete a procedure).

tonic-clonic a seizure that features rhythmic back-and-forth motion of an extremity and body stiffness.

torsades de pointes a specific type of ventricular tachycardia characterized by a wide QRS complex tachycardia that has a varying axis and is especially sensitive to treatment with magnesium.

totally implanted device a catheter totally implanted and not visible to the eye.

trachea a cylindrical cartilaginous tube from the larynx to the bronchial tubes. It extends from the 6th cervical to the 5th dorsal vertebra, where it divides at a point called the carina into two bronchi, one leading to each lung.

tracheitis an inflammation of the trachea.

tracheostomy operation of incising the skin over the trachea and making a surgical wound in the trachea in order to permit an airway during tracheal obstruction.

tracheostomy tube a tube inserted into the trachea in children who cannot breathe or maintain a clear airway on their own.

transdermal through the skin.

transient not lasting; of brief duration.

transmucosal to pass across a mucous membrane (e.g., the absorption of a toxin or pharmaceutical agent across the mucous membranes of the mouth).

transport officers the individual in charge of the transportation sector in a mass-casualty incident, who assigns patients from the treatment area to waiting ambulances in the transportation area.

traumatic brain injury (TBI) the preferred term for head trauma.

tripoding an abnormal position to keep the airway open; it involves leaning forward onto two arms stretched forward.

trismus tonic contraction of the muscles of mastication.

tympanic temperature body temperature measurement made by the use of a device which measures the reflectance of infrared light from the tympanic membrane (ear drum).

umbilical catheterization placing a cannula into the umbilical artery or vein.

umbilical cord the attachment connecting the fetus with the placenta.

universal precautions protective measures that have traditionally been developed by the Centers for Disease Control and Prevention (CDC) for use in dealing with objects, blood, body fluids, or other potential exposure risks of communicable disease.

universal standards for pediatric emergency care standards of care agreed upon and promoted by experts in pediatric emergency care and the organizations they represent for the management of children throughout the emergency medical system.

uterus an organ in the female reproductive system for containing and nourishing the embryo and fetus from the time the fertilized egg is implanted to the time of birth of the fetus.

vagal pertaining to the vagus

vaginal introitus the vaginal opening.

vagus nerve the cranial nerve (X) that provides motor functions to the soft palate, pharynx, and larynx and carries taste bud fibers from the posterior tongue, sensory fibers from the inferior pharynx, larynx, thoracic, and abdominal organs, and parasympathetic fibers to thoracic and abdominal organs.

varicella (chicken pox) an acute viral disease with mild constitutional symptoms (headache, fever, malaise) followed by an eruption appearing in crops and characterized by macules, papules, and vesicles.

vascular tone the amount of constriction in a blood vessel or more generally, the overall amount of constriction in the blood vessels of the body. This is a reflection of the acute cardiovascular health of the patient. Patients in shock often have marked vasoconstriction in an attempt to increase their vascular tone and blood pressure to maximize perfusion to vital organs. When there is a loss of vascular tone (e.g., in sepsis or spinal shock) there is often generalized vasodilatation and severe hypotension.

vasculitis inflammation of the blood vessels which usually is associated with pain, swelling, and often leakage of fluid and blood from the vessels into other organs. When this occurs in the skin a purpuric rash often develops.

vasoconstriction decrease in the caliber of blood vessels.

vasodilatation dilatation of blood vessels.

vasomotor pertaining to the nerves having muscular control of the blood vessel walls.

vasopressor agent a drug that increases vascular tone and increases blood pressure.

ventilation-perfusion mismatch a pathologic state where the oxygen going into the lungs is not mixing appropriately with the blood circulating through the lungs.

ventilator a mechanical device for artificial ventilation of the lungs.

ventricle one of two (right and left) lower chambers of the heart. The left ventricle receives blood from the left atrium (upper chamber) and delivers blood to the aorta. The right ventricle receives blood from the right atrium and pumps it into the pulmonary artery.

ventricular fibrillation disorganized, ineffective twitching of the ventricles, resulting in no blood flow and a state of cardiac arrest.

ventricular tachycardia a rapid heart rhythm in which the electrical impulse begins in the ventricle (instead of the atrium), which may result in inadequate blood flow and eventually deteriorate into cardiac arrest.

vertebral bodies the 33 bones that make up the spinal column.

vertex pertaining to the very top of the skull and head. In obstetrical care, a baby who has a vertex presentation is one whose head has lead the child's way down the birth canal.

vesicants blister agents; the primary route of entry for vesicants is through the skin.

viral myocarditis a viral infection of the heart which frequently leads to dysrhythmias, especially ventricular dysrhythmias and poor muscle function which produces congestive heart failure.

visual analogue scores scales generated by asking a patient or subject to quantify the amount of a sensation they are feeling (usually pain) by pointing to where on a line their sensation is. By measuring how far along the line the patient points one can use this as a measure of that sensation. A frequently used technique for the measurement of pain in research studies.

vital signs the key signs that are used to evaluate the patient's overall condition, including respirations, pulse, blood pressure, level of consciousness, and skin characteristics.

vocal cords two small folds of tissue in the larynx which vibrate as air moves across them to produce sound.

volume resuscitation replenishing the blood volume.

wheezing production of whistling sounds during expiration such as occurs in asthma and bronchiolitis.

womb uterus; female organ for containing, protecting, and nourishing the fetus.

work of breathing an indicator of oxygenation and ventilation. Work of breathing reflects the child's attempt to compensate for hypoxia.

Index

A

Additional Credits

Chapter 1

Opener: © Comstock Images/Getty Images; 1-3 © Photos.com; 1-4; 1-8; 1-16 Courtesy Health Resources and Services Administration, Maternal and Child Health Bureau, Emergency Medical Services for Children Program; 1-5; 1-7 Courtesy of Dena Brownstein, MD; 1-8 Courtesy of the National EMSC Slideset; 1-14 Source: Wong D.L., Hockenberry-Eaton M., Wilson D., Schwartz P.: Wong's Essentials of Pediatric Nursing, ed. 6, St. Louis, 2001, p. 1301. Copyrighted by Mosby, Inc. Reprinted by permission

Chapter 2

Opener: © Momentum Creative Group/Alamy Images; 2-1 © Linda Gheen; 2-2 Courtesy of Thomas P. Garcia, MD, FACEP; 2-4 © Photodisc/Getty Images; 2-5 Courtesy of Ron Deickmann, MD; 2-8 © Photos.com; 2-10 © Stockbyte/Creatas; 2-12 © Photos.com

Chapter 3

Opener: © Stockbyte/Creatas; 3-1 Courtesy Health Resources and Services Administration, Maternal and Child Health Bureau, Emergency Medical Services for Children Program; 3-4 Courtesy of Dena Brownstein, MD; 3-18 © Jones and Bartlett Publishers. Photographed by Kimberly Potvin

Chapter 4

Opener: © Patrick Olear/PhotoEdit; 4-1; 4-2a,b; 4-3 Courtesy of Ron Deickmann, MD; 4-4 Courtesy of James L. Horwitz, MD/Rainbow Pediatrics; 4-5 Courtesy of Lisa Wise; 4-7 Courtesy of Susan Fuchs, MD; 4-8 Courtesy of Thomas P. Garcia, MD, FACEP; 4-10 Courtesy of Philips Medical Systems. All rights reserved; 4-13 Courtesy of the Maryland Institute of Emergency Medical Services Systems

Chapter 5

Opener: © Eddie M. Sperling; 5-3 The Ascensia Contour Blood Glucose Meter. Photo courtesy of Bayer HealthCare LLC © 2004 Bayer HealthCare LLC; 5-4 © Stock Connection Distribution/Alamy Images; 5-5 Courtesy of Ron Deickmann, MD

Chapter 6

Opener: © Steve L. Smith; 6-12 Courtesy of North Carolina EMSC Prehospital; 6-17 © Charles Stewart & Associates; 6-18 Courtesy of Allied Healthcare Products, Inc; 6-21 Courtesy of Ron Deickmann, MD

Chapter 7

Opener: © SuperStock/Alamy Images; 7-1 © Creasource/PictureQuest

Chapter 8

Opener: Courtesy of Mark Wolfe/FEMA News Photo; 8-1 Courtesy of Dave Saville/FEMA; 8-2 Courtesy of Harald Richter/National Severe Storms Laboratory (NSSL)/NOAA; 8-3 © Ivan Sekretarev/AP Photo; 8-4 © 2002 Lou Romig, MD, FAAP, FACEP; 8-5 Courtesy Dr. John P. Noble, Jr./CDC

Chapter 9

Opener: © Davis Barber/PhotoEdit; 9-15 Courtesy of David J. Burchfield, MD; 9-16 Reproduced with permission from the American Heart Association. ©2003 Pediatric Advanced Life Support

Chapter 10

Opener: © Jeff Greenberg/age fotostock; 10-1 Courtesy of Dr. Hudson/CDC; 10-12 © Craig Jackson/In the Dark Photography

Chapter 11

Opener: © Glen E. Ellman; 11-2 © Photos.com; 11-3 © Glen E. Ellman; 11-4 © Sean O'Brien/Custom Medical Stock Photo

Chapter 12

Opener: Courtesy of Moose Jaw Police Service; 12-1; 12-2 © Jones and Bartlett Publishers. Photographed by Kimberly Potvin; 12-3; 12-4; 12-5; 12-6; 12-7 Courtesy of Ron Deickmann, MD; 12-8; 12-9 Courtesy of the American Academy of Pediatrics

Chapter 13

Opener: © Steve Hamblin/Alamy Images; 13-1 © Eddie M. Sperling; 13-3 Courtesy of the State of California, Emergency Medical Services Authority; 13-4 © Mike Heller/911 Pictures

Chapter 14

Opener: © Frank Whitney/Brand X Pictures/Alamy Images

Chapter 15

Opener: © Ryan McVay/Photodisc/Getty Images; 15-3 © Thinkstock/Getty Images; 15-4 © LiquidLibrary; 15-7 © Photos.com; 15-8 © Comstock Images/Getty Images

Photographs and illustrations also supplied by the American Academy of Orthopaedic Surgeons and Jones and Bartlett Publishers.